Advances in Cardiovascular Imaging: An Exciting Future to Revolutionize the Diagnosis and Management of Cardiovascular Disease

Advances in Cardiovascular Imaging: An Exciting Future to Revolutionize the Diagnosis and Management of Cardiovascular Disease

Guest Editor

Zhonghua Sun

MDPI

Basel • Beijing • Wuhan • Barcelona • Belgrade • Novi Sad • Cluj • Manchester

Guest Editor
Zhonghua Sun
Discipline of Medical
Radiation Science
Curtin University
Perth
Australia

Editorial Office
MDPI AG
Grosspeteranlage 5
4052 Basel, Switzerland

This is a reprint of the Special Issue, published open access by the journal *Journal of Cardiovascular Development and Disease* (ISSN 2308-3425), freely accessible at: https://www.mdpi.com/journal/jcdd/special_issues/Q4Q8C331QA.

For citation purposes, cite each article independently as indicated on the article page online and as indicated below:

Lastname, A.A.; Lastname, B.B. Article Title. *Journal Name* **Year**, *Volume Number*, Page Range.

ISBN 978-3-7258-5597-1 (Hbk)
ISBN 978-3-7258-5598-8 (PDF)
https://doi.org/10.3390/books978-3-7258-5598-8

Contents

About the Editor

Zhonghua Sun

Zhonghua Sun is a John Curtin Distinguished Professor of Curtin Medical School at Curtin University. His research interests include diagnostic radiology, 3D medical image visualization and processing, in particular, cardiovascular CT imaging, 3D printing, virtual reality/mixed reality, and artificial intelligence in cardiovascular disease. His significant contributions lie in his excellent track record of utilizing the latest technologies (3D printing, virtual reality and AI) to assist clinical diagnosis and management of patients with cardiovascular diseases. He is included in the "World Top 2% Scientist list in the field of cardiovascular disease" since 2019. In 2024, he was named as a highly ranked scholar by ScholarGPS in the specialty of computed tomography angiography (in the top 0.05% of scholars in the Specialty worldwide). His total career publications include >400 refereed journal articles, 5 books, and 14 book chapters, with a total citation of more than 10,000 and an H-index of 55 (Google Scholar).

Journal of
Cardiovascular
Development and Disease

MDPI

Editorial

Advances in Cardiovascular Imaging: A Platform to Share Recent Research Findings Through Utilization of Advanced Imaging Technologies

Zhonghua Sun [1,2]

1 Curtin Medical School, Curtin University, Perth 6845, Australia; z.sun@curtin.edu.au
2 Curtin Medical Research Institute (Curtin MRI), Curtin University, Perth 6845, Australia

Clinical diagnosis of cardiovascular disease has undergone revolutionary changes over the last decades thanks to rapid developments in medical imaging modalities significantly enhancing the diagnostic performance of cardiac imaging in cardiovascular disease. The diagnostic value of standard cardiac imaging examinations, such as computed tomography (CT), magnetic resonance imaging (MRI), echocardiography, and nuclear medicine technologies including positron emission tomography (PET) and PET-CT, has been augmented by recent advancements, which include the increasing use of three-dimensional (3D) visualizations, namely 3D-printed models, and virtual reality (VR) and mixed reality (MR). Furthermore, the widespread use of artificial intelligence (AI), machine learning (ML), and deep learning (DL), as well as CT-derived fractional flow reserve (FFR-CT), has further expanded the applications of cardiac imaging modalities by delivering more precise or personalized medicine and providing both anatomical and physiological assessment of cardiovascular disease, primarily helping to improve diagnostic assessment of coronary artery lesions. Hence, this Special Issue has been developed to showcase high-quality articles written by researchers from different regions and share the latest research findings in cardiovascular imaging.

This Special Issue includes nine published articles, and though these articles span different study designs, they are all based on the authors' experiences of using a range of technologies in cardiovascular disease. Four of them are original studies documenting the use of cardiac CT, MRI, PET/CT and 3D visualizations/methodologies in the diagnosis and prediction of cardiovascular diseases [1–4]. Of the remaining five articles, three are review articles providing an overview of the clinical applications of various imaging modalities in the diagnosis of acute pulmonary embolism [5], chronic total coronary occlusions [6], and FFR-CT and its applications in coronary artery disease [7]. Another review article is a systematic review of AI applications in cardiac MRI in coronary artery disease [8], and the final article is a communication reporting authors' experience of using mixed reality in guiding cardiac surgery [9]. The following sections summarize key findings from the articles published in this Special Issue.

Nappi et al. reported their experience of using whole-body PET-CT imaging in 109 oncology patients to assess the correlation between coronary artery calcium (CAC) and epicardial adipose tissue (EAT) in these patients without known coronary artery disease (CAD) [1]. Total CAC scores were estimated for three main coronary arteries, while EAT volume was measured and quantified through image processing from the level of the pulmonary trunk to the inferior diaphragmatic surface of the heart by manually tracing pericardial borders. Their results showed that the EAT volume was significantly higher in patients with CAC than in those without CAC ($p < 0.005$). Patient's age, body mass index

(BMI), hypertension, and CAC were significantly associated with increasing EAT values ($p < 0.005$). Based on the multivariable analysis model, only age and BMI were found to be independent factors associated with increasing EAT ($p < 0.001$). This study discusses the feasibility and cost effectiveness of evaluating cancer status and atherosclerotic burden in a single imaging examination in oncologic patients with optimization of radiation dose.

Cardiac magnetic resonance (CMR) is a well-established diagnostic tool for evaluation of patients with suspected myocarditis, and CMR-feature tracking (FT) further advances CMR's diagnostic accuracy by enabling both morphological and function assessment of myocardial strain. Despite the reported impact of atrial and ventricular functions in patients with acute myocarditis (AM), there is a lack of evidence on the clinical value of CMR-FT in patients with preserved ejection fraction (EF). Cau et al. addressed this research gap by determining the impact of combining atrial and ventricular strain functions using CMR in patients with AM [2]. In this retrospective study based on a single center experience, they reviewed 126 patients with AM with preserved EF, including another 52 age- and sex-matched patients as the control group. Univariable and multivariable logistic regression analysis was used to determine the relationship between left atrial (LA) and left ventricular (LV) functions and presence of AM with preserved EF. LA and LV myocardial strain parameters were found to be significantly associated with impaired function between the AM and control groups ($p < 0.005$). Integration of LA and LV strain parameters into the diagnostic approach improved the diagnostic accuracy of CMR, with the model integrating the global longitudinal strain with the conduit strain achieving the highest area under the curve (0.77). This study highlights how diagnostic performance can be improved by using a combined analysis of both atrial and ventricular functions in patients with AM.

Lee et al. compared four visualization modalities—3D-printed heart models, VR, 3D portable document format files (PDFs), and original digital imaging and communications in medicine (DICOM) images—with regard to their clinical value for diagnostic assessment and preoperative planning of congenital heart disease (CHD) [3]. Cardiac CT images of three CHD cases including ventricular septal defect, double outlet right ventricle, and tetralogy of Fallot were selected, and 3D personalized models were generated from these CT images (Figure 1). These four modalities were presented to 17 participants (13 cardiologists, 3 cardiac surgeons, and 1 radiologist) for assessment of the clinical value of each visualization modality. The participants completed a questionnaire which allowed them to rank the usefulness of these modalities in three main areas, namely pre-surgical planning, medical education, and patient communication. The results showed the superiority of VR and 3D-printed models over 3D PDFs and DICOM images in almost all categories that were assessed in the study, with VR being ranked as the best tool for assessment of anatomical locations, understanding the spatial relationships between cardiac structures and assisting pre-surgical planning. Three-dimensionally printed models were ranked as the best tool for medical education and patient communication, while 3D PDFs and DICOM images have limited value in these areas.

Hashemizadehkolowri et al. proposed a 3D method based on measuring the vessel wall thickness with the aim of overcoming the limitations of 2D techniques [4]. They adopted the Laplacian method, which allows for accurate and reproducible measurements of vessel wall thickness compared to conventional 2D approaches. To achieve their research objectives, the authors conducted a series of experiments based on 2D digital phantoms, 2D histology images (from two carotid artery samples), 3D digital phantoms, and black-blood MR images (from a healthy female volunteer) and measured the vessel wall thickness for comparisons. Their results showed the superiority of the Laplacian method over the current 2D-centric approaches in vessel wall measurements, as it provided accurate 3D thickness measurements based on 2D and 3D digital phantoms. In patient's MR data analysis, close alignment was observed in the 3D vessel thickness measurements between the baseline and follow-up scans, showing a high level of reproducibility with use of their 3D method, the adapted Laplacian method. Furthermore, the 3D thickness measurements derived from using the Laplacian method are consistent with other morphological features, especially the normalized wall volume index.

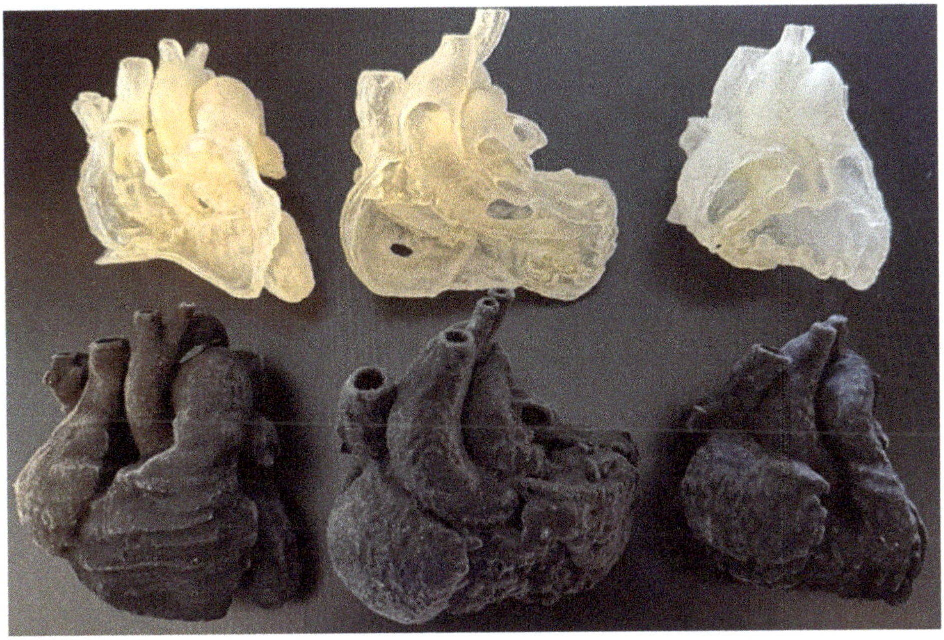

Figure 1. Models were printed with a flexible material, Agilus 30 (Objective 3D, Stratasys, Melbourne, VIC, Australia). VSD (ventricular septal defect) in the left column, DORV (double outlet right ventricle) in the middle column, and ToF (Tetralogy of Fallot) in the right column. Reprinted with permission under open access from Lee et al. [3].

Of the four review articles included in this Special Issue, three of them are narrative reviews overviewing various imaging modalities in the context of cardiovascular disease diagnosis. Cellina et al. reviewed the latest developments of diagnostic imaging techniques, including interventional radiology in acute pulmonary embolism (APE) [5]. Among the standard imaging modalities, they first reviewed the use of high-pitch CT pulmonary angiography (CTPA) with low radiation dose (1.04 mSv), followed by dual-energy CT with higher diagnostic accuracy when compared to single-energy CT in APE detection. They then reviewed the diagnostic value of photon counting CTPA in APE, with reported accuracy of more than 95% according to recent studies. Furthermore, photon counting CT offers superior spatial and contrast resolution, and with the use of virtual monoenergetic images, its diagnostic accuracy is further enhanced for APE detection. Dynamic digital radiography (DDR) is an emerging method for assessing pulmonary perfusion with low radiation dose (0.2 mSv) without use of contrast medium. However, it is mainly used in chronic thromboembolic disease, and its clinical value in APE is not yet validated. DL-based APE detection on CTPA was also reviewed with sensitivity and specificity over 90% according to several systematic reviews and meta-analyses. Finally, they also reviewed therapeutic strategies for managing patients with APE, including catheter-directed thrombolysis, mechanical thrombectomy, and thrombus aspiration.

Kasaeian et al. reviewed the clinical applications of FFR-CT in coronary artery disease [6]. FFR-CT has been increasingly reported in the literature to yield improved accuracy in guiding patient management compared to standard coronary CT angiography (CTA). Real-world evidence of using FFR-CT in clinical practice has been validated by a number of multicenter trials proving that FFR-CT serves as a gatekeeper to invasive coronary angiography by reducing a significant number of unnecessary invasive procedures (Figures 2 and 3). FFR-CT is associated with significantly lower all-cause mortality, so it can guide confidential clinical decision-making. Judicious use of FFR-CT to guide coronary CTA interpretation was discussed alongside distal-to-lesion FFR-CT measurement, showing improved concordance with invasive FFR, hence further enhancing diagnostic precision. In this study, the limitations of FFR-CT are highlighted, along with the impact of high-quality coronary CTA image acquisition and coronary calcium scores on FFR-CT performance. Future potential applications of FFR-CT, such as its implementation in the evaluation of coronary artery anomalies (Figure 4) and plaque characterization, are also reviewed. These authors also reviewed the role of FFR-CT as a reliable tool to plan percutaneous coronary intervention (PCI) and identify suitable patients undergoing coronary artery bypass grafting. Finally, they summarized the role of FFR-CT combined with risk stratification as a gatekeeper to the catheterization lab to reduce unnecessary invasive procedures without comprising clinical outcomes.

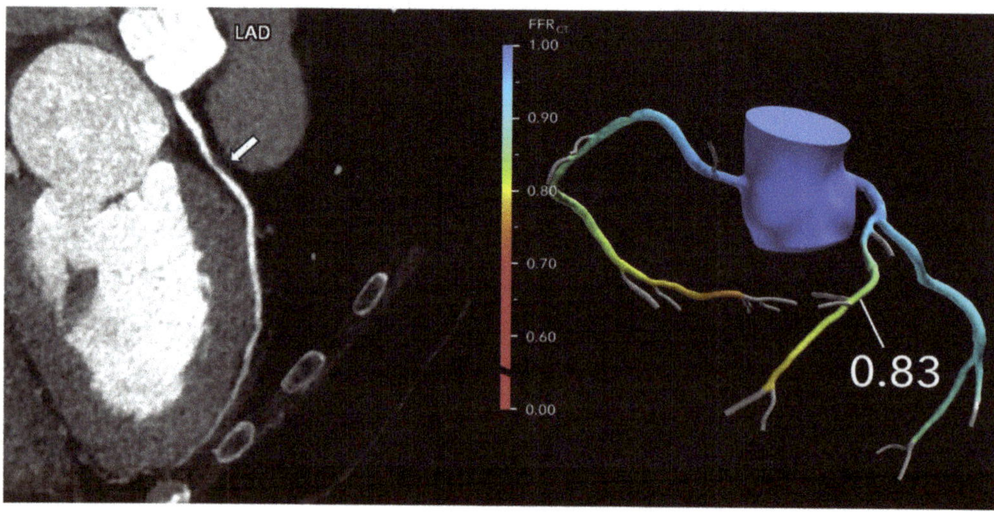

Figure 2. Optimizing treatment decisions with FFR-CT: (**Left**): A curved multiplanar reformatted coronary CTA image of the left anterior descending (LAD) in a 62-year-old man with atypical chest pain reveals severe stenosis (>70%) in the proximal LAD (arrow). (**Right**): The FFR-CT image demonstrates a value of 0.83 measured 2 cm distal to the lesion, indicating normal flow. As a result, invasive coronary angiography was deferred, and the patient was managed with medical therapy. Reprinted with permission under open access from Kasaeian et al. [6].

Panuccio et al. provide an overview of current coronary artery imaging modalities for diagnosis of chronic total occlusion (CTO), focusing on CTO-PCI. They discuss the strengths and limitations of each modality considered [7]. Optical coherence tomography (OCT), intravascular ultrasound (IVUS), and coronary CT angiography (CCTA) are reviewed in terms of their clinical value in assessment of CTO lesions. Despite the inherent superior spatial resolution (10–20 μm) allowing for detailed assessment of coronary wall and plaque morphology, OCT is limited by its penetration depth and invasive nature. In contrast, IVUS has several applications in CTO-PCI procedures, as it can be applied in proximal cap ambiguity, support in antegrade dissection and re-entry, support in reverse controlled antegrade and retrograde tracking, and integrated into stent deployment and optimization. IVUS-guided CTO-PCI is associated with higher procedural success rates, significantly lower procedural times, and a significantly lower risk of stent thrombosis. As a non-invasive imaging modality with the advantage of providing 3D visualizations, CCTA provides accurate assessment of plaque features and an overall vessel architecture (Figure 5). Furthermore, CCTA-based scores have shown better predictive performance than ICA-based scores. The authors of this article also discuss the future prospects of CTO interventions, including the use of AI/ML algorithms for automatic image segmentation and plaque quantification and the development of fusion imaging techniques consisting of combining CCTA with real-time fluoroscopy to provide real-time guidance during CTO-PCI procedures.

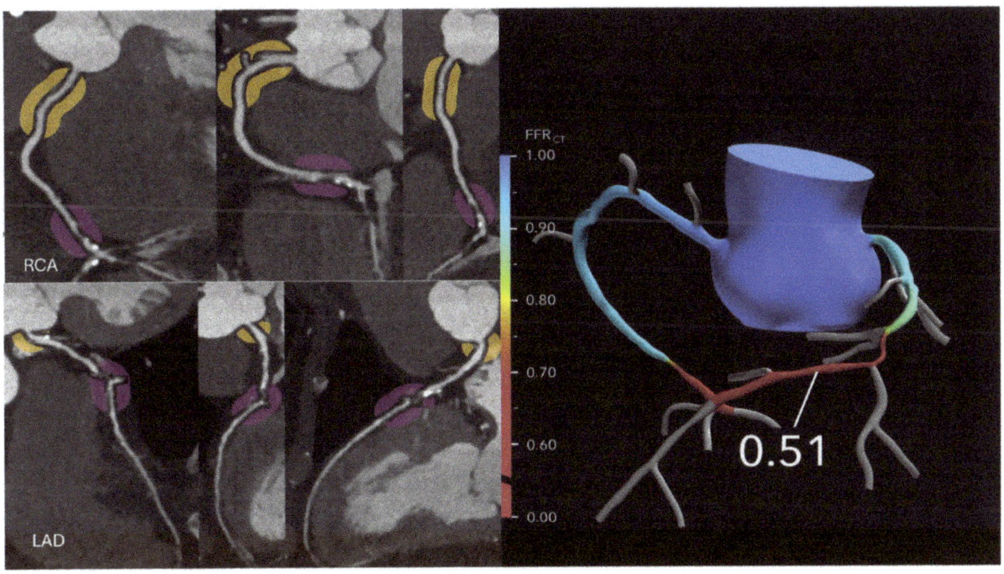

Figure 3. Optimizing treatment decisions with FFR-CT: (**Left**): A curved multiplanar reformatted coronary CTA image in a 64-year-old man with stable chest pain reveals severe stenoses in the mid left anterior descending (LAD) artery and distal right coronary artery. (**Right**): The corresponding FFR-CT image shows a value of 0.51 measured 2 cm distal to the lesion, indicating severely reduced flow. Based on these findings, the patient proceeded to invasive coronary angiography, followed by intervention. Please refer to Figure 4's caption for the degree of stenosis in relation to different colors. Reprinted with permission under open access from Kasaeian et al. [6].

The final review article is a systematic review of AI applications in CMR for CAD diagnosis [8]. Jimenez-Jara and colleagues searched three databases and identified 106 studies on the use of AI in the analysis of CMR images in patients with CAD. Forty-six studies documented the applications of AI in the classification of CMR images for diagnostic and prognostic purposes in CAD patients. They reviewed the characteristics of these studies by considering several aspects, including classification between healthy volunteers and patients with cardiovascular diseases, risk stratification for major adverse cardiovascular events and patients with arrhythmia-induced mortality, early detection of left ventricular remodeling, identification of normal and infarcted myocardial segments, and other less-studied factors, such as left ventricular paradoxical pulsation. Forty-one studies focused on the segmentation of different cardiac structures, including the myocardium, myocardial infarction scar, myocardial edema, the coronary artery, or adipose tissue, via CMR images. These studies used the Dice similarity coefficient (DSC) to determine AI performance compared to the ground truth, with high performance in AI segmentation of myocardium and infarcted regions being achieved, although there existed large variability in segmentation accuracy due to differences in MR imaging sequences. The remaining 19 studies reported the use of ML algorithms to extract radiomic features from CMR images for the differentiation of CAD patients. Despite showing great potential in improving diagnostic and prognostic accuracy in CAD, further improvements to the radiomics approach combined with AI models are needed before they are implemented into clinical practice.

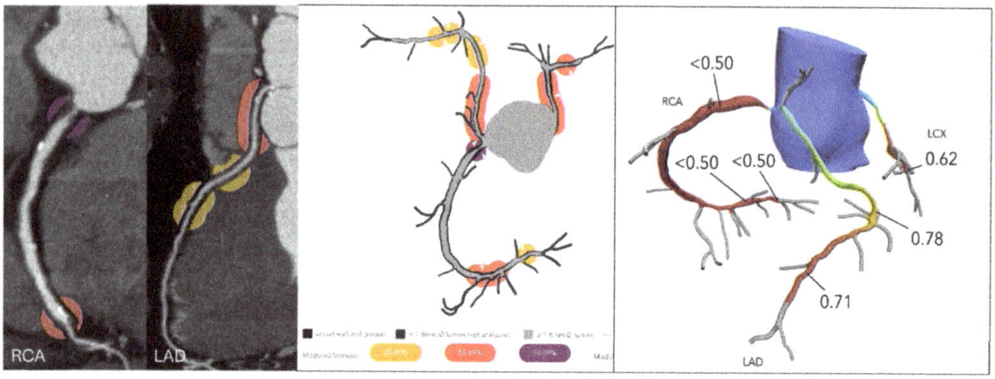

Figure 4. Anomalous aortic origin of the left coronary artery. (**Left**): Curved multiplanar reformatted coronary CT angiography (CTA) images in a 65-year-old male patient demonstrate severe stenosis at the ostium of the right coronary artery (RCA) and moderate stenosis at the ostium of the left anterior descending (LAD) artery, both originating from the right coronary cusp. (**Right**): Corresponding fractional flow reserve computed tomography (FFR-CT) images show a value of 0.50 at 2 cm distal to the RCA ostial lesion, indicating significantly reduced flow. The mid LAD displays a value of 0.78, and the distal LAD shows a value of 0.71, suggesting a high likelihood of hemodynamic significance. Based on these findings, the patient proceeded to invasive coronary angiography and subsequent intervention for both lesions. Reprinted with permission under open access from Kasaeian et al. [6].

The last study in this Special Issue is a communication on the application of mixed reality-guided minimally invasive cardiac surgery (MICS). Aye et al. [9] reported their initial experience of using HoloLens® 2 to guide preoperative planning and for real-time intraoperative guidance in three cases requiring MICS, including aortic value replacement via right anterior small thoracotomy (Figure 6), off-pump coronary artery bypass grafting surgery via left anterior small thoracotomy, and pulmonary valve replacement. The case series showed that mixed reality (HoloLens® 2) optimized ergonomics by superimposing the virtual model on the surgical field, and it provided more appropriate access to the operating field, leading to a mean reduction in cardiac surgical procedures by 34.3 ± 3.2 min. Regarding the use of mixed reality in surgery, positive responses were received from the clinical team. Despite the studied benefits of using mixed reality in MICS intraoperative visualization, further studies on a large cohort with inclusion of different cardiac anomalies and more complexities in cardiac disease are warranted.

In summary, this Special Issue showcases researchers' experiences of utilizing the latest imaging and innovative technologies in the diagnosis of cardiovascular disease. The findings of these nine studies encompass results that could have wide-ranging implications for cardiovascular disease diagnosis, from standard imaging modalities to the latest technologies, including FFR-CT, mixed reality, and artificial intelligence. This Special Issue serves as a useful resource for readers to learn more about the current status and future development of advanced imaging techniques in cardiovascular disease.

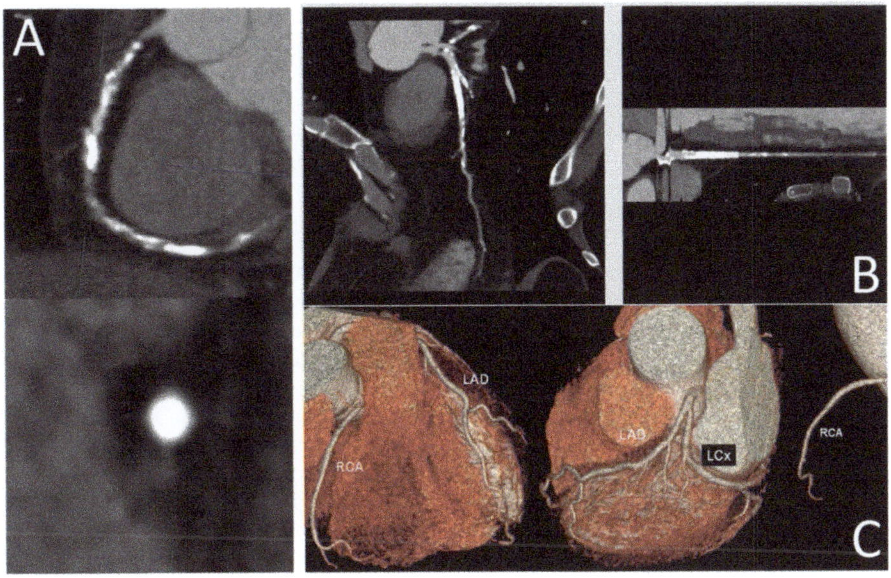

Figure 5. (**A**) Visualization of a high-calcified CTO plaque of a right coronary artery with the slab maximum intensity projection (MIP) technique; (**B**) curved and stretched multiplanar reconstruction of a left anterior descending CTO; (**C**) three-dimensional reconstruction of coronary arteries through the volume rendering approach. Reprinted with permission under open access from Panuccio et al. [7].

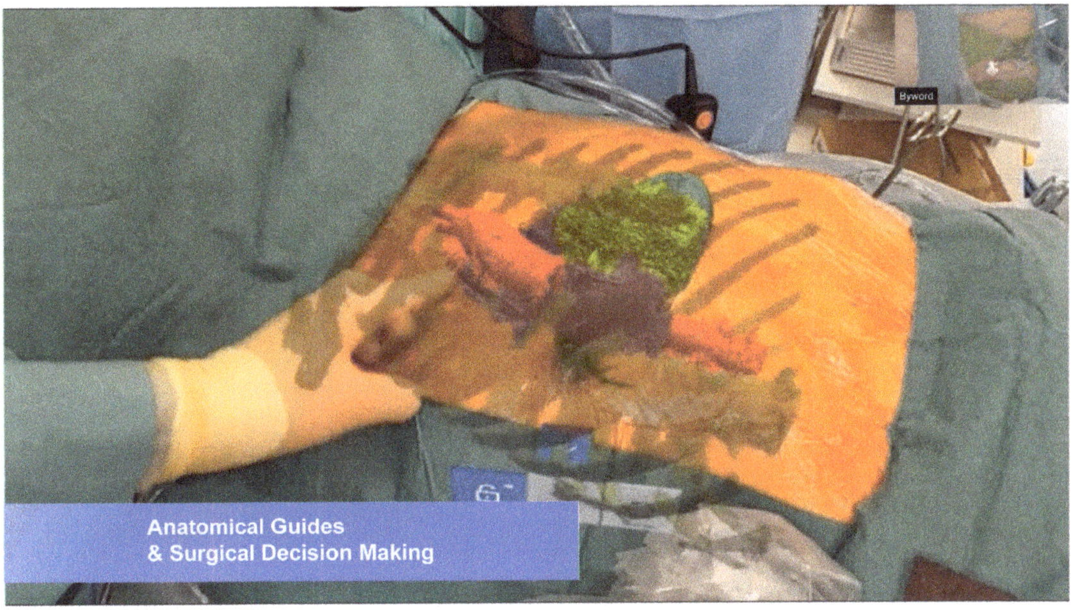

Figure 6. HoloLens® 2-guided minimally invasive surgery for aortic valve replacement. The colors indicate the virtual model overlaying the surgical field. Reprinted with permission under open access from Aye et al. [9].

Funding: This research received no external funding.

Conflicts of Interest: The author declares no conflicts of interest.

List of Contributions:

1. Nappi, C.; Ponsiglione, A.; Vallone, C.; Lepre, R.; Basile, L.; Green, R.; Cantoni, V.; Mainolfi, C.G.; Imbriaco, M.; Petretta, M.; et al. Association of cardiovascular risk factors and coronary calcium burden with epicardial adipose tissue volume obtained from PET-CT imaging in oncologic patients. *J. Cardiovasc. Dev. Dis.* **2024**, *11*, 331.
2. Cau, R.; Pisu, F.; Muscogiuri, G.; Suri, J.S.; Montisci, R.; Saba, L. Atrial and ventricular involvement in acute myocarditis patients with preserved rejection fraction: A single-centre cardiovascular magnetic resonance study. *J. Cardiovasc. Dev. Dis.* **2024**, *11*, 191.
3. Lee, S.; Squelch, A.; Sun, Z. Investigation of the clinical value of four visualization modalities for congenital heart disease. *J. Cardiovasc. Dev. Dis.* **2024**, *11*, 278.
4. Hashemizadehkolowri, S.; Akcicel, E.Y.; Akcicek, H.; Ma, X.; Ferguson, M.; Balu, N.; Hatsukami, T.S.; Yuan, C. Efficient and accurate 3D thickness measurement in vessel wall imaging: Overcoming limitations of 2D approaches using the Laplacian method. *J. Cardiovasc. Dev. Dis.* **2024**, *11*, 249.
5. Cellina, M.; Pavan, M.; Finardi, N.; Cicchetti, F.; Ce, M.; Biondetti, P.; Lanza, S.; Carrafiello, G. Advancement in acute pulmonary embolism diagnosis and treatment: A narrative review of emerging imaging techniques and intravascular interventions. *J. Cardiovasc. Dev. Dis.* **2025**, *12*, 333.
6. Kasaeian, A.; Ahmadzade, M.; Hoffmann, T.; Ghasemi-Rad, M.; Ayyappan, A.P. Fractional flow reserve from coronary CT: Evidence, applications and future directions. *J. Cardiovasc. Dev. Dis.* **2025**, *12*, 279.
7. Panucio, G.; Abdelwahed, Y.S.; Carabetta, N.; Landmesser, U.; De Rosa, S.; Torella, D. The role of coronary imaging in chronic total occlusions: Applications and future possibilities. *J. Cardiovasc. Dev. Dis.* **2024**, *11*, 295.
8. Jimenez-Jara, C.; Salas, R.; Diaz-Navarro, R.; Chabert, S.; Andia, M.E.; Vega, J.; Urbina, J.; Uribe, S.; Sekine, T.; Raimondi, F.; et al. AI applied to cardiac magnetic resonance for precision medicine in coronary artery disease: A systematic review. *J. Cardiovasc. Dev. Dis.* **2025**, *12*, 345.
9. Aye, W.M.M.; Kiraly, L.; Kumar, S.S.; Kasivoishvanaath, A.; Gao, Y.; Kofidis, T. Mixed reality (Holography)-guided minimally invasive cardiac surgery-A novel comparative feasibility study. *J. Cardiovasc. Dev. Dis.* **2025**, *12*, 49.

References

1. Nappi, C.; Ponsiglione, A.; Vallone, C.; Lepre, R.; Basile, L.; Green, R.; Cantoni, V.; Mainolfi, C.G.; Imbriaco, M.; Petretta, M.; et al. Association of cardiovascular risk factors and coronary calcium burden with epicardial adipose tissue volume obtained from PET-CT imaging in oncologic patients. *J. Cardiovasc. Dev. Dis.* **2024**, *11*, 331. [CrossRef] [PubMed]
2. Cau, R.; Pisu, F.; Muscogiuri, G.; Suri, J.S.; Montisci, R.; Saba, L. Atrial and ventricular involvement in acute myocarditis patients with preserved rejection fraction: A single-centre cardiovascular magnetic resonance study. *J. Cardiovasc. Dev. Dis.* **2024**, *11*, 191. [PubMed]
3. Lee, S.; Squelch, A.; Sun, Z. Investigation of the clinical value of four visualization modalities for congenital heart disease. *J. Cardiovasc. Dev. Dis.* **2024**, *11*, 278. [CrossRef] [PubMed]
4. Hashemizadehkolowri, S.; Akcicel, E.Y.; Akcicek, H.; Ma, X.; Ferguson, M.; Balu, N.; Hatsukami, T.S.; Yuan, C. Efficient and accurate 3D thickness measurement in vessel wall imaging: Overcoming limitations of 2D approaches using the Laplacian method. *J. Cardiovasc. Dev. Dis.* **2024**, *11*, 249. [CrossRef] [PubMed]
5. Cellina, M.; Pavan, M.; Finardi, N.; Cicchetti, F.; Ce, M.; Biondetti, P.; Lanza, S.; Carrafiello, G. Advancement in acute pulmonary embolism diagnosis and treatment: A narrative review of emerging imaging techniques and intravascular interventions. *J. Cardiovasc. Dev. Dis.* **2025**, *12*, 333. [CrossRef]
6. Kasaeian, A.; Ahmadzade, M.; Hoffmann, T.; Ghasemi-Rad, M.; Ayyappan, A.P. Fractional flow reserve from coronary CT: Evidence, applications and future directions. *J. Cardiovasc. Dev. Dis.* **2025**, *12*, 279. [CrossRef] [PubMed]
7. Panucio, G.; Abdelwahed, Y.S.; Carabetta, N.; Landmesser, U.; De Rosa, S.; Torella, D. The role of coronary imaging in chronic total occlusions: Applications and future possibilities. *J. Cardiovasc. Dev. Dis.* **2024**, *11*, 295. [CrossRef] [PubMed]

8. Jimenez-Jara, C.; Salas, R.; Diaz-Navarro, R.; Chabert, S.; Andia, M.E.; Vega, J.; Urbina, J.; Uribe, S.; Sekine, T.; Raimondi, F.; et al. AI applied to cardiac magnetic resonance for precision medicine in coronary artery disease: A systematic review. *J. Cardiovasc. Dev. Dis.* **2025**, *12*, 345. [CrossRef]
9. Aye, W.M.M.; Kiraly, L.; Kumar, S.S.; Kasivoishvanaath, A.; Gao, Y.; Kofidis, T. Mixed reality (Holography)-guided minimally invasive cardiac surgery-A novel comparative feasibility study. *J. Cardiovasc. Dev. Dis.* **2025**, *12*, 49. [CrossRef] [PubMed]

Journal of
Cardiovascular Development and Disease

MDPI

Article

Atrial and Ventricular Involvement in Acute Myocarditis Patients with Preserved Ejection Fraction: A Single-Center Cardiovascular Magnetic Resonance Study

Riccardo Cau [1,*], Francesco Pisu [1], Giuseppe Muscogiuri [2,3], Jasjit S. Suri [4], Roberta Montisci [5] and Luca Saba [1,*]

1 Department of Radiology, Azienda Ospedaliero Universitaria (A.O.U.), di Cagliari—Polo di Monserrato s.s. 554 Monserrato (Cagliari), 09045 Cagliari, Italy; fra.pisu1@gmail.com
2 School of Medicine and Surgery, University of Milano-Bicocca, 20126 Milan, Italy; g.muscogiuri@gmail.com
3 Department of Radiology, IRCCS Istituto Auxologico Italiano, San Luca Hospital, 20149 Milan, Italy
4 Stroke Monitoring and Diagnostic Division, AtheroPoint™, Roseville, CA 95661, USA; jsuri@comcast.net
5 Department of Cardiology, Azienda Ospedaliero Universitaria (A.O.U.), di Cagliari—Polo di Monserrato s.s. 554 Monserrato (Cagliari), 09045 Cagliari, Italy; rmontisci@unica.it
* Correspondence: riccardocau00@gmail.com (R.C.); lucasaba@tiscali.it (L.S.)

Abstract: Cardiac magnetic resonance (CMR) is commonly employed to confirm the diagnosis of acute myocarditis (AM). However, the impact of atrial and ventricular function in AM patients with preserved ejection fraction (EF) deserves further investigation. Therefore, the aim of this study was to explore the incremental diagnostic value of combining atrial and strain functions using CMR in patients with AM and preserved EF. This retrospective study collected CMR scans of 126 consecutive patients with AM (meeting the Lake Louise criteria) and with preserved EF, as well as 52 age- and sex-matched control subjects. Left atrial (LA) and left ventricular (LV) strain functions were assessed using conventional cine-SSFP sequences. In patients with AM and preserved EF, impaired ventricular and atrial strain functions were observed compared to control subjects. These impairments remained significant even in multivariable analysis. The combined model of atrial and ventricular functions proved to be the most effective in distinguishing AM patients with preserved ejection fraction from control subjects, achieving an area under the curve of 0.77 and showing a significant improvement in the likelihood ratio. These findings suggest that a combined analysis of both atrial and ventricular functions may improve the diagnostic accuracy for patients with AM and preserved EF.

Keywords: myocarditis; atrial strain; ventricular strain; preserved ejection fraction

1. Introduction

Acute myocarditis (AM) is an inflammatory disease of the myocardium with different clinical presentations and outcomes [1–4]. The heterogeneous clinical presentation makes the diagnosis challenging, mainly in patients with preserved ejection fraction (EF), in which the disease may go undetected (EF) [5,6]. However, the ITAMY study demonstrated that even patients with myocarditis and preserved EF developed major adverse cardiac events with an incidence of about 8% [6]. In this scenario, cardiovascular magnetic resonance (CMR) is the diagnostic tool of choice for patients with suspected myocarditis, allowing for an accurate morphological and functional cardiac assessment [2,7–10]. CMR has shown to be useful for the evaluation of myocardial strain, enabling the assessment of subclinical systolic and diastolic impairment [9,11]. Among strain acquisition techniques, CMR feature tracking (CMR-FT) is an emerging non-contrast quantitative method to evaluate both atrial and ventricular myocardial deformation using routinely acquired cine-CMR images [8,9,11–14]. This method utilizes optical flow to identify features within the image and subsequently tracks them through successive images in the sequences [11]. Myocardial strain measures the rate of myocardial deformation between relaxed and contracted states during a cardiac cycle [11,15–17]. The myocardium is composed of different layers with varied orientations of myofibers in each layer. Longitudinal strain indicates the shortening of the subendocardial fibers along the longitudinal axis from the base to the apex, and it is denoted by negative values. Circumferential strain measures the concentric myocardial shortening of subepicardial fibers on a short axis-view, and it is expressed by a negative value. Radial strain evaluates myocardial thickening and thinning of both subepicardial and subendocardial in the radial direction towards the center of the LV, and it is represented by a positive value [11,15,16]. Due to the distinctive orientations and thinness of the atrial wall, typically only the longitudinal strain is measured at the atrial level. Left atrial (LA) function can be divided into three consecutive phases, namely (1) reservoir, reflecting atrial filling during systole; (2) conduit, a measurement of the passive left atrium emptying during ventricular diastole; and (3) booster, representing atrial contractility [9]. Several studies investigated the impact of atrial and ventricular functions in patients with AM, reporting atrial and ventricular dysfunction during the acute phase of AM [18–20]. Conversely, there is a paucity of data with controversial results on CMR-FT in patients with AM patients and preserved EF. Gatti et al. demonstrated no differences in global longitudinal (GLS), global circumferential strain (GCS), and global radial strain (GRS) of the LV between AM patients with preserved EF and healthy subjects [21]. On the other hand, Meindl et al. reported a significant reduction in LV myocardial strain function compared to control subjects [22]. An echocardiography study of 30 patients with acute myocarditis and preserved EF, confirmed by CMR according to the Lake Louise criteria, demonstrated atrial impairment over LV dysfunction [23]. The aim of this study was to evaluate the impact of atrial and ventricular strain dysfunction and the benefit of multi-chamber investigation over the course of acute myocarditis with preserved EF.

2. Materials and Methods

2.1. Study Population

In this retrospective, longitudinal, observational, single-center study, all consecutive patients with acute myocarditis who underwent CMR and fulfilled the modified Lake Louise Criteria between 3 March 2019 and 7 August 2022 were included. Clinically suspected AM was defined based on the recent European Society of Cardiology position paper [2]. In particular, symptomatic patients with chest pain who fulfilled at least one diagnostic criterion (new electrocardiogram modification, elevated troponin, wall motion abnormalities with preserved LVEF on echocardiography) were considered to have suspected AM. A definitive diagnosis of AM was established using the current Lake Louise Criteria via CMR [7]. Endomyocardial biopsy (EMB) was not performed in our hospital in this low-risk population according to international statement [2]. Ejection fraction was assessed via CMR in each subject. In total, 52 healthy age- and gender-matched subjects were recruited to serve as a control group.

Exclusion criteria included subjects <18 years old; patients with reduced LVEF; previous myocardial infarction; pre-existing cardiomyopathy; and suspected or known prior irreversible myocardial damage.

The Institutional Review Board's approval for this retrospective, cross-sectional study was obtained, and patients' consent was waived because of the retrospective nature of this study.

A flowchart demonstrating the application of inclusion and exclusion criteria is provided in Figure 1.

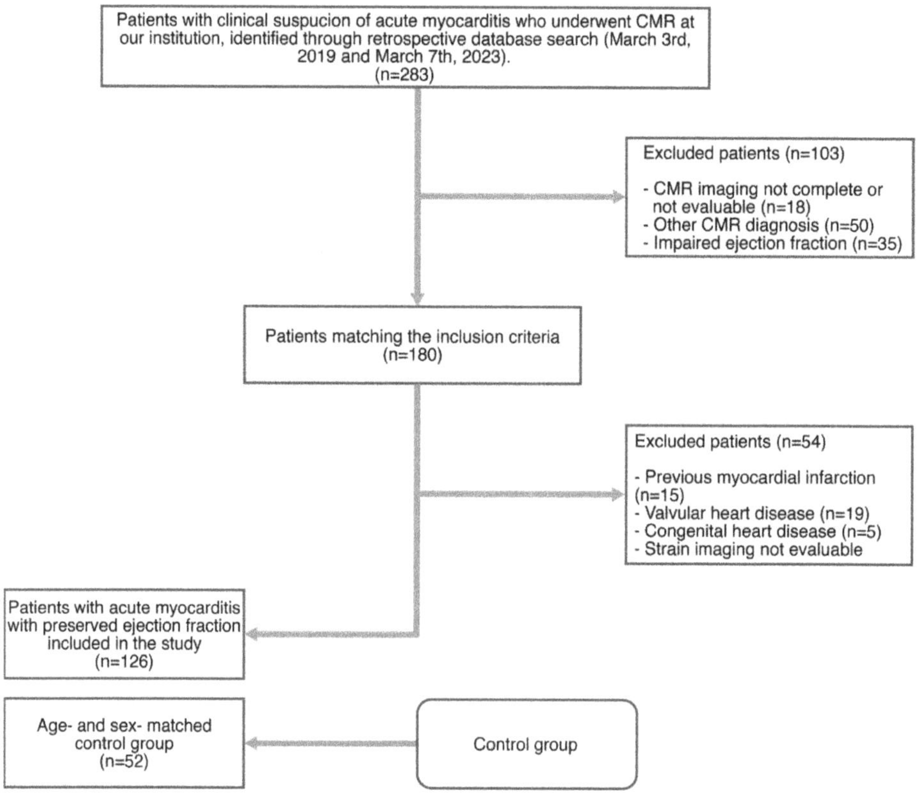

Figure 1. Flowchart of this study.

2.2. CMR Acquisition

CMR scans were performed at 4.1 ± 2.6 days (median = 1 day, range = 1–10 days) after admission to the hospital by using a Philips Achieva dStream 1.5 T scanner system (Philips Healthcare, Best, The Netherlands). Anterior coil arrays were used. All cine-images were acquired using a balanced steady-state free precession and retrospective gating during expiratory breath-hold maneuvers (TE: 1.7 ms; TR: 3.4 ms/flip-angle: 45°, section thickness = 8 mm) in both long-axis (two-, three- and four-chamber view) as well as short-axis planes with whole ventricular coverage from base to apex.

T2 mapping was acquired before the administration of contrast-media on three representative short-axis slices (at the base, mid-ventricular, and apex, respectively) using a single-breath-hold, black-blood prepared ECG-triggered, spin-echo multiecho sequence.

Late gadolinium enhancement (LGE) imaging was performed in both long- and short-axis slices 10–12 min minutes after contrast media injection (Gadovist, Bayer Healthcare, Berlin, Germany) with a dose of 0.15 mL per kg body weight using phase-sensitive inversion recovery sequences (PSIR) (TE: 2.0 ms; TR: 3.4 ms; flip-angle: 20°, section thickness = 8 mm) with an inversion time determined using the Look–Locker technique.

2.3. CMR Image Post-Processing

We used the commercially available software system Circle CVI42 (CV42 6.0, CVI42, Circle Cardiovascular Imaging Inc., Calgary, AB, Canada) for CMR-FT data analysis. Offline CMR feature tracking analyses were conducted for evaluation of peak global longitudinal strain, global radial strain, and global circumferential strain in a 16-segment software-generated 2D model. Concerning longitudinal strain, data on myocardial strain were derived from two-, three-, and four-chamber long-axis views. Regarding radial strain and circumferential strain, data on myocardial strain were derived from apical, mid-ventricular, and basal short-axis views in all patients. On all images, the epi- and endocardial borders were traced in end-diastole. After that, an automatic computation was triggered, by which the applied software algorithm automatically outlined the border throughout the cardiac cycle.

Similarly, CMR-FT analyses of atrial deformation were conducted offline. On all the acquired images, LA endocardial borders were manually traced in long view of the cine-images when the atrium was at its minimum volume. In particular, the four-, three-, and two-chamber views were used to derive LA longitudinal strain. LA appendage and pulmonary veins were excluded from segmentation.

After that, with an automatic computation, the software algorithm automatically tracked the myocardial borders throughout the cardiac cycle. The quality of the tracking and contouring was visually validated and manually corrected when needed. There are three peaks in the strain curve, including reservoir, conduit, and booster strain, as shown in Figure 2.

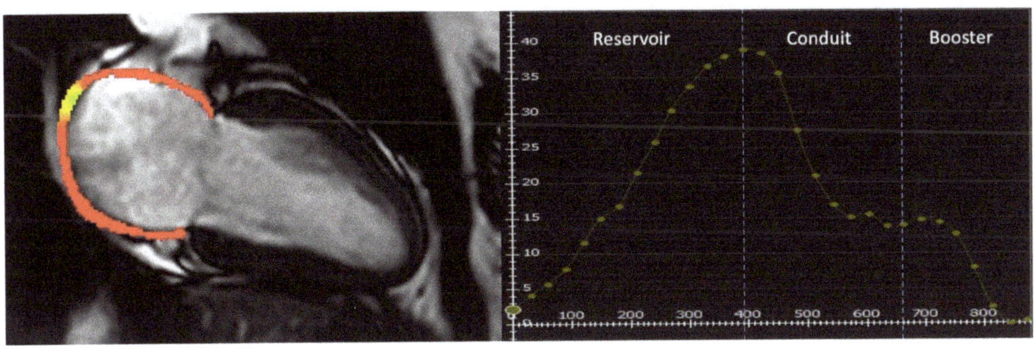

Figure 2. Examples of LA strain parameters in patient with AM. The endo- and epicardial borders of the LA were manually depicted, and the curves of the LA function were automatically obtained. Corresponding LA reservoir, conduit, and booster strain curves are shown.

Accordingly, their corresponding strain rate parameters were included. The quality of the tracking and contouring of atrial and ventricular function was visually validated and manually corrected by a radiologist with 4 years of experience in cardiac imaging.

The extent and location of LGE were assessed using both qualitative and quantitative methods. Qualitatively, the evaluation involved counting and determining the location of affected myocardial segments. Quantitatively, the extent of LGE was measured by tracing the epicardial and endocardial contours in each short-axis image. A region of interest (ROI) was manually placed in the myocardium without LGE to serve as a reference. LGE was defined as myocardium with a mean signal intensity exceeding the reference ROI by more than 5 standard deviations.

2.4. Statistical Analysis

Continuous variables are presented as mean $\pm$ standard deviation. Comparisons of continuous data were performed using the independent samples t-test or Mann–Whitney U test; Kolmogorov–Smirnov tests were used to assess the normality of residuals. Categorical variables were compared by using the chi-squared test or Fisher's exact test, as appropriate.

The association of LA and LV function parameters with the presence of AM with preserved EF was assessed by using univariable and multivariable logistic regression analysis. The univariable regression models included the presence of AM as the dependent variable and each LA and LV strain parameter as an independent variable. A subset of

CMR parameters that showed a p value < 0.05 in univariable analysis was further examined in multivariable analysis. All multivariable models were adjusted for age, sex, and LVEF.

To investigate the incremental value of considering both atrial and ventricular involvement, we compared multivariable models using the log-likelihood ratio (LR) test. Concretely, we compared models of ventricular or atrial parameters considered alone (base models) with models that included both parameters (complex models). The diagnostic accuracy of statistically significant parameters was further evaluated using receiver operating characteristics analysis. Confidence intervals (CIs) around the median area under the curve (AUC) were computed with 5000 bootstrap iterations.

A p value < 0.05 was considered statistically significant. All statistical analyses were performed using IBM SPSS Statistics version 22 (SPSS Inc., Chicago, IL, USA) and R (R Foundation for Statistical Computing, Vienna, Austria, version 4.1.0).

3. Results

3.1. Patient Demographics, Clinical Data, and CMR Data

Table 1 shows the characteristics of this study population. A total of 126 patients with AM and preserved EF, consisting of males (99, 78%) and females (27, 21%) with a mean age of 44.72 ± 18.22 years, as well as 52 age- and sex-matched control subjects, were included. There was no difference in the cardiovascular risk profile between the groups under study, except for some participants having a family history of coronary artery diseases (p = 0.001).

Table 1. Baseline characteristics and CMR parameters of included patients. The data are presented as mean ± standard deviation (SD) for quantitative variables and n (%) for qualitative variables.

	AM Subjects with Preserved EF (n = 126)	Control Subjects (n = 52)	p Value
Age, y	44.72 ± 18.22	46.73 ± 15.38	0.490
Male, n (%)	99 (78%)	43 (82%)	0.536
Weight, kg	71.53 ± 12.53	70.38 ± 17.31	0.778
Height, cm	170.70 ± 6.73	165.07 ± 10.57	0.136
BSA, m^2	1.82 ± 0.17	1.83 ± 0.16	0.187
Hypertension, n (%)	22 (17%)	11 (21%)	0.567
Dyslipidemia, n (%)	13 (10%)	6 (11%)	0.727
Obesity, n (%)	15 (12%)	3 (6%)	0.255
Smoke, n (%)	19 (15%)	8 (16%)	0.857
Diabetes, n (%)	5 (4%)	3 (6%)	0.559
Family history of CAD, n (%)	22 (17%)	1 (2%)	**0.001**
Elevated troponin, n (%)	126 (100%)	/	/
LVEF, %	56.48 ± 5.99	60.52 ± 5.54	**0.008**
LVEDV/BSA, mL/m^2	83.07 ± 15.15	80.37 ± 17.25	0.322
LVESV/BSA, mL/m^2	34.59 ± 13.23	32.22 ± 9.06	0.119
LVSV/BSA, mL/m^2	50.27 ± 10.15	48.18 ± 9.47	0.226
LV mass/BSA, g/m^2	62.87 ± 15.57	60.10 ± 10.70	0.216
LGE presence, n (%)	121 (96%)	/	/
LGE extent, %	7.81 ± 4.23	/	/
Reservoir, %	31.21 ± 11.88	36.09 ± 7.68	**0.001**
Reservoir rate, s^{-1}	1.42 ± 0,58	1.46 ± 0.42	0.597

Table 1. *Cont.*

	AM Subjects with Preserved EF (n = 126)	Control Subjects (n = 52)	p Value
Conduit, %	17.87 ± 9.77	21.61 ± 6.52	**0.004**
Conduit rate, s^{-1}	−1.91 ± 1.00	−1.73 ± 0.60	0.214
Booster, %	13.22 ± 4.99	13.52 ± 4.17	0.711
Booster rate, s^{-1}	−1.69 ± 0.60	−1.82 ± 0.62	0.218
GLS, %	−13.60 ± 3.25	−16.03 ± 2.35	0.001
GCS, %	−14,60 ± 3.91	−17.69 ± 3.27	0.001
GRS, %	22.48 ± 9.00	30.23 ± 8.08	0.001

Abbreviations: AM, acute myocarditis; CAD, coronary artery disease, EDV, end-diastolic volume; ESV, end-systolic volume; SV, stroke volume; EF, ejection fraction; BSA, body surface area; GLS, global longitudinal strain; GCS, global circumferential strain; GRS, global radial strain. Bold indicates statistical significance.

The median time from symptom onset to CMR was 5 days (interquartile range 2–7 days). Ejection fraction was preserved in the myocarditis group as well as in the control group (56.48% ± 5.99 vs. ± 60.52% ± 5.54, p = 0.008, Table 1). No differences were found in LV volumes and sizes quantified according to CMR imaging between the AM and control subjects.

Regarding LV myocardial strain parameters, GLS (−13.60% ± 3.25 vs. −16.03 ± 2.35, p = 0.001), GCS (−14.60% ± 3.91 vs. −17.69 ± 3.27, p = 0.001), and GRS (22.48% ± 9.00 vs. ± 30.23 ± 8.08, p = 0.001) demonstrated impaired function between the AM group and control subjects.

The LA reservoir mechanism was reduced in patients with myocarditis compared to control subjects (31.21 ± 11.88 vs. 36.09 ± 7.68, p = 0.001). Also, the LA conduit function was impaired in the myocardium compared to the control group (17.87 ± 9.77 vs. 21.61 ± 6.52, p = 0.004). In contrast, there was no difference in the LA reservoir strain rate, LA conduit strain rate, and contractile booster pump function between the groups under analysis.

3.2. Association of LA and LV Strain Mechanism with AM

Table 2 summarizes the findings of univariable and multivariable logistic regression analyses, which were conducted to examine the association between the AM, LA, and LV strain parameters. There was a significant association between the reservoir phase, conduit phase, and the presence of AM (odds ratio [OR] = 1.043, 95% CI 1.010–1.076, p = 0.009 and OR = 1.048, 95% CI 1.009–1.089, p = 0.001; respectively). In the model adjusted for traditional cardiovascular risk factors and LVEF, the association remained significant (OR = 1.044, 95% CI 1.006–1.083, p = 0.021 and OR = 1.069, 95% CI 1.016–1.125, p = 0.010; respectively).

Moreover, there was a significant association between GLS (OR = 0.738, 95% CI 0.642–0.849, p = 0.001), GCS (OR = 0.776, 95% CI 0.692–0.869, p = 0.001), GRS (OR = 1.117, 95% CI 1.065–1.171, p = 0.001), and the presence of AM. In the fully adjusted model, the association remained significant (GLS, OR = 0.726, 95% CI 0.611–0.842, p = 0.001; GCS OR = 0. 801, 95% CI 0.699–0.917, p = 0.001; GRS OR = 1.104, 95% CI 1.042–1.170, p = 0.001; respectively). Association of LVEF as a primary factor with AM was also statistically significant.

Table 2. Univariable and multivariable logistic regression analysis of CMR variables for discrimination between AM patients and controls. Each multivariable model was adjusted for age, sex, and left ventricle ejection fraction. Multivariable model for LVEF was adjusted for age and sex. Abbreviations are the same as in Table 1.

	Univariable Analysis		Multivariable Analysis	
	OR (95% CI)	*p* Value	OR (95% CI)	*p* Value
Reservoir, %	1.043 (1.010–1.076)	0.009	1.044 (1.006–1.083)	0.021
Conduit, %	1.048 (1.009–1.089)	0.001	1.069 (1.016–1.125)	0.010
GLS	0.738 (0.642–0.849)	0.001	0.726 (0.611–0.842)	0.001
GCS	0.776 (0.692–0.869)	0.001	0. 801 (0.699–0.917)	0.001
GRS	1.117 (1.065–1.171)	0.001	1.104 (1.042–1.170)	0.001
LVEF	0.918 (0.870–0.966)	0.001	0.921 (0.872–0.968)	0.002

3.3. Added Value of LA and LV Strain Parameters in Combination for Diagnosing AM

The diagnostic performance of LA and LV strain parameters alone versus their integrated models were evaluated using the LR test. The results showed that integrating LV and LA strain parameters resulted in a systematically better diagnostic accuracy than either parameter alone (Table 3). The integration of GLS, GCS, and GRS with the conduit resulted in a better discrimination ability (LR 31.73, 34.42 and 35.91, respectively) than the conduit (LR 23.37) diagnosing AM alone ($p = 0.004$, $p < 0.001$ and $p < 0.001$, respectively). Including GLS, GCS, and GRS in addition to the reservoir significantly improved the discrimination ability for diagnosing AM (LR 30.95, 32.70 and 34.73, respectively, vs. LR 21.96 for reservoir alone; $p = 0.003$, $p = 0.001$ and $p < 0.001$, respectively). The diagnostic performance of LVEF alone compared to the integrated models of LVEF and atrial and ventricular strain parameters is shown in Supplementary Table S1.

Table 3. Incremental value of combining ventricular and atrial strain measurements to identifying AM patients with preserved ejection fraction. All multivariable logistic regression models include age, sex, and left ventricle ejection fraction. Base models of conduit and reservoir strain are updated with one atrial strain measurement at a time, and these updated models are compared with the corresponding base model using a Likelihood ratio test. LR indicates log-likelihood ratio; Df, degrees of freedom. Other abbreviations are the same as in Table 1.

	Adjusted R^2 [a]	LR	Δ LR	Df	*p* Value [b]
Conduit [c]	0.175	23.37		5	<0.001
+GLS	0.233	31.73	8.36	6	0.004
+GCS	0.251	34.42	11.05	6	<0.001
+GRS	0.261	35.91	12.54	6	<0.001
Reservoir [c]	0.166	21.96		5	<0.001
+GLS	0.228	30.95	8.99	6	0.003
+GCS	0.239	32.70	10.74	6	0.001
+GRS	0.252	34.73	12.77	6	<0.001

[a] McFadden pseudo R^2. [b] *p* value by Likelihood ratio test. [c] base models of conduit and reservoir strains are compared with the null model.

In ROC analysis, the model that integrated GLS with the conduit strain outperformed both the LA and LV strain parameters in diagnosing AM, as indicated by the higher AUC (0.77, 95% CI 0.68–0.84, Figure 3). All other combined models are reported in Supplementary Figures S1 and S2. The ROC analysis for LVEF models is presented in Supplementary

Figure S3. LVEF models have lower AUCs compared to models of conduit and global ventricular strains.

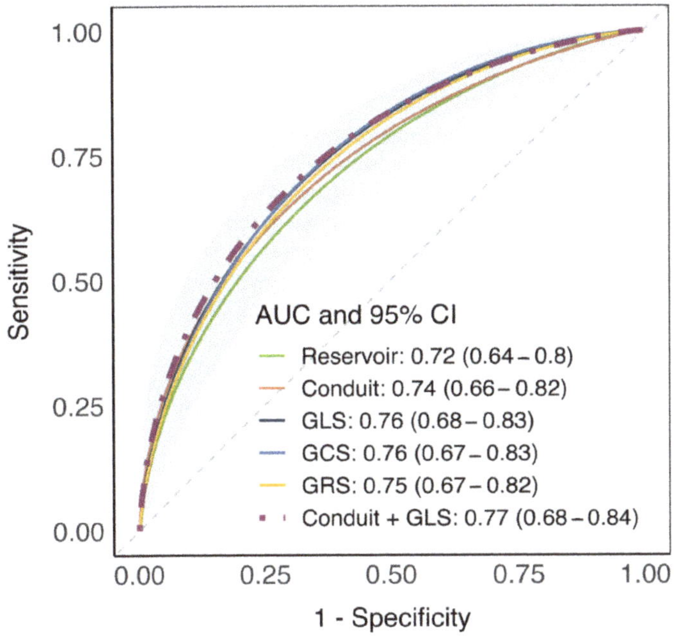

Figure 3. Receiver operating characteristics analysis reporting diagnostic performance of logistic regression models using atrial and ventricular strain measurements. The best performing model is reported with a violet, dashed line. The median area under curve and 95% confidence interval are reported for each model. Abbreviations are the same as in Table 1.

4. Discussion

Our data support the hypothesis that atrial and ventricular strain impairment is present in AM patients despite a preserved EF, suggesting subtle systolic and diastolic impairment. The main results of the current study can be summarized as follows: (1) a subtle ventricular impairment of all three myocardial layers was present despite normal EF, (2) besides ventricular dysfunction, the LA reservoir and conduit are significantly reduced, and (3) a multi-chamber approach improves the diagnostic accuracy, providing insights into the physiological communication between LV cardiac chambers in AM.

Previous studies evaluated the ventricular mechanism in AM patients with preserved EF with controversial results [20,21,24]. We found alterations of longitudinal, circumferential, and radial strain parameters in comparison with previous studies that reported no significant differences or involvement of longitudinal myocardial fiber alone during the acute stage of AM with preserved EF. These differences may be explained by the cut-off values used for normal EF. In particular, we decided to use a cut-off value for normal EF of 50% according to the 2022 AHA/ACC/HFSA Guideline for the Management of Heart Failure [25]. In addition, we included only a selected group of AM patients who fulfilled the modified Lake Louise Criteria [7].

Studies comparing left atrial mechanisms in patients with myocarditis have demonstrated reservoir and conduit impairment with preserved booster pump mechanisms in AM patients [19,20]. LA is an active cardiac chamber that plays a central role in cardiac output through an interaction with LV across the entire cardiac cycle [9,13].

However, little is known about the impact of the LA mechanism in AM patients with preserved EF. Given the relationship between LA dysfunction and adverse outcomes in various cardiovascular diseases [9,26,27], identifying atrial impairment in patients with preserved EF may aid in risk stratification. Meindl et al. investigated the diagnostic value of LV and LA myocardial strains in AM patients with preserved EF using speckle tracking echocardiography, demonstrating reservoir and conduit dysfunction in patients with acute myocarditis compared to healthy controls [23]. Similarly, Lee et al. showed impaired reservoir and conduit mechanisms in AM patients using CMR [28]. Our data confirmed these results, supporting the hypothesis of abnormalities in atrial compliance and diastolic impairment throughout the course of AM, despite preserved EF.

Overall, our results suggest abnormalities in both atrial and ventricular mechanisms in AM patients, emphasizing the physiological "communication" between left cardiac chambers during the course of the disease. Indeed, LA strain parameters depend on LV systolic function, especially subendocardial fibers, which can be evaluated by LV GLS [29].

Inoue et al. investigated LA strains as markers of LV diastolic impairment in a multicenter cohort of 322 patients with cardiovascular disease of different etiologies, reporting that the strongest determinant of LA strain parameters was LV GLS [30]. In addition, the authors demonstrated that the correlation between LA strain and LV diastolic dysfunction was more limited in patients with preserved EF (AUC of 0.67) or preserved GLS (AUC of 0.58) compared to those with impaired EF (AUC of 0.80) [30]. Similar results were also reported by Carluccio et al., supporting the significant contribution of LV impairment to LA dysfunction in patients with impaired EF [31].

Given this intrinsic relationship between LA and LV chambers, the LA strain may be a sub-optimal stand-alone marker of LV diastolic dysfunction in patients with normal EF [29], highlighting the importance of a comprehensive approach that includes both atrial and ventricular strain parameters. In particular, combining GLS and conduit mechanisms enhanced the diagnostic performance of CMR in AM patients compared to using atrial and ventricular strain parameters alone.

4.1. Clinical Implications

Our data emphasize the importance of evaluating multi-chamber strain parameters as a supportive non-contrast CMR diagnostic feature in AM patients, even with preserved EF. The integration of these parameters does not require additional CMR sequences and can be routinely acquired in standard CMR protocols, requiring only short post-processing examinations. This approach may be particularly helpful for patients who would benefit from abbreviated CMR protocols due to the inability to undergo lengthy CMR examinations or contrast media administrations. Confirming these results in a larger cohort of AM patients may facilitate a more in-depth understanding of multi-chamber involvement in AM patients with preserved EF. Indeed, the assessment of atrial and ventricular strains could potentially carry significant clinical implications, indicating that AM patients with preserved EF and impaired atrial and ventricular strains may constitute a distinct subgroup with subtle systolic and diastolic dysfunction. This finding ideally encourages therapeutic approaches to be applied earlier, potentially leading to improved outcomes for these patients.

4.2. Limitations

The current study's limitations should be acknowledged. Firstly, the relatively small sample size and the retrospective nature of this study are limitations. However, we exclusively enrolled very homogenous AM patients with preserved EF. The promising results of our study could prompt further prospective trials, including a larger number of patients, to confirm our findings.

Second, AM is more common in men. This prevalence of AM may influence the analysis of myocardial strain. To avoid bias, we matched the two groups under analysis for age and sex and used a multivariable regression model that included age and sex to account for their potential confounding effects. Although we observed significant differences in LVEF between these groups in both univariable and multivariable analyses,

LVEF demonstrated lower AUC values compared to models incorporating conduit and global ventricular strains. This highlights the need for future studies to incorporate a wider range of variables to account for potential confounding factors and to provide a more robust understanding of the relationship between myocardial strain and LVEF in AM patients. Third, there was no systematic endomyocardial biopsy to detect acute myocarditis. Finally, this study was cross-sectional in design, and we did not assess the predictive value of myocardial strain parameters for adverse cardiovascular events in AM patients, nor did we examine the data on patients' treatments during follow-up.

In our single-center study, we evaluated AM patients with the same CMR scanner and protocol, which may limit the reproducibility of our results. Externally validated multi-center longitudinal studies are needed to assess the association of these CMR parameters with patient outcomes.

5. Conclusions

Besides the dysfunction of ventricular strain parameters, patients with AM and preserved EF demonstrated impaired reservoir and conduit mechanisms. By combining atrial and ventricular mechanisms, CMR-FT can serve as a useful tool for assessing cardiac function and for gaining insights into multi-chamber dysfunction in the context of AM.

Supplementary Materials: The following supporting information can be downloaded at: https://www.mdpi.com/article/10.3390/jcdd11070191/s1, Supplementary Figure S1. Receiver operating characteristics analysis reporting diagnostic performance of logistic regression models using conduit and global ventricular strain measurements; Supplementary Figure S2. Receiver operating characteristics analysis reporting diagnostic performance of logistic regression models using reservoir and global ventricular strain measurements. Supplementary Figure S3. Receiver operating characteristics analysis reporting diagnostic performance of logistic regression models using left ventricle ejection fraction and atrial and global ventricular strain measurements. The best performing model is reported with a dark blue, dashed line. The median area under curve and 95% confidence interval are reported for each model. Supplementary Table S1. Incremental value of combining left ventricle ejection fraction (LVEF, primary factor) with ventricular and atrial strain measurements in identifying acute myocarditis patients with preserved ejection fraction. All multivariable logistic regression models include age and sex as adjustment factors. Base models of LVEF are updated with one atrial and ventricular strain measurement at a time, and these updated models are compared with the corresponding base model using a Likelihood ratio test. LR indicates log-likelihood ratio; Df, degrees of freedom. Other abbreviations are the same in Table 1 in the main text.

Author Contributions: Conceptualization, R.C. and F.P.; methodology, R.C. and F.P.; software, F.P.; validation, J.S.S., G.M., R.M., J.S.S. and L.S.; formal analysis, R.C. and F.P.; investigation, R.C. and F.P.; resources, R.C. and F.P.; data curation, L.S.; writing—original draft preparation, R.C. and F.P.; writing—review and editing, J.S.S., G.M., R.M. and L.S.; visualization, L.S.; supervision, L.S.; project administration, L.S. All authors have read and agreed to the published version of the manuscript.

Funding: This research received no external funding.

Institutional Review Board Statement: This study was conducted in accordance with the Declaration of Helsinki and approved by the Institutional Review Board of University of Cagliari NP/2023/1759, 19 April 2023.

Informed Consent Statement: Patient consent was waived due to the retrospective nature of this study.

Data Availability Statement: The data underlying this article cannot be shared publicly due to the privacy of the individuals that participated in this study. The data may be shared upon reasonable request from the corresponding author.

Conflicts of Interest: Jasjit S. Suri was employed by the company AtheroPoint^{TM}. The remaining authors declare that the research was conducted in the absence of any commercial or financial relationships that could be construed as a potential conflict of interest.

Abbreviations

AM, acute myocarditis; CMR, cardiovascular magnetic resonance; CMR-FT, cardiovascular magnetic resonance feature tracking; EF, ejection fraction; GCS, global circumferential strain; GLS, global longitudinal strain; GRS, global radial strain; LGE, late gadolinium enhancement; LR, log-likelihood ratio; LV, left ventricle; ROC, receiver operating characteristics; RV, right ventricle.

References

1. Ammirati, E.; Frigerio, M.; Adler, E.D.; Basso, C.; Birnie, D.H.; Brambatti, M.; Friedrich, M.G.; Klingel, K.; Lehtonen, J.; Moslehi, J.J.; et al. Management of Acute Myocarditis and Chronic Inflammatory Cardiomyopathy: An Expert Consensus Document. *Circ. Heart Fail.* **2020**, *13*, e007405. [CrossRef]
2. Caforio, A.L.P.; Pankuweit, S.; Arbustini, E.; Basso, C.; Gimeno-Blanes, J.; Felix, S.B.; Fu, M.; Heliö, T.; Heymans, S.; Jahns, R.; et al. Current state of knowledge on aetiology, diagnosis, management, and therapy of myocarditis: A position statement of the European Society of Cardiology Working Group on Myocardial and Pericardial Diseases. *Eur. Heart J.* **2013**, *34*, 2636–2648. [CrossRef]
3. Tschöpe, C.; Ammirati, E.; Bozkurt, B.; Caforio, A.L.P.; Cooper, L.T.; Felix, S.B.; Hare, J.M.; Heidecker, B.; Heymans, S.; Hübner, N.; et al. Myocarditis and inflammatory cardiomyopathy: Current evidence and future directions. *Nat. Rev. Cardiol.* **2021**, *18*, 169–193. [CrossRef]
4. Caforio, A.L.P.; Marcolongo, R.; Basso, C.; Iliceto, S. Clinical presentation and diagnosis of myocarditis. *Heart* **2015**, *101*, 1332–1344. [CrossRef]
5. Adiyaman, A.; Mouden, M. Cardiac magnetic resonance strain imaging in acute myocarditis with preserved ejection fraction: Promising and evolving. *Int. J. Cardiovasc. Imaging* **2022**, *38*, 1863–1864. [CrossRef]
6. Aquaro, G.D.; Perfetti, M.; Camastra, G.; Monti, L.; Dellegrottaglie, S.; Moro, C.; Pepe, A.; Todiere, G.; Lanzillo, C.; Scatteia, A.; et al. Cardiac MR with Late Gadolinium Enhancement in Acute Myocarditis with Preserved Systolic Function: ITAMY Study. *J. Am. Coll. Cardiol.* **2017**, *70*, 1977–1987. [CrossRef]
7. Ferreira, V.M.; Schulz-Menger, J.; Holmvang, G.; Kramer, C.M.; Carbone, I.; Sechtem, U.; Kindermann, I.; Gutberlet, M.; Cooper, L.T.; Liu, P.; et al. Cardiovascular Magnetic Resonance in Nonischemic Myocardial Inflammation: Expert Recommendations. *J. Am. Coll. Cardiol.* **2018**, *72*, 3158–3176. [CrossRef]
8. Xu, J.; Yang, W.; Zhao, S.; Lu, M. State-of-the-art myocardial strain by CMR feature tracking: Clinical applications and future perspectives. *Eur. Radiol.* **2022**, *32*, 5424–5435. [CrossRef]
9. Cau, R.; Bassareo, P.; Suri, J.S.; Pontone, G.; Saba, L. The emerging role of atrial strain assessed by cardiac MRI in different cardiovascular settings: An up-to-date review. *Eur. Radiol.* **2022**, *32*, 4384–4394. [CrossRef]
10. Cau, R.; Muscogiuri, G.; Pisu, F.; Mannelli, L.; Sironi, S.; Suri, J.S.; Pontone, G.; Saba, L. Effect of late gadolinium enhancement on left atrial impairment in myocarditis patients. *Eur. Radiol.* **2024**, *34*, 1846–1853. [CrossRef]
11. Scatteia, A.; Baritussio, A.; Bucciarelli-Ducci, C. Strain imaging using cardiac magnetic resonance. *Heart Fail. Rev.* **2017**, *22*, 465–476. [CrossRef]
12. Kebed, K.Y.; Addetia, K.; Lang, R.M. Importance of the Left Atrium: More Than a Bystander? *Heart Fail. Clin.* **2019**, *15*, 191–204. [CrossRef]
13. Pambianchi, G.; Marchitelli, L.; Cundari, G.; Ruoli, L.; Conia, L.; Catalano, C.; Galea, N. Takotsubo syndrome: Left atrial and ventricular myocardial strain impairment in the subacute and convalescent phases assessed by CMR. *Eur. Radiol. Exp.* **2024**, *8*, 34. [CrossRef] [PubMed] [PubMed Central]
14. Cau, R.; Loewe, C.; Cherchi, V.; Porcu, M.; Ciet, P.; Suri, J.S.; Saba, L. Atrial Impairment as a Marker in Discriminating between Takotsubo and Acute Myocarditis Using Cardiac Magnetic Resonance. *J. Thorac. Imaging* **2022**, *37*, W78–W84. [CrossRef]
15. Rajiah, P.S.; Kalisz, K.; Broncano, J.; Goerne, H.; Collins, J.D.; François, C.J.; Ibrahim, E.-S.; Agarwal, P.P. Myocardial Strain Evaluation with Cardiovascular MRI: Physics, Principles, and Clinical Applications. *RadioGraphics* **2022**, *42*, 968–990. [CrossRef]
16. Cau, R.; Bassareo, P.; Cademartiri, F.; Cadeddu, C.; Balestrieri, A.; Mannelli, L.; Suri, J.S.; Saba, L. Epicardial fat volume assessed with cardiac magnetic resonance imaging in patients with Takotsubo cardiomyopathy. *Eur. J. Radiol.* **2023**, *160*, 110706. [CrossRef]
17. Cau, R.; Muscogiuri, G.; Palmisano, V.; Porcu, M.; Pintus, A.; Montisci, R.; Mannelli, L.; Suri, J.S.; Francone, M.; Saba, L. Base-to-apex Gradient Pattern Assessed by Cardiovascular Magnetic Resonance in Takotsubo Cardiomyopathy. *J. Thorac. Imaging* **2023**. [CrossRef]
18. Luetkens, J.A.; Schlesinger-Irsch, U.; Kuetting, D.L.; Dabir, D.; Homsi, R.; Doerner, J.; Schmeel, F.C.; Fimmers, R.; Sprinkart, A.M.; Naehle, C.P.; et al. Feature-tracking myocardial strain analysis in acute myocarditis: Diagnostic value and association with myocardial oedema. *Eur. Radiol.* **2017**, *27*, 4661–4671. [CrossRef]
19. Dick, A.; Schmidt, B.; Michels, G.; Bunck, A.C.; Maintz, D.; Baeßler, B. Left and right atrial feature tracking in acute myocarditis: A feasibility study. *Eur. J. Radiol.* **2017**, *89*, 72–80. [CrossRef]
20. Doerner, J.; Bunck, A.C.; Michels, G.; Maintz, D.; Baeßler, B. Incremental value of cardiovascular magnetic resonance feature tracking derived atrial and ventricular strain parameters in a comprehensive approach for the diagnosis of acute myocarditis. *Eur. J. Radiol.* **2018**, *104*, 120–128. [CrossRef]

21. Gatti, M.; Palmisano, A.; Faletti, R.; Benedetti, G.; Bergamasco, L.; Bioletto, F.; Peretto, G.; Sala, S.; De Cobelli, F.; Fonio, P.; et al. Two-dimensional and three-dimensional cardiac magnetic resonance feature-tracking myocardial strain analysis in acute myocarditis patients with preserved ejection fraction. *Int. J. Cardiovasc. Imaging* **2019**, *35*, 1101–1109. [CrossRef]
22. Meindl, C.; Paulus, M.; Poschenrieder, F.; Zeman, F.; Maier, L.S.; Debl, K. Patients with acute myocarditis and preserved systolic left ventricular function: Comparison of global and regional longitudinal strain imaging by echocardiography with quantification of late gadolinium enhancement by CMR. *Clin. Res. Cardiol.* **2021**, *110*, 1792–1800. [CrossRef]
23. Meindl, C.; Paulus, M.; Poschenrieder, F.; Hamer, O.W.; Zeman, F.; Maier, L.S.; Debl, K. Left atrial strain parameters derived by echocardiography are impaired in patients with acute myocarditis and preserved systolic left ventricular function. *Int. J. Cardiovasc. Imaging* **2023**, *39*, 1157–1165. [CrossRef]
24. André, F.; Stock, F.T.; Riffel, J.; Giannitsis, E.; Steen, H.; Scharhag, J.; Katus, H.A.; Buss, S.J. Incremental value of cardiac deformation analysis in acute myocarditis: A cardiovascular magnetic resonance imaging study. *Int. J. Cardiovasc. Imaging* **2016**, *32*, 1093–1101. [CrossRef]
25. Heidenreich, P.A.; Bozkurt, B.; Aguilar, D.; Allen, L.A.; Byun, J.J.; Colvin, M.M.; Deswal, A.; Drazner, M.H.; Dunlay, S.M.; Evers, L.R.; et al. 2022 AHA/ACC/HFSA Guideline for the Management of Heart Failure: A Report of the American College of Cardiology/American Heart Association Joint Committee on Clinical Practice Guidelines. *Circulation* **2022**, *145*, e895–e1032. [CrossRef]
26. Chamsi-Pasha, M.A.; Zhan, Y.; Debs, D.; Shah, D.J. CMR in the Evaluation of Diastolic Dysfunction and Phenotyping of HFpEF: Current Role and Future Perspectives. *JACC Cardiovasc. Imaging* **2020**, *13*, 283–296. [CrossRef]
27. Cau, R.; Pisu, F.; Porcu, M.; Cademartiri, F.; Montisci, R.; Bassareo, P.; Muscogiuri, G.; Amadu, A.; Sironi, S.; Esposito, A.; et al. Machine learning approach in diagnosing Takotsubo cardiomyopathy: The role of the combined evaluation of atrial and ventricular strain, and parametric mapping. *Int. J. Cardiol.* **2023**, *373*, 124–133. [CrossRef]
28. Lee, J.; Choo, K.S.; Jeong, Y.J.; Lee, G.; Hwang, M.; Abraham, M.R.; Lee, J.W. Left Atrial Strain Derived from Cardiac Magnetic Resonance Imaging Can Predict Outcomes of Patients with Acute Myocarditis. *Korean J. Radiol.* **2023**, *24*, 512–521. [CrossRef]
29. Nagueh, S.F.; Khan, S.U. Left Atrial Strain for Assessment of Left Ventricular Diastolic Function: Focus on Populations with Normal LVEF. *JACC Cardiovasc. Imaging* **2023**, *16*, 691–707. [CrossRef]
30. Inoue, K.; Khan, F.H.; Remme, E.W.; Ohte, N.; García-Izquierdo, E.; Chetrit, M.; Moñivas-Palomero, V.; Mingo-Santos, S.; Andersen, Ø.S.; Gude, E.; et al. Determinants of left atrial reservoir and pump strain and use of atrial strain for evaluation of left ventricular filling pressure. *Eur. Heart J.-Cardiovasc. Imaging* **2022**, *23*, 61–70. [CrossRef]
31. Carluccio, E.; Biagioli, P.; Mengoni, A.; Francesca Cerasa, M.; Lauciello, R.; Zuchi, C.; Bardelli, G.; Alunni, G.; Coiro, S.; Ambrosio, G.; et al. Left Atrial Reservoir Function and Outcome in Heart Failure with Reduced Ejection Fraction. *Circ. Cardiovasc. Imaging* **2018**, *11*, e007696. [CrossRef]

Journal of
Cardiovascular
Development and Disease

MDPI

Article

Efficient and Accurate 3D Thickness Measurement in Vessel Wall Imaging: Overcoming Limitations of 2D Approaches Using the Laplacian Method

SeyyedKazem HashemizadehKolowri [1,*,†], Ebru Yaman Akcicek [1], Halit Akcicek [1], Xiaodong Ma [1], Marina S. Ferguson [2], Niranjan Balu [2], Thomas S. Hatsukami [3] and Chun Yuan [1,2]

1 Department of Radiology and Imaging Sciences, University of Utah, Salt Lake City, UT 84108, USA; ebru.akcicek@utah.edu (E.Y.A.); halit.akcicek@utah.edu (H.A.); xiaodong.ma@hsc.utah.edu (X.M.); chun.yuan@hsc.utah.edu (C.Y.)
2 Department of Radiology, University of Washington, Seattle, WA 98195, USA; msf2@uw.edu (M.S.F.); ninja@uw.edu (N.B.)
3 Department of Surgery, Division of Vascular Surgery, University of Washington, Seattle, WA 98195, USA; tomhat@uw.edu
* Correspondence: s.hashemizadehkolowri@utah.edu
† Current address: The Utah Center for Advanced Imaging Research (UCAIR), 729 Arapeen Dr., Salt Lake City, UT 84108, USA.

Abstract: The clinical significance of measuring vessel wall thickness is widely acknowledged. Recent advancements have enabled high-resolution 3D scans of arteries and precise segmentation of their lumens and outer walls; however, most existing methods for assessing vessel wall thickness are 2D. Despite being valuable, reproducibility and accuracy of 2D techniques depend on the extracted 2D slices. Additionally, these methods fail to fully account for variations in wall thickness in all dimensions. Furthermore, most existing approaches are difficult to be extended into 3D and their measurements lack spatial localization and are primarily confined to lumen boundaries. We advocate for a shift in perspective towards recognizing vessel wall thickness measurement as inherently a 3D challenge and propose adapting the Laplacian method as an outstanding alternative. The Laplacian method is implemented using convolutions, ensuring its efficient and rapid execution on deep learning platforms. Experiments using digital phantoms and vessel wall imaging data are conducted to showcase the accuracy, reproducibility, and localization capabilities of the proposed approach. The proposed method produce consistent outcomes that remain independent of centerlines and 2D slices. Notably, this approach is applicable in both 2D and 3D scenarios. It allows for voxel-wise quantification of wall thickness, enabling precise identification of wall volumes exhibiting abnormal wall thickness. Our research highlights the urgency of transitioning to 3D methodologies for vessel wall thickness measurement. Such a transition not only acknowledges the intricate spatial variations of vessel walls, but also opens doors to more accurate, localized, and insightful diagnostic insights.

Keywords: vessel wall imaging; vessel wall 3D thickness measurement; Laplace's equation; convolutions

1. Introduction

Cardiovascular disease remains a prominent cause of morbidity and mortality worldwide, necessitating the development of precise diagnostic and preventive strategies. The connection between vessel wall thickness and cardiovascular outcomes has been extensively established [1–9], underscoring the clinical importance of accurately measuring and characterizing arterial wall thickness. While various imaging techniques have been developed for this purpose, the fundamentally three-dimensional (3D) nature of vessel wall thickness measurement has often been overlooked in existing approaches.

B-mode ultrasound, a widely employed method [1,5,10,11], offers real-time imaging and non-invasiveness, allowing accurate vessel wall thickness measurement at relatively low cost. Magnetic resonance imaging (MRI), another modality for vessel wall imaging, provides exceptional soft tissue contrast and spatial resolution, yielding precise vessel wall thickness measurements with high reproducibility [12–14]. Recent advancement in imaging technologies has led to the emergence of various techniques for imaging vessel walls and characterizing atherosclerotic lesions, potentially improving risk assessment and patient management [15–18]. Additionally, recent progress in deep learning methodologies, has improved lumen and outer wall segmentation accuracy [19–21], highlighting the potential for enhanced vessel wall thickness measurement methodologies.

Traditionally, vessel wall thickness measurement has relied on two-dimensional (2D) approaches [14,22–27], which involve extracting 2D slices from 3D volumetric data. While these techniques allow calculation of standardized parameters, such as mean/maximum wall thickness and the normalized wall index, they inherently neglect the complete 3D nature of vessel walls [28]. Overlooking wall thickness variations in all three spatial directions, limits capacity of these methods to capture the holistic 3D characteristics of vessel walls, leading to inherent limitations that hinder the full clinical potential of vessel wall imaging techniques. A primary limitation of existing approaches is their reliance on the extracted 2D slices. In the case of straight vessels, the thickness measurement using cross-sectional 2D slices is reasonable; however, twisted arteries require extraction of cross-sectional slices that are perpendicular to luminal centerlines. Even with perfect centerline calculation, it is not always possible to extract cross-sectional slices perpendicular to vessel walls at all locations in highly tortuous vessels (see Figure 1a). Additionally, the lumen and outer wall boundaries in the extracted cross-sectional slices might be very complex (see Figure 1c), which makes wall thickness measurement very challenging even only in two dimensions. Furthermore, existing methods often only measure wall thickness at the lumen boundary, disregarding vital information about thickness variations across the entire vessel wall volume. As a result, comprehensive evaluations of wall thickness distribution throughout the entire wall volume remain elusive using conventional 2D techniques.

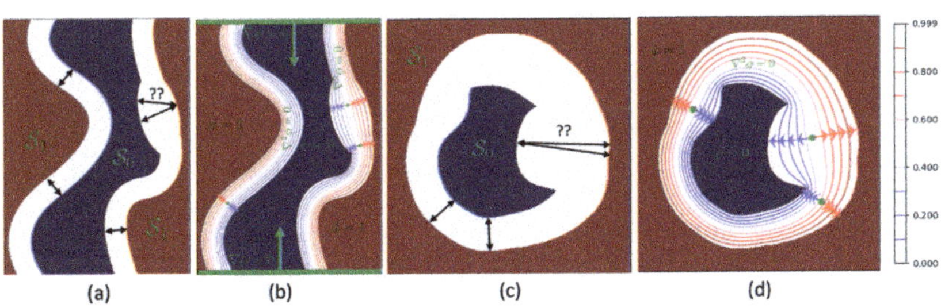

Figure 1. (**a**,**c**) Thickness measurement for parallel (double arrows) versus non-parallel (double arrows with ??) boundaries. (**b**,**d**) Subdividing the space between the two boundaries into smaller regions using parallel sublayers. By summing up the distances between these parallel sublayers, the thickness can be computed. The Laplace's Equation ($\nabla^2\phi = 0$), and Dirichlet ($\phi|_{S_0} = 0.00, \phi|_{S_1} = 1.00$) and Neumann ($\nabla\phi|_{\text{caps}} = \vec{0}$) boundary conditions are shown. At any given point, the thickness is determined by the summation of the lengths of two paths: a positive path (illustrated in red) extending from the specified point to the boundary with the higher potential, and a negative path (depicted in blue) extending from the specified point to the boundary with the lower potential.

To address these limitations and advance vessel wall thickness assessment, this study proposes adopting the Laplacian method [29] as an alternative measurement technique. By relying on the 3D geometric properties of vessel walls, the Laplacian method offers accurate and reproducible measurements while providing crucial localization insights into regions exhibiting abnormal wall thickening. Notably, this approach can be efficiently and expeditiously executed on deep learning (DL) platforms utilizing graphics processing units (GPUs), facilitating its integration into clinical workflows. The Laplacian method introduced in this study confers several advantages over existing approaches. First, it uses all available spatial dimensions in measuring the wall thickness. Second, its applicability spans both 2D and 3D scenarios, ensuring seamless transition between imaging modalities and offering adaptability in clinical settings. Third, by enabling voxel-wise measurements of arterial wall thickness, the Laplacian method captures thickness variations not only at lumen boundaries, but at the entire vessel wall volume. This allows for the 3D identification of regions with abnormal wall thickness, enabling precise localization of pathological changes and refining risk stratification.

In the subsequent sections, we will detail the Laplacian method's implementation through convolutions, demonstrating its efficient execution on DL platforms with GPU acceleration. Additionally, we will present experimental results showcasing the accuracy, reproducibility, and localization capabilities of this proposed approach, emphasizing its potential for enhanced cardiovascular risk diagnosis and prevention.

2. Theory

Thickness is a commonly employed concept that describes the distance separating two boundaries of an object or material. Typically, when dealing with 2D and 3D objects, their boundaries are specified using 1D curves and 2D surfaces, respectively. Consequently, the measurement of thickness becomes equivalent to measuring the distance between two 1D curves or two 2D surfaces. In cases where the boundaries are parallel, determining the distance (and thus, the thickness) is straightforward, as the distance between the two boundaries remains unchanged at all locations. However, when dealing with non-parallel boundaries, establishing a generalized and self-consistent definition of thickness becomes less straightforward, as depicted in Figure 1a,c.

Fortunately, for most practical applications, including the measurement of vessel wall thickness, the space between the two boundaries of interest can be subdivided into smaller regions using numerous infinitesimally proximate sublayers, all of which are parallel, as illustrated in Figure 1b,d. By summing up the distances between these parallel sublayers, the overall distance between the two original boundaries can be computed. To establish a mathematical formalization of this process, we denote the two boundaries by $\mathcal{S}_0$ and $\mathcal{S}_1$. To identify the parallel sublayers, we assign a scalar or a potential field ϕ to the space between $\mathcal{S}_0$ and $\mathcal{S}_1$, and assign different values (e.g., $\phi|_{\mathcal{S}_0} = 0.00$ and $\phi|_{\mathcal{S}_1} = 1.00$) to the boundaries to distinguish between them. By imposing a constraint on the divergence of the potential field, such that $\nabla^2\phi = 0$ within the space between the two boundaries, the resulting contours or equipotential surfaces of the potential field do not diverge at any point, thereby forming parallel sublayers. A brief overview of the Laplacian operator and its application is presented in the Supporting Information. Consequently, the problem of thickness measurement reduces to solving the following partial differential equation:

$$\nabla^2\phi = 0 \quad \text{s.t.} \quad \phi|_{\mathcal{S}_0} = 0.00, \quad \phi|_{\mathcal{S}_1} = 1.00. \tag{1}$$

The above equation and boundary conditions are referred to as Laplace's equation and Dirichlet conditions, respectively. Laplace's equation is encountered in a wide array of mathematical and physical problems. Another type of boundary condition commonly associated with Laplace's equation is known as the Neumann boundary condition, which imposes restrictions on the gradients of the potential field. In the context of measuring vessel wall thickness, the Neumann conditions, i.e., $\nabla\phi|_{\text{caps}} = \vec{0}$, can be applied to the end caps of the vessels, assuming that the vessels are extend uniformly when measuring the thickness at the end caps. After finding the solution to Equation (1), the normalized gradient vector field in the space between two boundaries can be obtained using $\vec{n} = \nabla\phi/\|\nabla\phi\|$. Given the normalized gradient vector field, the thickness at a specific location, $\vec{P}$, can be determined by adding lengths of two distinct paths, as visually depicted in Figure 1b,d. One path is characterized by a positive trajectory originating from $\vec{P}$ and extending towards the boundary with the higher potential. The other path represents a negative trajectory proceeding from $\vec{P}$ and terminating at the boundary with the lower potential. Notably, both paths are oriented perpendicularly to the potential field. The procedure for this thickness measurement can be realized following the steps outlined in Algorithm 1. In this algorithm, T is the measured thickness at point $\vec{P}$, T^+ is the length of the positive path which is equal to the distance to the outer wall, T^- is the length of the negative path which is equal to the distance to the lumen, and γ is the step size which is set to be smaller than a voxel size, e.g., $h/4$.

Algorithm 1: Computing the thickness

Input: $\mathcal{S}_0$, $\mathcal{S}_1$, $\vec{n}$, $\vec{P}$, γ(the step size)
Output: thickness at location $\vec{P}$

$\vec{P}^+_{\text{old}} := \vec{P}, T^+ := 0$ // positive path initialization
while $\vec{P}^+_{\text{old}} \notin \mathcal{S}_1$ **do**
    $\vec{P}^+_{\text{new}} := \vec{P}^+_{\text{old}} - \gamma\vec{n}(\vec{P}^+_{\text{old}})$
    $T^+ := T^+ + \gamma$
    $\vec{P}^+_{\text{old}} := \vec{P}^+_{\text{new}}$
$\vec{P}^-_{\text{old}} := \vec{P}, T^- := 0$ // negative path initialization
while $\vec{P}^-_{\text{old}} \notin \mathcal{S}_0$ **do**
    $\vec{P}^-_{\text{new}} := \vec{P}^-_{\text{old}} + \gamma\vec{n}(\vec{P}^-_{\text{old}})$
    $T^- := T^- + \gamma$
    $\vec{P}^-_{\text{old}} := \vec{P}^-_{\text{new}}$
return $T = T^+ + T^-$

In order to solve partial differential equations such as the Laplace's equation stated in Equation (1), numerical methods are commonly utilized. These techniques predominantly involve estimating partial derivatives of the potential field by employing finite difference approximations on either regular or non-regular grids. In the context of medical images, the boundaries of pixels/voxels within the image can be employed as a regular Cartesian grid for the purpose of finite difference approximation. In the case of a two-dimensional image, the Laplacian operator applied to the potential field, denoted by $\nabla^2\phi$, can be approximated using the five-point stencil finite difference formula [30], which is expressed as follows:

$$\nabla^2\phi(x,y) = \frac{1}{h^2}[\phi(x-h,y) + \phi(x+h,y) + \phi(x,y+h) + \phi(x,y-h) - 4\phi(x,y)] \quad (2)$$

where h represents the grid spacing. For image processing applications, we assign $h = 1$ to reflect a one-pixel spacing. Consequently, Equation (2) can be reformulated using a simpler notation as follows:

$$\nabla^2\phi_{0,0} = \phi_{-1,0} + \phi_{1,0} + \phi_{0,1} + \phi_{0,-1} - 4\phi_{0,0}. \quad (3)$$

To obtain a numerical solution for Laplace's equation, as stated in Equation (1), it is possible to set the right-hand side of Equation (3) to zero. By iteratively enforcing this condition along with the boundary conditions, convergence towards a solution can be achieved. To be more precise, the potential field in the i-th iteration can be updated using the following recursive expression:

$$\phi^{(i+1)}_{0,0} = \frac{1}{4}[\phi^{(i)}_{-1,0} + \phi^{(i)}_{1,0} + \phi^{(i)}_{0,1} + \phi^{(i)}_{0,-1}]. \quad (4)$$

The above equation demonstrates the updating process of an individual pixel. To apply this process to the entire potential field, denoted by ϕ and represented as a 2D image, a 2D convolution operation can be utilized in the following manner:

$$\phi^{(i+1)} = \frac{1}{4}\begin{bmatrix} 0 & 1 & 0 \\ 1 & 0 & 1 \\ 0 & 1 & 0 \end{bmatrix} \circledast \phi^{(i)} = K_{5\text{-pt}} \circledast \phi^{(i)} \tag{5}$$

We note that modern deep learning platforms facilitate rapid and efficient computation of convolutions by leveraging GPU resources. Consequently, Equation (5) enables the implementation of thickness measurement in an efficient manner. To start solving Equation (5), the potential field can be initialized as the average value between the two potential values at the boundaries. Moreover, the attainment of convergence can be evaluated by examining the change in total energy of the potential field, as expressed by the following equation:

$$E^{(i+1)} = \|\phi^{(i+1)} - \phi^{(i)}\| \tag{6}$$

By consolidating all the aforementioned information, the solution to Laplace's equation can be derived by following the procedural steps outlined in Algorithm 2.

Algorithm 2: Solving the Laplace's equation using convolutions

Input: $\mathcal{S}_0, \mathcal{S}_1, \phi_0 = 0.0, \phi_1 = 1.0, \epsilon = 10^{-5}$(convergence threshold)
Output: solution to Laplace's equation, ϕ

$i := 0, r := 1, \phi^{(0)} := [(\phi_0 + \phi_1)/2]$, // algorithm initialization
$\phi^{(0)}|_{\mathcal{S}_0} = \phi_0, \phi^{(0)}|_{\mathcal{S}_1} = \phi_1, E^{(0)} := \|\phi^{(0)}\|$
while $r \geq \epsilon$ **do**
  $\phi^{(i+1)} := K_{5\text{-pt}} \circledast \phi^{(i)}$
  $\phi^{(i+1)}|_{\mathcal{S}_0} = \phi_0, \phi^{(i+1)}|_{\mathcal{S}_1} = \phi_1$
  set the Neumann conditions for $\phi^{(i+1)}$ if applicable
  $E^{(i+1)} := \|\phi^{(i+1)} - \phi^{(i)}\|$
  $r := \frac{E^{(i)} - E^{(i+1)}}{E^{(i)}}$
  $i := i + 1$
return $\phi = \phi^{(i)}$

We note that for thickness measurement, as demonstrated in Algorithm 1, the potential field's gradient is needed. The computation of the gradient of the potential field can be accomplished efficiently by employing the Sobel–Feldman operator [31] and implementing it using convolutions, as follows:

$$\phi_x = \frac{1}{8}\begin{bmatrix} 1 & 0 & -1 \\ 2 & 0 & -2 \\ 1 & 0 & -1 \end{bmatrix} \circledast \phi = G_x \circledast \phi \tag{7a}$$

$$\phi_y = \frac{1}{8}\begin{bmatrix} 1 & 2 & 1 \\ 0 & 0 & 0 \\ -1 & -2 & -1 \end{bmatrix} \circledast \phi = G_y \circledast \phi \tag{7b}$$

The extension of the aforementioned algorithms for 3D thickness measurement is straightforward and accomplished by substituting 2D operations with their corresponding 3D counterparts as discussed in Appendix A. Furthermore, enhancing the robustness of the Laplacian and gradient operators can be achieved by employing alternative kernels in the convolutions. These modifications are elaborated upon in greater detail in Appendix B.

3. Materials and Methods

In this section, we present a series of experiments crafted to assess the accuracy and reproducibility of the proposed Laplacian method for measuring vessel wall thickness. By conducting a variety of experiments that encompass both 2D and 3D scenarios, our aim is to evaluate the effectiveness of the Laplacian method across different imaging modalities and clinical situations.

3.1. Thickness Measurement of 2D Digital Phantoms

In the first experiment, digital phantoms with circular and elliptical ring geometries were employed to simulate vessel wall thickness measurements in 2D scenarios. The circular ring had an inner radius of $r = 1.5\,\text{mm}$ with a uniform thickness of $d = 1.5\,\text{mm}$. The elliptical ring, showcasing a more complex geometry, had a major axis of $r_1 = 1.5\,\text{mm}$ and a minor axis of $r_2 = 1\,\text{mm}$ with a uniform thickness of $d = 1.5\,\text{mm}$. Thickness measurements using the Laplacian method were conducted at isotropic spatial resolutions of 2, 5, 10, 20, 50, 100, and 200 pixels/mm, respectively.

3.2. Outer Wall Thickness Measurement in 2D Histology Images

In the second experiment, we utilized histology images from two carotid artery samples. After obtaining informed consent, specimens from carotid endarterectomy were acquired. The specimens underwent formalin fixation, formic acid decalcification, and paraffin embedding. Serial Sections (10 µm thick) were made at specific intervals in the common carotid artery (CCA) and internal carotid artery (ICA) and stained with hematoxylin and eosin (H&E). An experienced research scientist, performed manual segmentation on 2D histology images, based on histopathologic classification, particularly following Stary et al.'s criteria [32], to identify outer wall and plaque compositional features.

Regions of interest, including lipid pools, necrotic cores, recent and late hemorrhages, calcifications, and loose extracellular matrices, were defined according to established criteria outlined by various authors [33–36]. Lipid pools, representing early lesions with distinct spaces composed of phospholipids and cholesterol, are visualized as acellular spaces through H&E. Necrotic cores, characterized by lipid and necrotic debris, may contain recent or late hemorrhage. Recent hemorrhages exhibit a mixture of intact and degenerating red cells, while late hemorrhages present eosinophilic material with cholesterol clefts. Calcifications show hydroxyapatite crystals, and loose extracellular matrices exhibit loosely organized fibers with smooth muscle cells and micro-vessels. These defined regions provided insights into carotid artery pathology.

The vessel wall thickness measurements using the Laplacian method were conducted on digital histology images with spatial resolutions of 100 and 180 pixel/mm, respectively. For each region of interest (ROI), the area, the normalized index, the mean and standard deviation of the wall thickness, as well as the mean and standard deviation of the distance to the lumen, were computed. The normalized index is defined as the area of ROI divided by the total vessel area. We note that the wall thickness and distance to lumen measurements are obtained using the Laplacian method, while the lumen area and the normalized wall index are computed directly from the manually drawn segmentation masks. On a CentOS server equipped with Intel® Xeon® E5-2620 v4 @2.10 GHz CPUs and two Nvidia® Tesla P40 GPUs, each with 24 GB of memory, the thickness measurement algorithm took 126 and 307 s to run for two different samples, respectively.

3.3. Thickness Measurements of 3D Digital Phantoms

In the third experiment, we utilized three digital phantoms, including a half-spherical shell, a half-ellipsoid shell, and a bent pipe, to simulate thickness measurements of 3D objects. The half-spherical shell had an inner radius of $r = 1.5\,\text{mm}$. The half-ellipsoid shell had a major axis of $r_1 = 2\,\text{mm}$ and minor axes of $r_2 = 1.5$ and $r_3 = 1\,\text{mm}$. The bent pipe had an inner radius of $r = 1.5\,\text{mm}$ and a quarter-circle axis with the radius of $R = 4.5\,\text{mm}$. All three phantoms had a uniform thickness of $d = 1.5\,\text{mm}$. The thickness measurements using the Laplacian method were performed for isotropic spatial resolutions of 2, 5, and 10 voxel/mm, respectively. We note that thickness measurements at higher spatial resolutions are not practically feasible because of huge computational requirements.

3.4. 3D Vessel Wall Thickness Measurement of Carotid Arteries in Black Blood MR Images

In the final experiment, we evaluated carotid vessel wall thickness measurements in MR images acquired using a 3D black blood contrast sequence. A healthy female volunteer aged 25 years, after providing informed consent and receiving institutional review board (IRB) approval, underwent scanning twice on a Siemens 3T MRI scanner (Prisma-fit, Erlangen, Germany). The follow-up scan took place one month after the baseline scan. For both scans, we utilized a custom-designed neck-shape-specific carotid coil (7 channels) [37], combined with a Siemens 20-channel head/neck coil. The black blood contrast was achieved using the 3D motion-sensitized driven equilibrium (MSDE), prepared rapid gradient echo (3D-MERGE) sequence [15], with the following parameters: field of view (FOV) = $250 \times 160 \times 42$ mm^3, acquistion voxel size = $0.82 \times 0.82 \times 0.82$ mm^3, interpolated voxel size = $0.41 \times 0.41 \times 0.41$ mm^3, TE/TR = 4.3/9.1 ms, preparation time = 22 ms, number of segments = 22, number of averages = 2, and scan time = 4 min and 35 s.

The 3D segmentation masks for the lumen and outer wall of the left and right carotid arteries were derived through processing of 3D MERGE imaging data using an in-house artificial intelligence (AI) framework [38,39]. This framework adopts a three-step methodology to process data from black blood vessel wall imaging data. Initially, it detects the locations of the right and left bifurcation slices. Subsequently, these identified slices are utilized to extract axial slices that encompass the bifurcation region, as well as the distal and proximal segments of the carotid arteries. In the next step, precise localization of the carotid arteries is achieved through 3D segmentation of their lumens by employing a 3D U-Net. Finally, the outcomes of this localization process are employed to extract 2D patches along the lumens of both the left and right carotid arteries, which are fed to 2D convolutional neural networks for the final lumen and outer wall segmentation. The segmentation outcomes were reviewed and manually corrected by trained reviewers using the ITK-SNAP 4.X software (Available online: http://www.itksnap.org/, accessed on 10 August 2024) [40], to ensure accuracy. Minor adjustments were made, if necessary, to refine the boundaries of the lumen and outer wall, improving overall segmentation quality.

To enhance thickness measurement accuracy, the segmentation masks were upsampled by a factor of 3 and smoothed using a 3D Gaussian filter before thickness measurement. Vessel wall thickness measurements utilizing the Laplacian method were subsequently performed. Using the same server mentioned in Section 3.2, the 3D thickness measurement algorithm took 227 and 212 s to run for the baseline and follow-up scans, respectively. For comparative analysis of thickness measurement results between the baseline and follow-up scans, the centerline and bifurcation coordinate system for the left and right carotid arteries were obtained using their lumen surfaces according to [41,42]. Lumen surfaces were extracted from the corresponding upsampled lumen masks using the marching cube algorithm. The centerline extraction and bifurcation coordinate system derivation methods have been implemented in an open-source Python package known as the vascular modeling toolkit (VMTK) (Available online: http://www.vmtk.org/, accessed on 10 August 2024) [43]. These routines enable robust extraction of the centerlines and associated metrics, including the centerline length parameter (abscissa) and the radius of the maximum inscribed sphere on the luminal surface. The bifurcation coordinate system establishes a non-uniform rectangular grid on the luminal surface of each branch within the carotid artery. The determination of coordinates involves partitioning the surface in the angular direction into sectors and in the longitudinal direction (along the centerline) into slabs.

Thickness measurement results were compared in two ways. In the first approach, vessel wall thickness was measured on the luminal surface and then averaged over rectangular patches forming the bifurcation coordinate system. In the second approach, vessel wall thickness was measured in all voxels within the outer wall volume, then averaged within a moving cylinder centered at each point along the centerline. The moving cylinder's axis coincided with the centerline, and its length was equal to the diameter of the maximum inscribed sphere to the luminal surface.

4. Results

4.1. Thickness Measurement of 2D Digital Phantoms

The results of the first experiment are shown in Figures 2 and 3. Figure 2 depicts circular and elliptical ring geometries (first row), solutions to the Laplace's Equation (second row), subsets of derived streamlines (third row), and the thickness maps (fourth row) corresponding to spatial resolutions of 2, 5, and 10 pixel/mm. We note that the second row displays a continuous potential field that increases from 0 to 1 as we move from the lumen to the outer wall, representing the solution to Laplace's equation obtained using Algorithm 2. The third row shows the trajectories of streamlines obtained using Algorithm 1. It is evident from Figure 2 that thickness maps exhibit a nearly uniform distribution around 1.5 mm, thereby affirming the uniform thickness of digital phantoms. Moreover, as the spatial resolution increases, thickness maps display enhanced uniformity, converging toward the 1.5 mm mark. This observation suggests that, at sufficiently high spatial resolutions, the Laplacian method yields accurate thickness measurements.

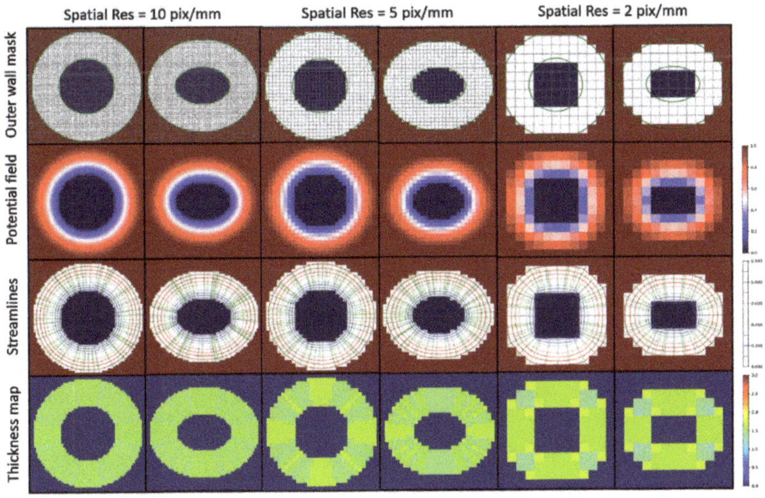

Figure 2. (First row) 2D digital phantoms with circular and elliptical ring geometries. (Second row) Solutions to the Laplace's Equation. (Third row) Subsets of derived streamlines. (Fourth row) Thickness maps.

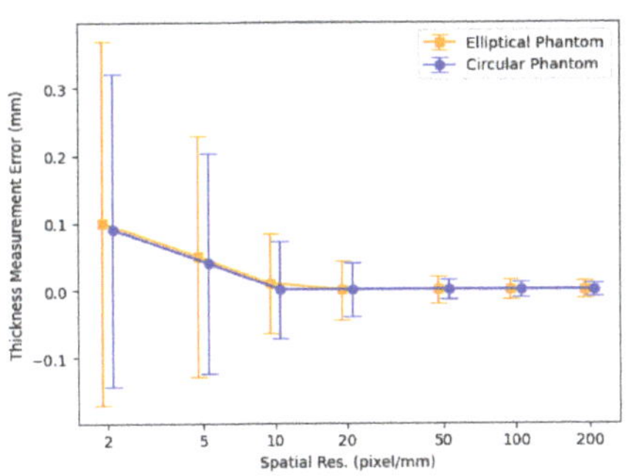

Figure 3. Thickness measurement errors for 2D digital phantoms as spatial resolution is increased.

Figure 3 displays thickness measurement errors for 2D digital phantoms as functions of spatial resolution. The plot reveals that, for higher spatial resolutions, thickness measurement biases approach zero, and the errors remain minimal. Conversely, as spatial resolution decreases, the errors exhibit a proportional increase with pixel size. Additionally, non-zero biases emerge, attributed to pixelation effects that prevent a precise realization of the ring geometry at lower spatial resolutions. Notably, the elliptical phantom manifests marginally higher errors compared to the circular phantom, implying that a more complex geometry tends to yield a larger thickness error compared to a simpler geometry.

4.2. Outer Wall Thickness Measurement in 2D Histology Images

The results from the second experiments are presented in Figure 4 and Table 1. In Figure 4, histology images of two carotid samples and manual annotation of ROIs (first column), vessel wall segmentation masks (second column), solutions to the Laplace's Equation (third column), contours of potential fields and subsets of corresponding streamlines (fourth column), the vessel wall thickness maps (fifth column), and the maps of distance to lumen (sixth column) are shown. We note that the Laplacian method, in addition to thickness measurement, allows for measuring the distance to lumen (length of the negative path in Algorithm 1) and the distance to outer wall (length of the positive path in Algorithm 1). We also see that the Laplacian method is capable of accurately measuring wall thickness for both regular, e.g., sample#1, and complex, e.g., sample#2, vessel wall morphologies. From thickness maps, it is evident that vessel wall regions with hemorrhage exhibit a notably increased wall thickness compared to other regions, which is consistent with the findings reported in previous studies. Additionally, we see that pathologies such as lipid pools are present in wall regions with both normal and abnormal thickness; however, most plaque features are observed in areas with abnormal wall thickening. This implies that diseased vessel walls may not be completely identifiable solely based on the wall thickness measurement; nevertheless, a strong correlation exists between the wall thickness and the presence of plaque components. Looking at distance-to-lumen maps, we see that plaque features are observed both in close proximity to the lumen and away from it, but distances of most plaque components to the lumen appear to be larger than the 1 mm threshold. This observation suggests that wall thickening attributed to plaque development predominantly occurs in areas closer to the outer wall boundary in these two histology samples.

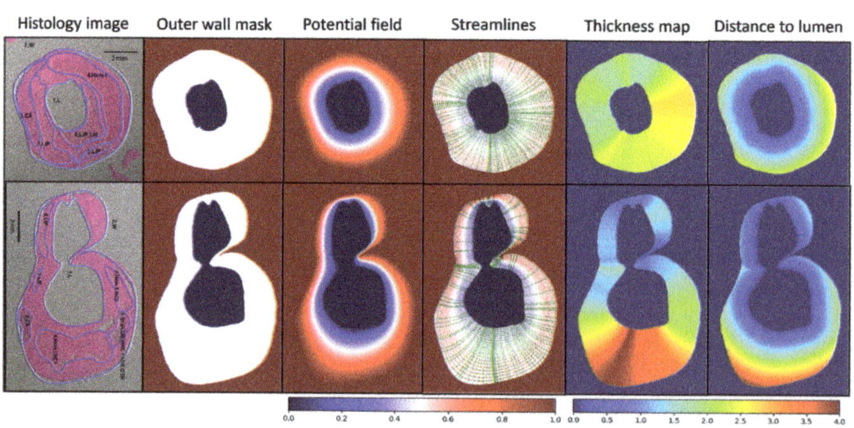

Figure 4. (First column) Histology images of two carotid samples and manual annotation of ROIs. (Second column) Vessel wall segmentation masks. (Third column) Solutions to the Laplace's Equation. (Fourth column) Contours of potential fields and subsets of corresponding streamlines. (Fifth column) Vessel wall thickness maps. (Sixth column) Distance-to-lumen maps.

Table 1. Morphological measurements form the histology images.

ROI #	ROI Type	ROI Area (mm^2)	Normalized Index	Wall Thickness (mm) (Mean ± Std)	Dist. to Lumen (mm) (Mean ± Std)
			Sample #1		
1	Lumen	5.64	0.14	-	-
2	Outer Wall	34.30	0.86	2.24 ± 0.31	1.29 ± 0.66
3	Calcification	3.80	0.09	1.93 ± 0.09	1.44 ± 0.23
4	Hemorrhage	9.05	0.22	2.30 ± 0.36	1.40 ± 0.41
5	Lipid Pool	0.85	0.02	2.42 ± 0.06	1.84 ± 0.17
6	Lipid Pool	3.74	0.09	2.49 ± 0.16	0.52 ± 0.29
7	Lipid Pool	4.69	0.12	2.11 ± 0.20	1.02 ± 0.56
			Sample #2		
1	Lumen	19.93	0.29	-	-
2	Outer Wall	49.77	0.71	2.31 ± 1.02	1.32 ± 0.96
3	Calcification	1.63	0.02	2.35 ± 0.25	1.86 ± 0.36
4	Hemorrhage	2.24	0.03	1.86 ± 0.23	1.15 ± 0.31
5	Loose Matrix	1.89	0.03	2.32 ± 0.28	1.41 ± 0.27
6	Hemorrhage	9.04	0.13	3.42 ± 0.30	1.61 ± 0.55
7	Lipid Pool	0.51	0.01	1.27 ± 0.08	0.81 ± 0.14
8	Lipid Pool	2.05	0.03	1.11 ± 0.11	0.63 ± 0.19

In Table 1, quantitative morphological measurements derived from histology images of carotid samples are presented. The two specimens manifest abnormal wall thickness, as evidenced by the overall mean wall thickness exceeding 2 mm. Additionally, the mean wall thickness within all ROIs corresponding to plaque components, excluding lipid pools, surpasses the threshold of normal wall thickness (1.5 mm). This affirmation aligns with our earlier observation in Figure 4, i.e., that a strong correlation exists between the vessel wall thickening and the presence of plaque. For both samples, ROIs featuring hemorrhage exhibit a relatively large mean wall thickness. Moreover, for all plaque components except lipid pools, the average distance-to-lumen exceeds 1 mm, corroborating the findings observed in Figure 4.

4.3. Thickness Measurements of 3D Digital Phantoms

The outcomes of the third experiment are presented in Figures 5 and 6. Figure 5 illustrates 3D volumes of three digital phantoms with isotropic spatial resolutions of 2, 5, and 10 voxel/mm in the first through third columns, respectively. Additionally, it displays equipotential surfaces of the potential fields, which are solutions to the Laplace's equation, and subsets of orthogonal streamlines for the spatial resolution of 10 voxel/mm in the fourth column. The fifth column shows thickness maps on the inner surfaces of phantoms for the spatial resolution of 10 voxel/mm. These results indicate that the Laplacian method, employed for measuring thickness in 3D objects, performs comparably well to its application in 2D scenarios. In particular, the fifth column in Figure 5 shows that thickness maps for all three phantoms have a nearly uniform distribution around a value of 1.5 mm. This observation affirms the uniform thickness of digital phantoms, and hence, implies that at a sufficiently high spatial resolution, the Laplacian method provides accurate 3D thickness measurements.

Figure 6 displays the 3D thickness measurement errors for the three digital phantoms, ploted as functions of spatial resolution. The plot indicates that, for the examined spatial resolutions, thickness measurement biases are nearly zero. Furthermore, as the spatial resolution is decreased, the errors demonstrate a proportional increase in accordance with voxel size. A comparison with the thickness measurement errors for 2D phantoms in Figure 3 reveals that biases are smaller in 3D scenarios. This might be attributed to less severe pixelation effects in three dimensions due to increased spatial degree of freedom.

Conversely, the measurement errors for 3D phantoms are larger than those of 2D phantoms, as an additional error term from the third dimension contributes to the overall thickness measurement error. We note that all three phantoms exhibit similar thickness measurement errors, suggesting the 3D geometrical complexity of these phantoms are comparable.

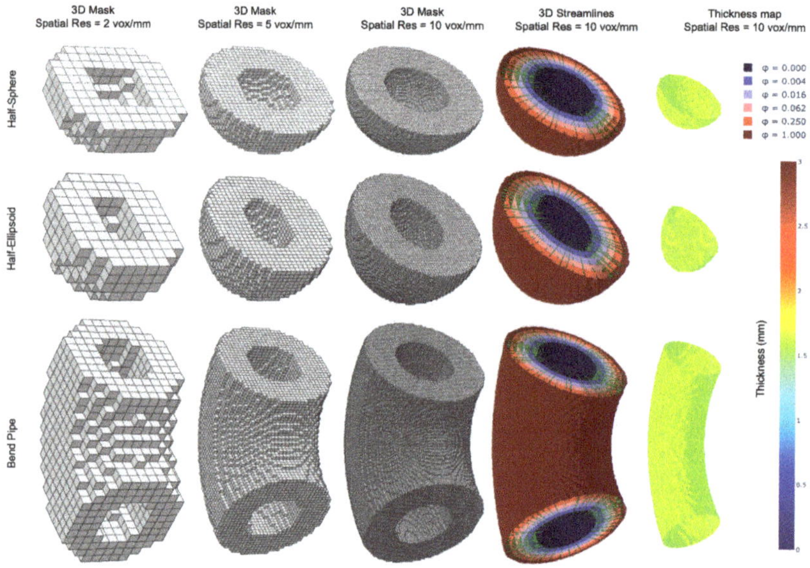

Figure 5. (First–third columns) 3D masks (volumes) of three digital phantoms with isotropic spatial resolutions of 2, 5, and 10 voxel/mm, respectively. (Fourth column) Equipotential surfaces of the potential field (solutions to the Laplace's equation) and subsets of corresponding orthogonal streamlines for a spatial resolution of 10 voxel/mm. (Fifth column) Thickness maps on the inner surfaces of the digital phantoms for a spatial resolution of 10 voxel/mm.

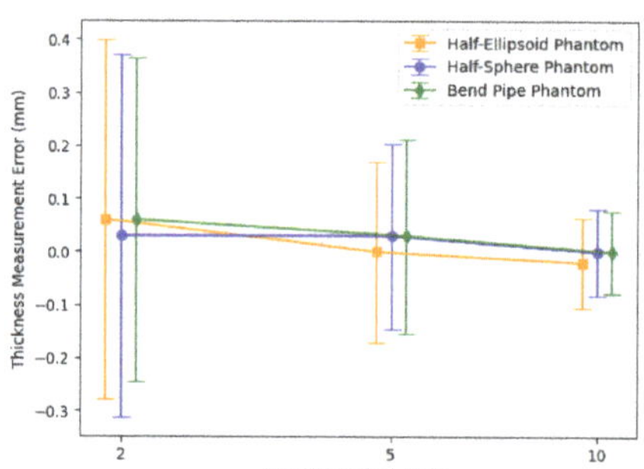

Figure 6. Thickness measurement errors for 3D digital phantoms as spatial resolution is increased.

4.4. 3D Vessel Wall Thickness Measurement of Carotid Arteries in Black Blood MR Images

The results from the final experiment are presented in Figures 7–9. In the left panel of Figure 7, axial views of 3D MERGE MR imaging data in the bifurcation region are shown for both baseline and follow-up scans (a,c). The vessel wall thickness maps superimposed on axial views are also shown (b,d). The axial images from the baseline and follow-up scans were meticulously chosen to represent identical anatomical regions; yet, the slices could not be fully aligned. The middle and right panels of Figure 7, illustrate extracted centerlines, bifurcation coordinate systems, and vessel wall thickness maps on luminal surfaces in baseline and follow-up scans for the right (e) and left (f) carotid arteries, respectively. We note that only CCA and ICA branches are considered. From the axial images shown, we see that image qualities in the bifurcation region for the baseline and follow-up scans are comparable; however, automated segmentation results reveal that the AI framework is not able to fully localize the distal CCA of the right carotid in the follow-up scan. This is due to signal-to-noise ratio (SNR) degradation occurring as one moves away from the bifurcation region, given that the carotid coils are conventionally centered around the carotid bulb.

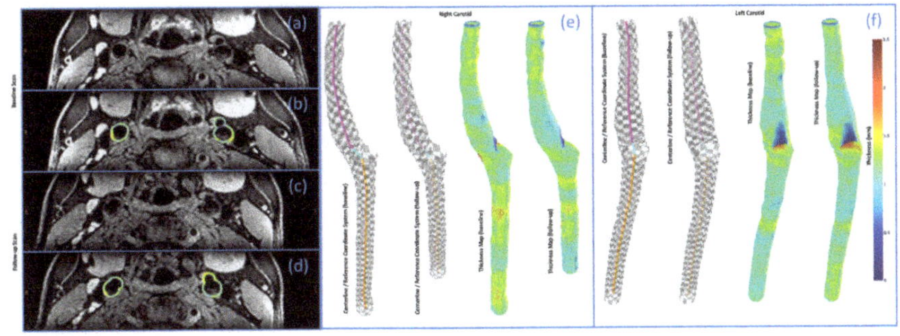

Figure 7. (**a**,**c**) Axial views of 3D MERGE MR imaging data for the baseline and follow-up scans. (**b**,**d**) The corresponding vessel wall thickness maps superimposed on the axial views. (**e**,**f**) Extracted centerlines, bifurcation coordinate systems, and vessel wall thickness maps on the luminal surfaces in baseline and follow-up scans for the right (**e**) and left (**f**) carotid arteries.

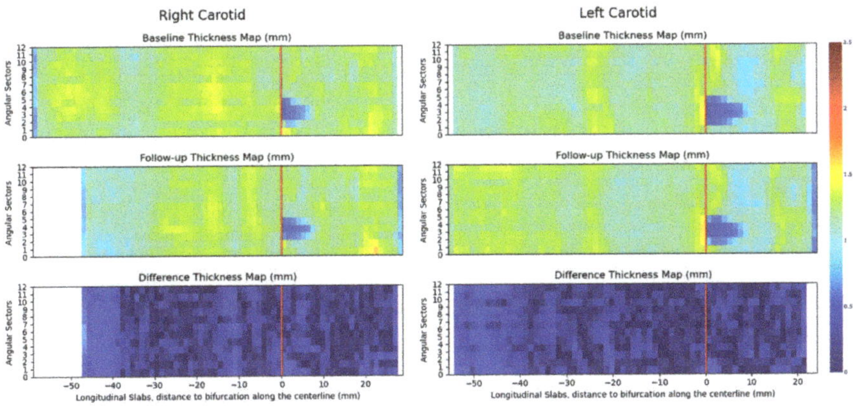

Figure 8. 3D vessel wall thickness measurements on luminal surfaces of the left and right carotid arteries in the baseline and follow-up scans. These regular 2D grids represent rectangular patches (derived from bifurcation coordinate system) on the luminal surfaces in an unwrapped and flattened format. Vertical red lines separate 2D grids associated with CCA and ICA branches. Each thickness value on the flattened grid is computed by averaging thickness measurements within the corresponding patch on the luminal surface.

Figure 8 compares the 3D vessel wall thickness measurements on luminal surfaces of the left and right carotid arteries between the baseline and follow-up scans. The luminal surfaces were partitioned into rectangular patches using bifurcation coordinate systems (see Figure 7e,f), subsequently unwrapped and flattened to generate regular 2D grids. Vertical red lines separate 2D grids associated with CCA and ICA branches. Each thickness value on the flattened grid is computed by averaging thickness measurements within the corresponding patch on the luminal surface. Using this approach, we can represent the thickness measurement results in a standardized structure, enabling quantitative and localized comparisons. This is achieved by computing the difference between flattened grids corresponding to baseline and follow-up scans, as demonstrated in Figure 8.

From Figure 8, it is evident that the wall thickness of both left and right carotid arteries predominantly falls within the range of 1 to 1.5 mm, with the exception of flow dividers in ICA branches. The latter can be readily identified on flattened thickness maps as dark blue spots. This observation implies a normal vessel wall condition for the subject under study, aligning with expectations for a healthy volunteer. The difference maps in Figure 8 demonstrate a close correspondence in thickness measurements between the baseline and follow-up scans. The small differences observed indicate a high reproducibility of the Laplacian method. Notably, the most significant differences manifest in the distal part of CCA branches, where the discrepancy may be attributed to inconsistent segmentation of the outer wall, potentially arising from the SNR degradation, as discussed previously.

Figure 9 compares the average 3D vessel wall thickness measurement, luminal radius, and the normalized wall volume index of the left and right carotid arteries along their respective centerlines between the baseline and follow-up scans. The solid-line curves correspond to the baseline, while the dash-line curves represent the follow-up scan. Carotid artery branches are color-coded, with orange indicating the CCA, magenta indicating the ICA, and cyan indicating the bifurcation region. From Figure 9, we see a close alignment between the 3D thickness measurements obtained from the baseline and follow-up scans, indicating a high level of reproducibility in 3D thickness measurements. Additionally, the reproducibility of the 3D thickness measurement, obtained using the Laplacian method, remains consistent with other morphological features, particularly the normalized wall volume index. The average vessel wall thickness for the subject under study falls within the range of 1 to 1.5 mm, while the normalized wall volume index ranges from 0.4 to 0.6, suggesting a normal vessel wall condition. In line with observations from Figures 7 and 8, the most significant deviation between baseline and follow-up measurements is observed in the distal part of the CCA branch.

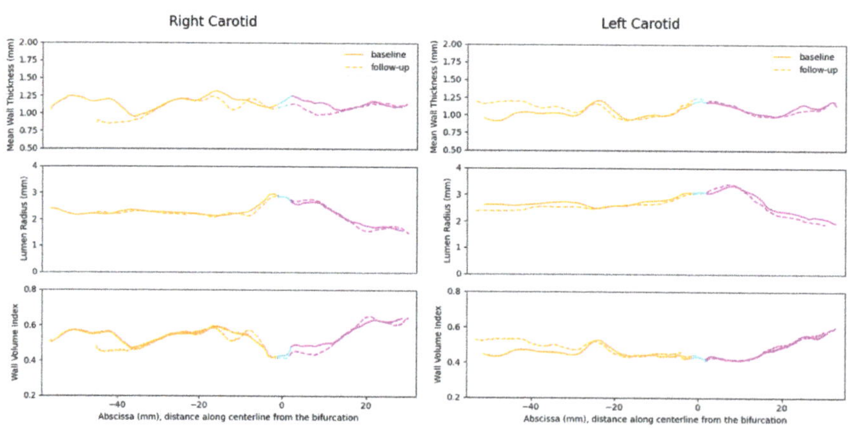

Figure 9. Average 3D vessel wall thickness measurement, luminal radius, and the normalized wall volume index of the left and right carotid arteries along their centerlines for the baseline and follow-up scans. The solid-line and dash-line curves correspond to the baseline and follow-up scans, respectively. Carotid artery branches are color-coded, with orange indicating the CCA, magenta indicating the ICA, and cyan indicating the bifurcation region.

5. Discussion

In this paper, we advocated for the recognition of vessel wall thickness measurement as inherently a 3D challenge and proposed the adoption of the Laplacian method to address this challenge in medical imaging applications. We argued that this method is capable of overcoming limitations associated with existing 2D-centric approaches. Specifically, the Laplacian method is versatile in its application to both 2D and 3D scenarios. It captures variations in vessel wall thickness across all dimensions, without reliance on the extraction of centerlines and 2D cross-sectional slices. This method provides localized wall thickness measurements, enabling precise 3D localization of regions manifesting increased wall thickness. Furthermore, it can be implemented efficiently by leveraging convolutions available in deep learning platforms and harnessing GPU resources. We also demonstrated the accuracy and reproducibility of the proposed method through multiple experiments involving digital phantoms and actual medical imaging data.

Throughout this paper, in both theoretical and experimental settings, the thickness measurement using the Laplacian method is explained in scenarios characterized by isotropic pixel/voxel dimensions. Generalization of this method to accommodate non-isotropic pixel/voxel dimensions is straightforward and can be achieved by incorporating scale factors corresponding to distinct spatial dimensions. An alternative solution is to resample the original object ensuring that the resultant pixels/voxels have isotropic dimensions, and then utilizing the implementation explained in this paper.

In the course of experiments involving digital phantoms, it was observed that increasing the spatial resolution leads to improved accuracy of thickness measurements utilizing the Laplacian method. In practical scenarios, increasing the spatial resolution of the binary mask of an object through upsampling can yield more precise thickness measurements. However, this also results in a heavier computational load associated with the Laplacian method. This effect is particularly noticeable in the case of 3D objects, where an upsampling by a factor of n translates into a volumetric increase in the number of voxels by n^3. The computational demand primarily arises from the number of pixels/voxels for which the thickness measurement is required. To address the computational burden in higher spatial resolution scenarios, one strategy involves measuring the thickness within a subset of pixels/voxels and subsequently extrapolating the entire thickness map. A more rigorous approach entails dynamically tracking the streamlines and storing information about voxels that share the same streamline, as they inherently have identical thickness measurements.

As previously mentioned, thickness describes the distance separating two boundaries of an object or material. When the boundaries of an object lack clear delineation, utilizing the Laplacian method for thickness measurements may yield inaccurate results. Therefore, particular attention should be paid towards regions where the boundaries of an object are not well-defined. In the context of measuring vessel wall thickness, this scenario may arise when two vessels appear to be in close proximity, leading to potential inaccuracies. For instance, the internal and external carotid arteries in the carotid bifurcation region often exhibit close spatial proximity, and the outer wall boundary in the flow divider section may remain invisible in the imaging data due to the inherent spatial resolution limitations of the imaging technique. In such instances, it is essential to correct the segmentation masks of the vessels to ensure an accurate separation of the outer wall boundaries of distinct vessels.

6. Conclusions

In this paper, we studied the vessel wall thickness measurement using the Laplacian method and demonstrated its efficient implementation using convolutions. Additionally, we showcased the application of this technique in 2D and 3D scenarios by conducting multiple experiments and investigating its accuracy, reproducibility, and localization capabilities. Overall, the method proposed in this research offers a promising avenue for accurate vessel wall thickness measurement, delivering heightened localization and comprehensive assessments in both 2D and 3D scenarios. By addressing the limitations inherent in existing techniques, this method holds the potential to advance the field of cardiovascular imaging, contributing to more precise risk evaluation and targeted interventions.

Supplementary Materials: The following supporting information can be downloaded at: https://www.mdpi.com/article/10.3390/jcdd11080249/s1, Section S1: Overview of the Laplacian Operator.

Author Contributions: Conceptualization, S.H.; methodology, S.H.; software, S.H.; validation, S.H., E.Y.A. and H.A.; formal analysis, S.H.; investigation, S.H.; resources, S.H., X.M., M.S.F., T.S.H. and C.Y.; data curation, E.Y.A., H.A., X.M. and M.S.F.; writing—original draft preparation, S.H.; writing—review and editing, S.H., E.Y.A., H.A., X.M., M.S.F., N.B., T.S.H. and C.Y.; visualization, S.H.; supervision, N.B., T.S.H. and C.Y.; project administration, S.H.; funding acquisition, X.M., M.S.F., T.S.H. and C.Y. All authors have read and agreed to the published version of the manuscript.

Funding: This study was supported in part by the 2023 Radiology Seed Grant at University of Utah and the National Institutes of Health [grant numbers R01-NS127317, R01-HL103609].

Institutional Review Board Statement: The study was conducted in accordance with the Declaration of Helsinki, and approved by the Institutional Review Board of The University of Utah (IRB_00162281, 25 January 2023).

Informed Consent Statement: Informed consent was obtained from all subjects involved in the study.

Data Availability Statement: The digital phantoms and implementation codes for the proposed thickness measurement method are available online at https://github.com/KazemHashemi/Vessel-Wall-3D-Thickness-Measurement.git (accessed on 1 August 2024).

Acknowledgments: During the preparation of this work, the authors used OpenAi/ChatGBT 3.5 in order to improve the language and grammar of the manuscript. After using this tool, the authors reviewed and edited the content as needed and take full responsibility for the content of the publication.

Conflicts of Interest: The authors declare no potential conflicts of interests.

Abbreviations

The following abbreviations are used in this manuscript:

2D	Two-dimensional
3D	Three-dimensional
MRI	Magnetic resonance imaging
DL	Deep learning
GPU	Graphics processing unit
ROI	Region of interest
CCA	Common carotid artery
ICA	Internal carotid artery
H&E	Hematoxylin and eosin
IRB	institutional review board
3T	Three Tesla
3D-MERGE	3D motion-sensitized rapid gradient echo
FOV	Field of view
AI	Artificial intelligence
VMTK	Vascular modeling toolkit
SNR	Signal-to-noise ratio

Appendix A. Extension to 3D

In the case of three-dimensional volume data, the Laplacian operator can be approximated by employing the seven-point stencil finite difference formula [44]. The formulation of this approximation is provided below:

$$\nabla^2\phi_{0,0,0} = \phi_{-1,0,0} + \phi_{1,0,0} + \phi_{0,1,0} + \phi_{0,-1,0} + \phi_{0,0,1} + \phi_{0,0,-1} - 6\phi_{0,0,0}. \tag{A1}$$

This leads to updating the potential field through a convolutional operation when iteratively solving the 3D Laplace's Equation (refer to line 4 of Algorithm 2):

$$\phi^{(i+1)} = \frac{1}{6}\left[\begin{bmatrix}0&0&0\\0&1&0\\0&0&0\end{bmatrix}\begin{bmatrix}0&1&0\\1&0&1\\0&1&0\end{bmatrix}\begin{bmatrix}0&0&0\\0&1&0\\0&0&0\end{bmatrix}\right] \circledast \phi^{(i)} = K_{7\text{-pt}} \circledast \phi^{(i)} \tag{A2}$$

Furthermore, the computation of the gradient of the potential field in three-dimensional space can be achieved through the utilization of the Sobel–Feldman operator, which is implemented using convolution operations. The process can be outlined as follows:

$$\phi_x = \frac{1}{32}\left[\begin{bmatrix} 1 & 0 & -1 \\ 2 & 0 & -2 \\ 1 & 0 & -1 \end{bmatrix}\begin{bmatrix} 2 & 0 & -2 \\ 4 & 0 & -4 \\ 2 & 0 & -2 \end{bmatrix}\begin{bmatrix} 1 & 0 & -1 \\ 2 & 0 & -2 \\ 1 & 0 & -1 \end{bmatrix}\right] \circledast \phi = G_x \circledast \phi \quad \text{(A3a)}$$

$$\phi_y = \frac{1}{32}\left[\begin{bmatrix} 1 & 2 & 1 \\ 0 & 0 & 0 \\ -1 & -2 & -1 \end{bmatrix}\begin{bmatrix} 2 & 4 & 2 \\ 0 & 0 & 0 \\ -2 & -4 & -2 \end{bmatrix}\begin{bmatrix} 1 & 2 & 1 \\ 0 & 0 & 0 \\ -1 & -2 & -1 \end{bmatrix}\right] \circledast \phi = G_y \circledast \phi \quad \text{(A3b)}$$

$$\phi_z = \frac{1}{32}\left[\begin{bmatrix} 1 & 2 & 1 \\ 2 & 4 & 2 \\ 1 & 2 & 1 \end{bmatrix}\begin{bmatrix} 0 & 0 & 0 \\ 0 & 0 & 0 \\ 0 & 0 & 0 \end{bmatrix}\begin{bmatrix} -1 & -2 & -1 \\ -2 & -4 & -2 \\ -1 & -2 & -1 \end{bmatrix}\right] \circledast \phi = G_z \circledast \phi \quad \text{(A3c)}$$

Appendix B. More Robust Kernels

The convolution operators employed in Equations (5) and (A2) utilize a minimal number of spatial points when computing the potential field's Laplacian. However, a more stable and isotropic approach to implementing the Laplacian necessitates incorporation of additional spatial points. In the context of 2D space, this can be accomplished by employing the nine-point stencil finite difference formula, as presented in [30], yielding the following formulation:

$$K_{9\text{-pt}} = \frac{1}{12}\begin{bmatrix} 1 & 2 & 1 \\ 2 & 0 & 2 \\ 1 & 2 & 1 \end{bmatrix} \quad \text{(A4)}$$

For 3D scenarios, more robust and isotropic implementation of the Laplacian operation can be attained through the utilization of the 19- or 27-point stencil finite difference formula [44], leading to the derivation of the following kernels:

$$K_{19\text{-pt}} = \frac{1}{24}\left[\begin{bmatrix} 0 & 1 & 0 \\ 1 & 2 & 1 \\ 0 & 1 & 0 \end{bmatrix}\begin{bmatrix} 1 & 2 & 1 \\ 2 & 0 & 2 \\ 1 & 2 & 1 \end{bmatrix}\begin{bmatrix} 0 & 1 & 0 \\ 1 & 2 & 1 \\ 0 & 1 & 0 \end{bmatrix}\right] \quad \text{(A5a)}$$

$$K_{27\text{-pt}} = \frac{1}{88}\left[\begin{bmatrix} 2 & 3 & 2 \\ 3 & 6 & 3 \\ 2 & 3 & 2 \end{bmatrix}\begin{bmatrix} 3 & 6 & 3 \\ 6 & 0 & 6 \\ 3 & 6 & 3 \end{bmatrix}\begin{bmatrix} 2 & 3 & 2 \\ 3 & 6 & 3 \\ 2 & 3 & 2 \end{bmatrix}\right] \quad \text{(A5b)}$$

The gradient kernels described in Equations (7) and (A3) exhibit two distinct types of filtering operations. Firstly, there is the central difference operation in the gradient direction, characterized by filter weights of $[1, 0, -1]/2$. Secondly, there are the smoothing (averaging) operations executed perpendicular to the gradient direction with filter weights of $[1, 2, 1]/4$. To enhance the rotational symmetry and numerical consistency of the gradient kernels, alternative smoothing operations can be employed. In [31], an optimization process is demonstrated to improve the gradient kernels. This optimization results in smoothing weights of $[47, 162, 47]/256$.

References

1. Hodis , H.N.; Mack, W.J.; LaBree, L.; Selzer, R.H.; Liu, C.-R.; Liu, C.-H.; Azen, S.P. The Role of Carotid Arterial Intima-Media Thickness in Predicting Clinical Coronary Events. *Ann. Intern. Med.* **1998**, *128*, 262–269. [CrossRef] [PubMed]
2. O'Leary, D.H.; Polak, J.F.; Kronmal, R.A.; Manolio, T.A.; Burke, G.L.; Wolfson, S.K. Carotid-Artery Intima and Media Thickness as a Risk Factor for Myocardial Infarction and Stroke in Older Adults. *N. Engl. J. Med.* **1999**, *340*, 14–22. [CrossRef] [PubMed]
3. Spence, J.D.; Eliasziw, M.; DiCicco, M.; Hackam, D.G.; Galil, R.; Lohmann, T. Carotid Plaque Area. *Stroke* **2002**, *33*, 2916–2922. [CrossRef] [PubMed]

4. Lorenz, M.W.; Markus, H.S.; Bots, M.L.; Rosvall, M.; Sitzer, M. Prediction of Clinical Cardiovascular Events with Carotid Intima-Media Thickness. *Circulation* **2007**, *115*, 459–467. [CrossRef]
5. Stein, J.H.; Korcarz, C.E.; Hurst, R.T.; Lonn, E.; Kendall, C.B.; Mohler, E.R.; Najjar, S.S.; Rembold, C.M.; Post, W.S. Use of Carotid Ultrasound to Identify Subclinical Vascular Disease and Evaluate Cardiovascular Disease Risk: A Consensus Statement from the American Society of Echocardiography Carotid Intima-Media Thickness Task Force Endorsed by the Society for Vascular Medicine. *J. Am. Soc. Echocardiogr.* **2008**, *21*, 93–111. [CrossRef]
6. Polak, J.F.; Pencina, M.J.; Pencina, K.M.; O'Donnell, C.J.; Wolf, P.A.; D'Agostino, R.B. Carotid-Wall Intima–Media Thickness and Cardiovascular Events. *N. Engl. J. Med.* **2011**, *365*, 213–221. [CrossRef] [PubMed]
7. Baldassarre, D.; Hamsten, A.; Veglia, F.; de Faire, U.; Humphries, S.E.; Smit, A.J.; Giral, P.; Kurl, S.; Rauramaa, R.; Mannarino, E.; et al. Measurements of Carotid Intima-Media Thickness and of Interadventitia Common Carotid Diameter Improve Prediction of Cardiovascular Events: Results of the IMPROVE (Carotid Intima Media Thickness IMT and IMT-Progression as Predictors of Vascular Events in a High Risk European Population) Study. *J. Am. Coll. Cardiol.* **2012**, *60*, 1489–1499. [CrossRef] [PubMed]
8. Touboul, P.J.; Hennerici, M.; Meairs, S.; Adams, H.; Amarenco, P.; Bornstein, N.; Csiba, L.; Desvarieux, M.; Ebrahim, S.; Hernandez Hernandez, R.; et al. Mannheim Carotid Intima-Media Thickness and Plaque Consensus (2004–2006–2011): An Update on Behalf of the Advisory Board of the 3rd, 4th and 5th Watching the Risk Symposia, at the 13th, 15th and 20th European Stroke Conferences, Mannheim, Germany, 2004, Brussels, Belgium, 2006, and Hamburg, Germany, 2011. *Cerebrovasc. Dis.* **2012**, *34*, 290–296. [CrossRef]
9. Bots, M.L.; Groenewegen, K.A.; Anderson, T.J.; Britton, A.R.; Dekker, J.M.; Engström, G.; Evans, G.W.; de Graaf, J.; Grobbee, D.E.; Hedblad, B.; et al. Common Carotid Intima-Media Thickness Measurements Do Not Improve Cardiovascular Risk Prediction in Individuals With Elevated Blood Pressure. *Hypertension* **2014**, *63*, 1173–1181. [CrossRef]
10. Pignoli, P.; Tremoli, E.; Poli, A.; Oreste, P.; Paoletti, R. Intimal plus medial thickness of the arterial wall: A direct measurement with ultrasound imaging. *Circulation* **1986**, *74*, 1399–1406. [CrossRef]
11. Wofford, J.L.; Kahl, F.R.; Howard, G.R.; McKinney, W.M.; Toole, J.F.; Crouse, J.R. Relation of extent of extracranial carotid artery atherosclerosis as measured by B-mode ultrasound to the extent of coronary atherosclerosis. *Arterioscler. Thromb. J. Vasc. Biol.* **1991**, *11*, 1786–1794. [CrossRef] [PubMed]
12. Underhill, H.R.; Kerwin, W.S.; Hatsukami, T.S.; Yuan, C. Automated measurement of mean wall thickness in the common carotid artery by MRI: A comparison to intima-media thickness by B-mode ultrasound. *J. Magn. Reson. Imaging* **2006**, *24*, 379–387. [CrossRef] [PubMed]
13. Harloff, A.; Zech, T.; Frydrychowicz, A.; Schumacher, M.; Schöllhorn, J.; Hennig, J.; Weiller, C.; Markl, M. Carotid intima-media thickness and distensibility measured by MRI at 3T versus high-resolution ultrasound. *Eur. Radiol.* **2009**, *19*, 1470–1479. [CrossRef] [PubMed]
14. Harteveld, A.A.; Denswil, N.P.; Van Hecke, W.; Kuijf, H.J.; Vink, A.; Spliet, W.G.; Daemen, M.J.; Luijten, P.R.; Zwanenburg, J.J.; Hendrikse, J.; et al. Ex vivo vessel wall thickness measurements of the human circle of Willis using 7T MRI. *Atherosclerosis* **2018**, *273*, 106–114. [CrossRef] [PubMed]
15. Balu, N.; Yarnykh, V.L.; Chu, B.; Wang, J.; Hatsukami, T.; Yuan, C. Carotid plaque assessment using fast 3D isotropic resolution black-blood MRI. *Magn. Reson. Med.* **2011**, *65*, 627–637. [CrossRef] [PubMed]
16. Qiao, Y.; Steinman, D.A.; Qin, Q.; Etesami, M.; Schär, M.; Astor, B.C.; Wasserman, B.A. Intracranial arterial wall imaging using three-dimensional high isotropic resolution black blood MRI at 3.0 Tesla. *J. Magn. Reson. Imaging* **2011**, *34*, 22–30. [CrossRef] [PubMed]
17. Li, M.L.; Xu, Y.Y.; Hou, B.; Sun, Z.Y.; Zhou, H.L.; Jin, Z.Y.; Feng, F.; Xu, W.H. High-resolution intracranial vessel wall imaging using 3D CUBE T1 weighted sequence. *Eur. J. Radiol.* **2016**, *85*, 803–807. [CrossRef] [PubMed]
18. Xie, Y.; Yang, Q.; Xie, G.; Pang, J.; Fan, Z.; Li, D. Improved black-blood imaging using DANTE-SPACE for simultaneous carotid and intracranial vessel wall evaluation. *Magn. Reson. Med.* **2016**, *75*, 2286–2294. [CrossRef] [PubMed]
19. Shi, F.; Yang, Q.; Guo, X.; Qureshi, T.A.; Tian, Z.; Miao, H.; Dey, D.; Li, D.; Fan, Z. Intracranial Vessel Wall Segmentation Using Convolutional Neural Networks. *IEEE Trans. Biomed. Eng.* **2019**, *66*, 2840–2847. [CrossRef]
20. Xie, M.; Li, Y.; Xue, Y.; Shafritz, R.; Rahimi, S.A.; Ady, J.W.; Roshan, U.W. Vessel lumen segmentation in internal carotid artery ultrasounds with deep convolutional neural networks. In Proceedings of the 2019 IEEE International Conference on Bioinformatics and Biomedicine (BIBM), San Diego, CA, USA, 18–21 November 2019, pp. 2393–2398. [CrossRef]
21. Chen, L.; Sun, J.; Canton, G.; Balu, N.; Hippe, D.S.; Zhao, X.; Li, R.; Hatsukami, T.S.; Hwang, J.N.; Yuan, C. Automated Artery Localization and Vessel Wall Segmentation Using Tracklet Refinement and Polar Conversion. *IEEE Access* **2020**, *8*, 217603–217614. [CrossRef]
22. Wendelhag, I.; Gustavsson, T.; Suurküla, M.; Berglund, G.; Wikstrand, J. Ultrasound measurement of wall thickness in the carotid artery: fundamental principles and description of a computerized analysing system. *Clin. Physiol.* **1991**, *11*, 565–577. [CrossRef] [PubMed]
23. Adame, I.M.; van der Geest, R.J.; Bluemke, D.A.; Lima, J.A.; Reiber, J.H.; Lelieveldt, B.P. Automatic vessel wall contour detection and quantification of wall thickness in in vivo MR images of the human aorta. *J. Magn. Reson. Imaging* **2006**, *24*, 595–602. [CrossRef] [PubMed]
24. Yuan, C.; Han, C.; Hatsukami, T.S. Computation of Wall Thickness. US Patent 7353117, 1 April 2008.

25. Shum, J.; DiMartino, E.S.; Goldhammer, A.; Goldman, D.H.; Acker, L.C.; Patel, G.; Ng, J.H.; Martufi, G.; Finol, E.A. Semiautomatic vessel wall detection and quantification of wall thickness in computed tomography images of human abdominal aortic aneurysms. *Med. Phys.* **2010**, *37*, 638–648. [CrossRef] [PubMed]
26. Suri, J.S. Vascular Ultrasound Intima-Media Thickness (IMT) Measurement System. US Patent 8313437, 20 November 2012.
27. van Hespen, K.M.; Zwanenburg, J.J.; Hendrikse, J.; Kuijf, H.J. Subvoxel vessel wall thickness measurements of the intracranial arteries using a convolutional neural network. *Med. Image Anal.* **2021**, *67*, 101818. [CrossRef] [PubMed]
28. Antiga, L.; Wasserman, B.; Steinman, D. On the overestimation of early wall thickening at the carotid bulb by black blood MRI, with implications for coronary and vulnerable plaque imaging. *Magn. Reson. Med.* **2008**, *60*, 1020–1028. [CrossRef] [PubMed]
29. Jones, S.E.; Buchbinder, B.R.; Aharon, I. Three-dimensional mapping of cortical thickness using Laplace's Equation. *Hum. Brain Mapp.* **2000**, *11*, 12–32. [CrossRef] [PubMed]
30. Nikolas, P.; Ken, E. *Phase-Field Methods in Material Science and Engineering*; Wiley-VCH: Weinheim, Germany, 2010.
31. Jähne, B.; Haussecker, H.; Geissler, P. *Handbook of Computer Vision and Applications*; Citeseer: Princeton, NJ, USA, 1999; Volume 2.
32. Stary, H.C.; Chandler, A.B.; Dinsmore, R.E.; Fuster, V.; Glagov, S.; Insull, W.; Rosenfeld, M.E.; Schwartz, C.J.; Wagner, W.D.; Wissler, R.W. A Definition of Advanced Types of Atherosclerotic Lesions and a Histological Classification of Atherosclerosis. *Circulation* **1995**, *92*, 1355–1374. [CrossRef] [PubMed]
33. Falk, E. Pathogenesis of Atherosclerosis. *J. Am. Coll. Cardiol.* **2006**, *47*, C7–C12. [CrossRef] [PubMed]
34. Virmani, R.; Burke, A.P.; Kolodgie, F.D.; Farb, A. Vulnerable Plaque: The Pathology of Unstable Coronary Lesions. *J. Interv. Cardiol.* **2002**, *15*, 439–446. [CrossRef]
35. Virmani, R.; Burke, A.P.; Farb, A.; Kolodgie, F.D. Pathology of the Vulnerable Plaque. *J. Am. Coll. Cardiol.* **2006**, *47*, C13–C18. [CrossRef]
36. Davies, K.J. Degradation of oxidized proteins by the 20S proteasome. *Biochimie* **2001**, *83*, 301–310. [CrossRef] [PubMed]
37. Beck, M.J.; Parker, D.L.; Bolster, B.D., Jr.; Kim, S.E.; McNally, J.S.; Treiman, G.S.; Hadley, J.R. Interchangeable neck shape–specific coils for a clinically realizable anterior neck phased array system. *Magn. Reson. Med.* **2017**, *78*, 2460–2468. [CrossRef] [PubMed]
38. HashemizadehKolowri, S.; Guo, Y.; Akcicek, E.Y.; Akcicek, H.; Ma, X.; Canton, G.; Balu, N.; Hatsukami, T.S.; Yuan, C. Automated 3D Localization and Segmentation of Carotid Arteries in Black Blood Vessel Wall Imaging. In Proceedings of the 35th Annual International Conference of Society for MR Angiography (SMRA), Sendai, Japan, 17–20 October 2023; p. 080.
39. HashemizadehKolowri, S.; Zanaty, N.; Canton, G.; Balu, N.; Hatsukami, T.S.; Yuan, C. Automated Localization of the Extracranial Carotid Artery in Black Blood Contrast MR Images Using a Deep Learning Approach. In Proceedings of the ISMRM & ISMRT Annual Meeting & Exhibition, Toronto, ON, Canada, 3–8 June 2023.
40. Yushkevich, P.A.; Piven, J.; Cody Hazlett, H.; Gimpel Smith, R.; Ho, S.; Gee, J.C.; Gerig, G. User-Guided 3D Active Contour Segmentation of Anatomical Structures: Significantly Improved Efficiency and Reliability. *Neuroimage* **2006**, *31*, 1116–1128. [CrossRef] [PubMed]
41. Antiga, L.; Steinman, D. Robust and objective decomposition and mapping of bifurcating vessels. *IEEE Trans. Med Imaging* **2004**, *23*, 704–713. [CrossRef] [PubMed]
42. Piccinelli, M.; Veneziani, A.; Steinman, D.A.; Remuzzi, A.; Antiga, L. A Framework for Geometric Analysis of Vascular Structures: Application to Cerebral Aneurysms. *IEEE Trans. Med Imaging* **2009**, *28*, 1141–1155. [CrossRef]
43. Antiga, L.; Steinman, D. The Vascular Modeling Toolkit. [Online]. Copyright ©2004–2024. Luca Antiga, David Steinman, Simone Manini, Richard Izzo. Available online: http://www.vmtk.org/ (accessed on 1 August 2024).
44. O'Reilly, R.C.; Beck, J.M. A family of large-stencil discrete Laplacian approximations in three-dimensions. *Int. J. Numer. Methods Eng.* **2006**, 1–16.

Journal of
Cardiovascular Development and Disease

MDPI

Article

Investigation of the Clinical Value of Four Visualization Modalities for Congenital Heart Disease

Shen-yuan Lee [1], Andrew Squelch [2] and Zhonghua Sun [1,3,*]

[1] Discipline of Medical Radiation Science, Curtin Medical School, Curtin University, Perth, WA 6845, Australia; shen-yuan.lee@postgrad.curtin.edu.au
[2] School of Earth and Planetary Sciences, Faculty of Science & Engineering, Curtin University, Perth, WA 6845, Australia; a.squelch@curtin.edu.au
[3] Curtin Health Innovation Research Institute (CHIRI), Curtin University, Perth, WA 6845, Australia
* Correspondence: z.sun@curtin.edu.au; Tel.: +61-8-9266-7509; Fax: +61-8-9266-2377

Abstract: Diagnosing congenital heart disease (CHD) remains challenging because of its complex morphology. Representing the intricate structures of CHD on conventional two-dimensional flat screens is difficult owing to wide variations in the pathologies. Technological advancements, such as three-dimensional-printed heart models (3DPHMs) and virtual reality (VR), could potentially address the limitations of viewing complex structures using conventional methods. This study aimed to investigate the usefulness and clinical value of four visualization modalities across three different cases of CHD, including ventricular septal defect, double-outlet right ventricle, and tetralogy of Fallot. Seventeen cardiac specialists were invited to participate in this study, which was aimed at assessing the usefulness and clinical value of four visualization modalities, namely, digital imaging and communications in medicine (DICOM) images, 3DPHM, VR, and 3D portable document format (PDF). Out of these modalities, 76.4% of the specialists ranked VR as the best for understanding the spatial associations between cardiac structures and for presurgical planning. Meanwhile, 94.1% ranked 3DPHM as the best modality for communicating with patients and their families. Of the various visualization modalities, VR was the best tool for assessing anatomical locations and vessels, comprehending the spatial relationships between cardiac structures, and presurgical planning. The 3DPHM models were the best tool for medical education as well as communication. In summary, both 3DPHM and VR have their own advantages and outperform the other two modalities, i.e., DICOM images and 3D PDF, in terms of visualizing and managing CHD.

Keywords: 3D printing; virtual reality; congenital heart disease; visualization; communication; modality

1. Introduction

The clinical management of congenital heart disease (CHD) poses significant challenges owing to its diverse morphologies that vary between individuals [1–5]. A comprehensive understanding of anomalous cardiac structures is crucial for successful surgical intervention, when necessary. However, current visualization methods based on cardiac computed tomography or magnetic resonance imaging with volume rendering lack realism as they fail to depict the actual depth of the object. Over the past two decades, three-dimensional (3D) printing has emerged as an important technique in cardiovascular medicine to demonstrate the geometric associations between intra- and extra-cardiac structures [6–10]. Recent research has established the utility of 3D-printed heart models (3DPHMs) in aiding surgical decision making in cases where conventional imaging provides inconclusive results [11]. However, despite the benefits in surgical planning, training, and education, the time and cost of producing 3DPHMs hinder their widespread application in the medical field [12]. Moreover, standardization and quality control processes are required because of the novelty of the technology in medical settings [13].

Virtual reality (VR) has transformed the medical field by offering innovative solutions for both education and patient care [14–16]. VR technology is making a groundbreaking impact in the management and understanding of CHD [17–20]. By creating detailed, immersive 3D heart and vascular models, VR allows cardiologists and cardiac surgeons to explore the unique anatomical complexities of each patient's heart condition in a way that was previously not possible with conventional imaging methods [21–23]. This enhanced visualization aids in accurate diagnosis, surgical planning, and simulation, enabling medical professionals to visualize the heart's structures and plan interventions with unprecedented precision [24]. For educational purposes, VR serves as an invaluable tool for training medical students and professionals, providing them with a hands-on experience of congenital heart defects without the need for invasive procedures. In addition, VR facilitates an enhanced understanding of CHD by patients and their families, thus fostering clear communication about the condition, treatment options, and expected outcomes. By leveraging the capabilities of VR, healthcare providers can improve surgical outcomes, reduce the risks associated with complex procedures, and enhance the quality of life for patients with CHD [25].

The introduction of 3D portable document format (PDF) technology in the medical field has revolutionized the sharing and visualization of medical information, offering considerable advantages in diagnostics, patient education, and collaborative care [26]. Unlike conventional two-dimensional images, 3D PDFs permit the interactive visualization of complex anatomical structures directly within a PDF document. Therefore, healthcare professionals are able to manipulate and examine patient-specific models in three dimensions.

This study aimed to investigate the usefulness and clinical value of four visualization modalities in three different cases of CHD, including ventricular septal defect (VSD), double-outlet right ventricle (DORV), and tetralogy of Fallot (ToF). The rationale of choosing these three case scenarios is that VSD represents a simple CHD condition, while DORV and ToF represent moderately complex CHD situations; thus, this allows us to determine the clinical value of these visualization modalities in assessing different congenital heart defects. The four visualization modalities comprised DICOM (digital imaging and communications in medicine) images, 3DPHM, 3D VR, and 3D PDF. To determine the clinical value of these four visualization modalities, cardiologists and cardiac surgeons were invited to compare their usefulness in presurgical planning, medical education, and communication with patients and their families.

2. Materials and Methods

2.1. Generation of Digital Heart Models

Anonymized DICOM formats of cardiac computed tomography angiography (CCTA) images with simple and complex CHD conditions were collected in this study. The Mimics Innovation Suite 22.0 (Materialise, Leuven, Belgium) was used for the postprocessing and segmentation of the images. DICOM images were imported into Mimics for segmentation based on thresholding and editing across multiple slices. Voxels within a certain range of Hounsfield units (HU) were isolated via thresholding by selecting different threshold ranges, allowing the creation of different masks to depict various anatomical features. The heart's blood pool was separated from other structures, with a 2 mm thickness layer applied externally to assist in the heart model's printing process. The 3-Matic software 22.0 (Materialise, Leuven, Belgium) was utilized to repair holes in the digital model using wrap and smooth functions. The standard tessellation language (STL) file was then transferred to Meshmixer 3.5 (Autodesk, San Rafael, CA, USA) for additional modifications. The 3D model was split into a two-part component to inspect the heart's internal structure and provide a clear view and assessment of each model's specific defect.

2.2. 3D Printing

STL files were transferred into Objet500 Connex3 (Objective 3D, Stratasys, Melbourne, VIC, Australia) for printing. The models were printed with a flexible material, Agilus 30

(Objective 3D, Stratasys, Melbourne, VIC, Australia), which has a shore hardness of 30 A (materials with softer, more flexible features similar to those of human tissues) in both clear and black color. The models were printed in two ways, as depicted in Figure 1. The cost of the whole heart model was approximately 350 AUD each and that of the plane-cut model was approximately 260 AUD each. The printing time was approximately 5 h for each model.

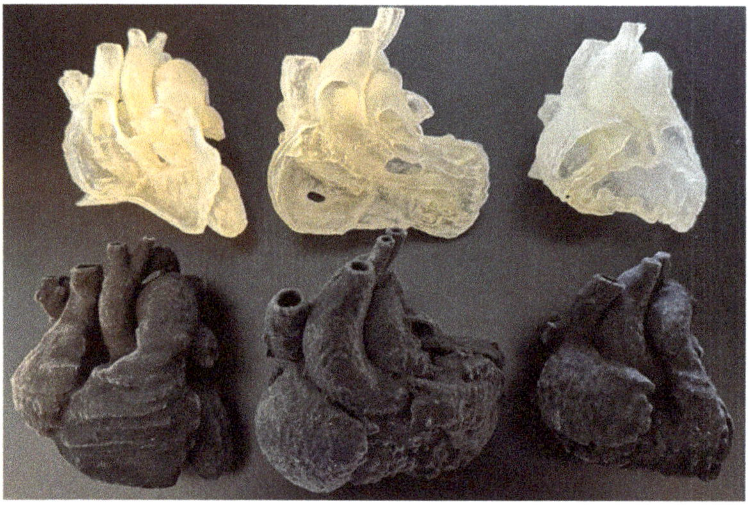

Figure 1. Models were printed with a flexible material, Agilus 30 (Objective 3D, Stratasys, Melbourne, VIC, Australia). VSD in the left column, DORV in the middle column, and ToF in the right column.

2.3. VR

Three-dimensional VR models were built using Unity 3D (Unity Technologies, San Francisco, CA, USA) with C# coding for additional functionality, such as for grabbing. Creating a VR project for the Oculus Quest 2 headset in the context of CHD using Unity involves several key steps to ensure an immersive and educational experience. Initially, the developers must install Unity with the appropriate VR development support packages and the Oculus Integration package from the Unity Asset Store, which includes essential tools, scripts, and prefabs for Oculus VR development. The digital heart model STL file can be imported using advanced 3D modeling software, Meshmixer 3.5 (Autodesk, San Rafael, CA, USA) and is then imported into Unity. Within Unity, script interactions and animations to simulate various heart conditions using VR hand tracking allow users to manipulate the view or interact with the model to better understand the heart's structure and function. Implementing user interface elements that provide educational content, such as turning on and off the body part and performing a live plane-cut of the heart, can enhance learning. To ensure a smooth and immersive experience, the VR environment for Oculus Quest 2 must be optimized by considering its processing capabilities to maintain high performance and visual quality. The VR project, including its three main functions, is shown in Figure 2. A video clip demonstrating how VR works in this study is presented in Supplementary File S1.

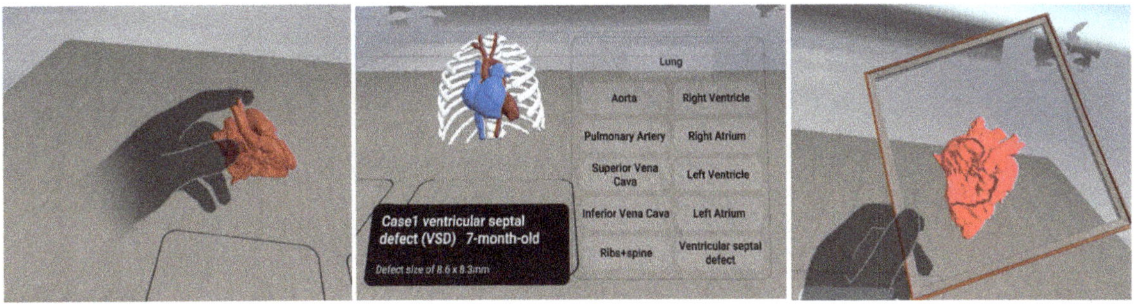

(**A**) (**B**) (**C**)

Figure 2. The three functions in VR visualization: (**A**) grabbing the model; (**B**) turning body parts on/off; and (**C**) plane-cutting of the heart.

2.4. 3D PDF

Adobe Acrobat Pro (Adobe Systems Incorporated, San Jose, CA, USA) was used to create 3D PDF for the three cases of CHD. The STL file of each case was imported into the PDF file with the case's details (Figure 3), for both the whole heart and the plane-cut heart. The "Add Default Views" function was used to select the view that would allow the participant to visualize the defect in each case. The cross-sectional property function was used to immediately display the cross-section of the 3D model, cutting it in half and looking inside, to determine the axis (x, y, or z) with which the cross-section was aligned.

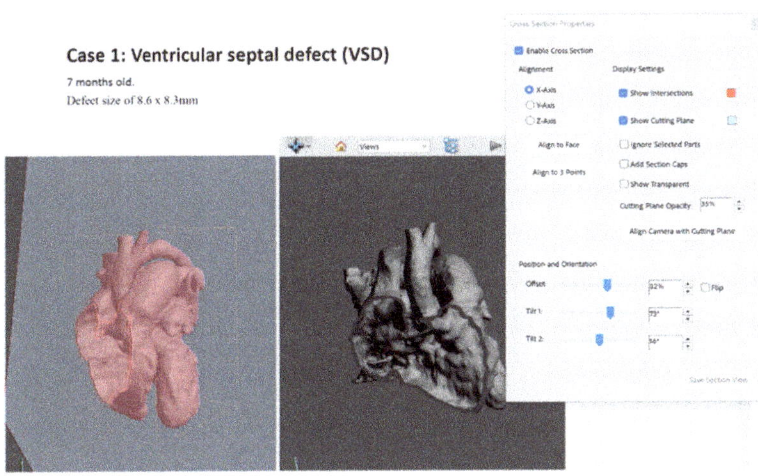

Figure 3. Three-dimensional PDF of the patient with VSD. The segmented volume data file in STL was used to generated the 3D PDF visualization.

2.5. Participant Recruitment and Data Collection

Seventeen cardiac professionals were recruited for this study from public and private hospitals in Western Australia. Each participant was involved in comparing and ranking the usefulness of the four visualization modalities across three different CHD cases, which took approximately 20 min (Figure 4). The 3DPHMs were printed using the flexible material Agilus30. The DICOM images and 3D PDFs were displayed on a 2D flat screen, whereas the 3D VR experiences were shown via a VR headset. An open-source DICOM viewer, RadiAnt (Medixant, Poznan, Poland), was used by the participants to view the DICOM images of each case on a laptop. Before evaluating the VR project, a tutorial video was shown to provide a better understanding of how to operate it with the VR headset. Questionnaires were distributed after demonstrating the four modalities, with questions based on ranking the usefulness in three major areas, namely, presurgical planning, medical education, and communication with patients and their families. The questionnaire is provided in Supplementary File S2. Each modality was ranked for each case, with 1 indicating the best and 4 indicating the worst modality.

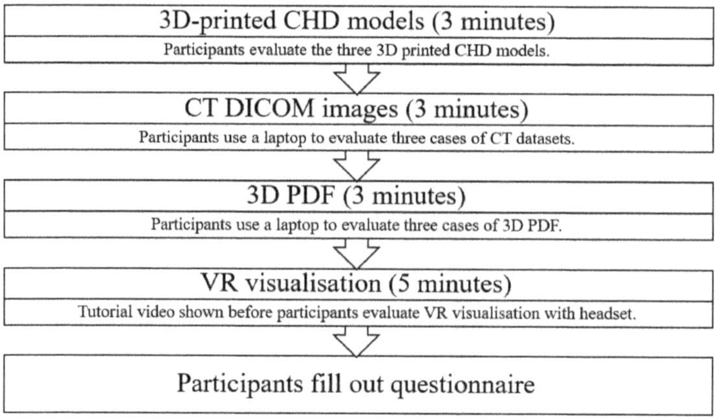

Figure 4. Process for each participant to visualize the 4 modalities and provide their ranking scores.

2.6. Statistical Analysis

Quantitative data from the questionnaire were analyzed using the IBM SPSS statistical package, version 26 (IBM Corp, Armonk, NY, USA). The normality of the data was evaluated using a normal probability plot, and skewness and kurtosis of the distribution were reported. A p-value of <0.05 was considered statistically significant.

3. Results

In total, 17 participants were included in this study, of which 12 were men and 11 had 10–20 years of working experience. There were 3 cardiac surgeons, 13 cardiologists, and 1 radiologist (Table 1).

Table 1. Characteristics of the study participants.

Variables	No. of Participants (%)
Sex	
Male	12 (70.6)
Female	5 (29.4)
Working Experience (years)	
Below 10	3 (17.6)
10 to 20	11 (64.8)
Above 20	3 (17.6)
Occupation	
Cardiac surgeon	3 (17.6)
Cardiologist	13 (76.5)
Radiologist	1 (5.9)

The mean rank of each modality for each question is presented in Table 2. The participants were requested to rank the modalities from 1 to 4, with 1 indicating the highest preference. Hence, a mean rank approaching 1 signified a favorable perception of the modality by the participants.

Table 2. The mean ranks of different modalities for each question.

Question	Modality	Ventricular Septal Defect			Double-Outlet Right Ventricle			Tetralogy of Fallot		
		Mean	SD	*p*-Value	Mean	SD	*p*-Value	Mean	SD	*p*-Value
Assessment of anatomicallocation and vessels	3DPHM	1.82	0.64	0.05	2.18	0.53	0.01	2.17	0.53	0.05
	VR	1.65	0.79		1.68	0.86		1.64	0.93	
	3D PDF	3.59	0.62		3.71	0.77		3.71	0.59	
	DICOM	2.82	1.19		2.47	1.12		2.47	1.17	
Spatial relationship between the cardiac structures	3DPHM	1.76	0.66	0.00	1.94	0.66	0.02	1.94	0.66	0.01
	VR	1.53	0.71		1.41	0.71		1.59	0.93	
	3D PDF	3.41	0.79		3.47	0.79		3.47	0.62	
	DICOM	3.29	0.77		3.18	0.81		3.12	1.06	
Visualize the heart defects	3DPHM	1.53	0.51	0.05	1.94	0.56	0.05	1.94	0.66	0.05
	VR	1.89	0.78		1.71	0.85		1.82	0.95	
	3D PDF	3.59	0.62		3.47	0.79		3.53	0.62	
	DICOM	2.94	1.09		2.88	1.22		2.71	1.26	
Learn about the pathology	3DPHM	1.65	0.51	0.00	1.71	0.59	0.01	1.76	0.56	0.01
	VR	1.59	0.79		1.53	0.72		1.65	0.93	
	3D PDF	3.41	0.62		3.53	0.62		3.68	0.61	
	DICOM	3.35	0.87		3.24	0.83		2.94	0.89	
Presurgical tool	3DPHM	2.18	0.53	0.00	1.82	0.53	0.03	1.88	0.49	0.03
	VR	1.41	0.71		1.35	0.71		1.47	0.94	
	3D PDF	3.59	0.87		3.71	0.59		3.65	0.61	
	DICOM	2.82	1.01		3.11	0.61		3.11	0.79	
Medical education	3DPHM	1.59	0.51	0.01	1.47	0.51	0.03	1.59	0.51	0.03
	VR	1.53	0.72		1.76	0.75		1.71	0.92	
	3D PDF	3.35	0.71		3.29	0.69		3.41	0.62	
	DICOM	3.53	0.53		3.47	0.79		3.29	0.85	
Communication tools	3DPHM	1.06	0.24	0.00	1.06	0.24	0.00	1.06	0.24	0.00
	VR	2.76	0.67		2.82	0.64		2.71	0.69	
	3D PDF	2.52	0.87		2.47	0.81		2.59	0.87	
	DICOM	3.65	0.61		3.71	0.59		3.65	0.61	
Reduce errors during the surgery	3DPHM	2.01	0.78	0.36	1.94	0.66	0.85	2.17	0.6	0.92
	VR	1.98	0.92		2.01	0.87		1.95	0.99	
	3D PDF	2.98	0.56		2.88	0.75		2.59	0.61	
	DICOM	2.65	0.86		2.65	0.79		2.82	0.95	

VR was the best modality for assessing the anatomical location and vessels. This method exhibited the lowest mean score across all heart defects, indicating that it provides the most accurate evaluation. The 3DPHM and DICOM modalities followed, with 3D PDF being the least effective. Furthermore, VR ranked the highest in spatial association among cardiac structures, with the lowest mean scores, which signified its superior performance in illustrating spatial relationships. The 3DPHM method was the most effective modality for visualizing heart defects, with the lowest mean scores. This method was followed by VR, DICOM, and 3D PDF. In learning about pathology, 3DPHM outperformed the other modalities, offering the clearest insights into pathology, with the lowest mean scores.

VR was the best presurgical tool, as inferred from its lowest mean scores. The 3DPHM, DICOM, and 3D PDF modalities came next, with 3D PDF being the least preferred. For medical education, 3DPHM and VR were highly effective, and both showed lower mean scores than DICOM and 3D PDF, with 3DPHM slightly surpassing the others in certain cases. The 3DPHM modality stood out as the best communication tool, with significantly lower mean scores, indicating its effectiveness.

The quality of visualization was quantified by the mean score, with a rating scale from 1 (well visualized) to 4 (not visualized), and the standard deviation (SD) implied the variability in the scores (Table 3). Across all anatomical structures, VR consistently showed excellent visualization capabilities, with low mean scores and minimal variability. DICOM was also effective, particularly for the aorta and pulmonary artery. The 3DPHMperformed well but was not as consistent as VR. Three-dimensional PDF was the least effective modality, especially for complex visualizations such as defects.

Table 3. The mean score of visualization of the anatomical locations.

Location	Modality	Mean	SD
Heart chamber	3DPHM	1.65	0.61
	VR	1.12	0.33
	3D PDF	2.06	0.65
	DICOM	1.29	0.47
Aorta	3DPHM	1.18	0.39
	VR	1.12	0.33
	3D PDF	1.41	0.62
	DICOM	1.05	0.24
Pulmonary artery	3DPHM	1.12	0.33
	VR	1.06	0.24
	3D PDF	1.41	0.61
	DICOM	1.06	0.24
Defect	3DPHM	1.29	0.47
	VR	1.18	0.39
	3D PDF	2.24	0.75
	DICOM	1.76	0.83

A rating scale of 1 = well visualized; 2 = visualized; 3 = poorly visualized; and 4 = not visualized was used.

Table 4 presents the mean scores of the different modalities for each question. The participants were requested to rate the modalities on a scale of 1–10 for each question, with 10 being the highest score. For presurgical planning, VR was rated as the most useful modality, with a mean score of 8.71 and an SD of 1.1. Thus, this method appears to have a high average usefulness, with moderate variability in the responses. 3DPHMfollowed closely, with a mean of 8.47 and a slightly lower SD of 1.07, alluding a similarly high level of usefulness but with slightly more consistent responses among the participants. In addition, DICOM demonstrated considerable usefulness, with a mean of 7.82 and the lowest SD of 0.95, indicating a more uniform perception among the respondents. Three-dimensional PDFs scored significantly lower in usefulness for presurgical planning, with a mean of 5.25 and the highest SD of 1.41, which implies both a lower perceived usefulness and a higher variability in the responses. In the context of educational tools for medical students or junior doctors, VR scored the highest at 9.12, which indicates its effectiveness in providing immersive learning experiences. The 3DPHM modality also scored highly at 8.94, emphasizing its value in tangible learning aids. DICOM, while still useful, scored lower at 7.18, and 3D PDFs were rated the least useful at 4.65, reflecting potentially limited engagement or interactivity compared to the other modalities.

Table 4. The mean scores of different modalities for each question.

Question	Modality	Mean	SD
Usefulness for presurgical planning	3DPHM	8.47	1.07
	VR	8.71	1.1
	3D PDF	5.25	1.41
	DICOM	7.82	0.95
Usefulness of educational tools for medical students or junior doctors	3DPHM	8.94	0.83
	VR	9.12	1.11
	3D PDF	4.65	1.77
	DICOM	7.18	0.88

Overall, VR and 3DPHM were consistently valued across both categories for their high engagement and effectiveness in medical education and planning, with VR having a slight advantage. Conversely, 3D PDFs were consistently rated as the least useful modality, which shows that more immersive or tangible technologies are preferred in these contexts. There were no significant differences in the scores given to these modalities under the three different CHD case scenarios.

Of the 17 participants, 14 (82%) and 15(88%) opined that the grabbing function and turn on/off option for the body parts in VR exhibited the greatest value in the education area, respectively. Moreover, 16 (94%) indicated that the live plane-cut function displayed the greatest value in the presurgical planning area (Figure 5). None of the participants provided "no" as the response to all three questions, which suggests the positive inclination of the participants toward this aspect.

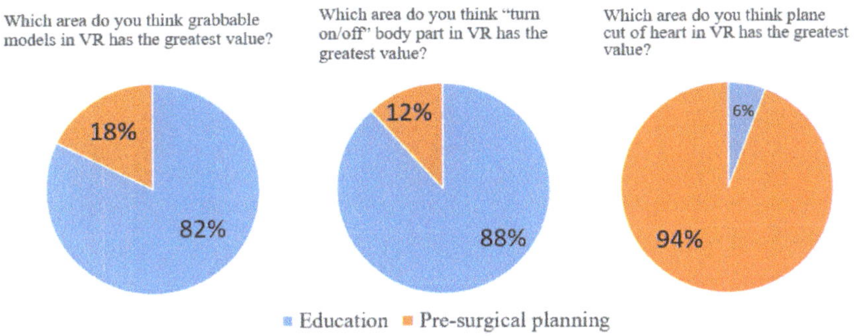

Figure 5. Responses from the participants regarding the usefulness of VR functions.

4. Discussion

The results of this study demonstrated the consistent superiority of 3DPHM and VR over 3D PDFs and DICOM in almost all evaluated categories. Feedback from cardiac specialists and physicians regarding the three CHD cases indicated promising outcomes for the four visualization modalities. VR emerged as the leading modality in assessing anatomical locations and vessels across all CHD types, implying its strength in providing clear and detailed visualizations for the accurate identification and understanding of complex heart structures. For comprehending the spatial associations between cardiac structures, VR exhibited superior performance, which showed its capability to offer an immersive experience that can augment the understanding of intricate spatial dynamics within the heart, which is crucial for both diagnostics and surgical planning.

Both VR and 3DPHM performed well in facilitating pathology learning, with VR having a slight edge. This finding highlights the potential of these techniques in medical education, providing interactive and engaging methods for studying and comprehending CHD pathologies. VR proved to be the most effective presurgical planning tool, which emphasizes its value in presurgical preparations owing to the benefit of 3D visualization and simulation. This capability could considerably influence surgical outcomes by enabling the use of precise and informed surgical strategies. In medical education, 3DPHM and VR showed immense promise, with 3DPHM slightly outperforming VR. The 3DPHM modality was the best communication tool, which indicates that physical models are particularly effective in explaining complex cardiac conditions to patients and their families. This modality can enhance patient understanding and involvement in the care process. This is consistent with similar recent reports, highlighting the usefulness of VR and 3DPHM in CHD [16,24].

The advent of 3D printing technology has substantially transformed the landscape of CHD management and has offered innovative approaches for diagnosis, surgical planning, medical education, and patient communication. In their study, Valverde et al. demonstrated that 3D-printed models of complex CHD cases facilitated an in-depth understanding of anatomical structures, thereby aiding in the identification of optimal surgical pathways and potential complications. These models enable surgeons to simulate and rehearse procedures, which can potentially reduce operative times and improve surgical precision, with surgical decisions being modified in 48% of CHD cases after the use of 3D-printed models [27]. Similarly, Kiraly et al. reported their multidisciplinary team experience of using 3D-printed models in managing complex CHD scenarios [23]. Personalized 3D-printed models were developed in 15 cases of patients with complex congenital cardiac defects, and the 3D-printed models were found to refine diagnosis in 13 cases and provide new information in 9 cases. With the aid of the 3D-printed models, intracardiac repair was modified in 13 cases.

The 3DPHM modality allows students and medical professionals to physically explore cardiac defects, which fosters a more intuitive understanding of congenital anomalies compared to conventional 2D imaging techniques. This interactive learning approach can improve knowledge retention and clinical skills among learners [28]. Furthermore, 3DPHM models have emerged as a powerful tool for patient education and communication. Healthcare providers can more effectively explain the nature of the disease, the proposed surgical interventions, and the expected outcomes to the patients and their families with the aid of physical models of heart defects. This approach not only enhances patient understanding but also facilitates informed decision making and augments patient satisfaction with the provided care [29]. The findings from this investigation suggest that 3DPHM is the best modality for communication with patients and their family.

The ability of VR technology to enhance diagnostic accuracy and surgical planning in CHD has been increasingly recognized. VR enables clinicians to visualize complex cardiac anomalies in ways that were hitherto not possible with standard 2D imaging techniques. Studies by Priya et al. demonstrated that VR-assisted preoperative planning could significantly improve the understanding of anatomical structures, thus aiding in the strategic planning of surgical interventions to potentially reduce operative times and improve patient outcomes [22]. Kieu et al. established the role of VR in enhancing the educational experience of medical students and professionals. Thus, VR can facilitate a more intuitive grasp of spatial relationships and surgical techniques, which can enhance the learning outcomes [17]. A study by Lim et al. reported that VR-based patient education can lead to higher satisfaction rates and a better understanding of medical conditions and treatments [25]. Moreover, studies documented the use of VR for preoperative planning, which allowed surgeons to explore patient-specific anatomy and devise surgical strategies for more precise and effective interventions [30]. However, the integration of VR in CHD care has its own limitations. Technical limitations, cost implications, and the need for specialized training are some of the factors that prevent its widespread adoption. In addition, there is a growing need for standardized protocols and validation studies to ensure the reliability and accuracy of VR models. In our study, VR was considered the best modality for presurgical planning as the live plane-cut function allows cardiac professionals to cut open the heart in any angle.

The findings of Lau et al. are similar to ours, with mixed-reality models ranking the best in preoperative planning and 3DPHM being the preferred tool in communication with patients [24]. The difference between the two studies is that our research compared 3D PDF with three other visualization modalities. Furthermore, the headset and VR environment and function were different. While Oculus Quest 2 was used in this study, HoloLens 2 was utilized in Lau's study.

One of main advantages of VR over the other three modalities lies in its ability to provide a 3D immersive environment, which significantly enhances user understanding of complex anatomical structures. This is especially important when dealing with complex congenital heart defects due to a wide range of complexity associated with different CHD conditions. VR was ranked the best tool for providing realistic 3D visualization of the spatial relationship between cardiac structures and defects; therefore, it plays an important role in guiding the presurgical planning of CHD surgeries, with potential reductions in the risks or complications that may arise from the challenging surgery procedures. This is consistent with a recent study comparing VR with 3D printing and 3D PDF in imaging patients with CHD [31]. Raimondi et al. compared VR models with 3D-printed models and 3D PDF in three different types of CHD conditions with regard to their performance in visualizing anatomical structures and congenital heart defects. VR was ranked to be advantageous in the following, compared to the other two 3D visualization modalities: demonstrating anatomical structures, easy navigation, faster, reproducible, and less prone to human errors.

The use of VR in CHD surgery or surgical planning is not well studied in the current literature. Priya and colleagues reported the application of VR for baffle planning in two CHD cases [22]. Their developed VR interface model allowed surgeons to simulate different baffle configurations, enhancing the baffle surgical planning process and the patient outcomes. Despite findings based on a few cases, these studies show that VR is a promising approach in CHD visualization and surgical planning. The results of our study also confirm these case reports regarding the potential value of VR in CHD surgical planning. Although our analysis is subjective due to its qualitative nature, it does provide insights into the participants (cardiac specialists)' experiences, perceptions, or opinions on the usefulness of VR versus other 3D modalities in CHD management. Thus, our findings lay a good foundation for further research on the utility of VR in guiding CHD surgical planning, in addition to its value in improving communication and comprehension among multidisciplinary teams. Furthermore, VR models allow cardiac surgeons to perform the real-time exploration of cardiac anatomy compared to physical and static 3D-printed models, thus assisting clinical decision making.

Another advantage of VR technology is its cost effectiveness and time efficiency compared to 3DPHM. In this study, we used an Oculus Quest 2 headset for the VR demonstration, which cost around 400–500 AUD. In contrast, each 3D-printed heart model cost about 300 AUD, with a total of 900 AUD for the three models in this study. Another limitation of using 3D printing technology is the time spent on printing and the cleaning process, which take much longer than VR visualization.

The main advantage of 3DPHM is that it provides a physical model for hands-on learning and training experience. Thus, it serves as a useful tool for medical education and clinical communication as 3D-printed personalized physical models provide direct views of the anatomical structures to enhance the learning experience and communication with patients or families, as well as clinical colleagues [32,33].

This study has certain limitations. First, the allocated time might have been insufficient for a complete evaluation of the modality, which might have potentially led to biased responses from the participants. Furthermore, we did not randomize the order of these modalities when presenting them to the participants; thus, we could not avoid the potential risk of biased opinions by the participants when ranking these modalities. This should be considered in future studies. Second, despite receiving a brief tutorial on the use of 3D PDFs, the participants faced challenges in navigating the 3D heart models on a flat 2D screen. Finally, the number of participants was small, and a sufficient number of cardiac surgeons were not available to assess the clinical value of these modalities. Future studies should seek opinions from more cardiac surgeons to further quantify these benefits and potentially explore the advantage of these tools in other areas of medical diagnosis and treatment for enhancing patient care. A further follow-up study is desirable to include two aspects that will further strengthen our study's outcomes: the inclusion of patients and their relatives, giving opinions on which modality helped them understand their condition best, and surgeons, giving their views on whether they changed their approach or strategy following a review of the case using these modalities. This will allow us to better understand how the selection of these modalities will change current practices and benefit patient care when planning CHD surgeries.

5. Conclusions

The findings from this study have established that, out of the four visualization modalities, VR is the best tool for assessing anatomical location and vessels, understanding the spatial relationships between cardiac structures, and conducting presurgical planning. The 3DPHM models are the best tool for medical education and communication. For the comprehensive and effective management of CHD, 3DPHM and VR are superior modalities, offering detailed and interactive ways to comprehend and address complex cardiac conditions. These tools hold immense promise for augmenting the outcomes in medical education, surgical planning, and patient communication.

Supplementary Materials: The following supporting information can be downloaded at https://www.mdpi.com/article/10.3390/jcdd11090278/s1: File S1: Video clip of VR; and File S2: Questionnaire.

Author Contributions: Conceptualization, S.-y.L. and Z.S.; methodology, S.-y.L., A.S. and Z.S.; formal analysis, S.-y.L.; investigation, S.-y.L., A.S. and Z.S.; data curation, S.-y.L. and Z.S.; writing—original draft preparation, S.-y.L. and Z.S.; writing—review and editing, all authors; visualization, S.-y.L.; supervision, A.S. and Z.S.; and project administration, Z.S. All authors have read and agreed to the published version of the manuscript.

Funding: This research received no external funding.

Institutional Review Board Statement: This study was conducted according to the guidelines of the Declaration of Helsinki and approved by the Human Research Ethics Committee of CURTIN UNIVERSITY (approval number: HRE2018-0799).

Informed Consent Statement: Patient consent was waived due to the use of anonymized data for 3D printing purposes, with no patient information identified.

Data Availability Statement: Data are contained within the article and Supplementary Materials.

Acknowledgments: The authors would like to express their gratitude to Carley Tillett for their invaluable assistance with the VR project. Additionally, they would like to extend their thanks to medical professionals from the clinical sites for their participation in this study.

Conflicts of Interest: The authors declare no conflicts of interest.

References

1. Morton, S.U.; Quiat, D.; Seidman, J.G.; Seidman, C.E. Genomic frontiers in congenital heart disease. *Nat. Rev. Cardiol.* **2022**, *19*, 26–42. [CrossRef]
2. Wu, W.; He, J.; Shao, X. Incidence and mortality trend of congenital heart disease at the global, regional, and national level, 1990–2017. *Medicine* **2020**, *99*, e20593. [CrossRef] [PubMed]
3. Bhatla, P.; Tretter, J.T.; Ludomirsky, A.; Argilla, M.; Latson, L.A.; Chakravarti, S.; Barker, P.C.; Yoo, S.-J.; McElhinney, D.B.; Wake, N. Utility and scope of rapid prototyping in patients with complex muscular ventricular septal defects or double-outlet right ventricle: Does it alter management decisions? *Pediatr. Cardiol.* **2017**, *38*, 103–114. [CrossRef] [PubMed]
4. Biglino, G.; Koniordou, D.; Gasparini, M.; Capelli, C.; Leaver, L.-K.; Khambadkone, S.; Schievano, S.; Taylor, A.M.; Wray, J. Piloting the use of patient-specific cardiac models as a novel tool to facilitate communication during cinical consultations. *Pediatr. Cardiol.* **2017**, *38*, 813–818. [CrossRef] [PubMed]
5. Loke, Y.-H.; Harahsheh, A.S.; Krieger, A.; Olivieri, L.J. Usage of 3D models of tetralogy of Fallot for medical education: Impact on learning congenital heart disease. *BMC Med. Educ.* **2017**, *17*, 54. [CrossRef] [PubMed]
6. Lee, S.; Squelch, A.; Sun, Z. Quantitative assessment of 3D printed model accuracy in delineating congenital heart disease. *Biomolecules* **2021**, *11*, 270. [CrossRef]
7. Tarca, A.; Woo, N.; Bain, S.; Crouchley, D.; McNulty, E.; Yim, D. 3D Printed Cardiac Models as an Adjunct to Traditional Teaching of Anatomy in Congenital Heart Disease—A Randomised Controlled Study. *Heart Lung Circ.* **2023**, *32*, 1443–1450. [CrossRef]
8. Karsenty, C.; Guitarte, A.; Dulac, Y.; Briot, J.; Hascoet, S.; Vincent, R.; Delepaul, B.; Vignaud, P.; Djeddai, C.; Hadeed, K. The usefulness of 3D printed heart models for medical student education in congenital heart disease. *BMC Med. Educ.* **2021**, *21*, 480. [CrossRef]
9. Gomez, A.; Gomez, G.; Simpson, J.; Valverde, I. 3D hybrid printed models in complex congenital heart disease: 3D echocardiography and cardiovascular magnetic resonance imaging fusion. *Eur. Heart J.* **2020**, *41*, 4214. [CrossRef]
10. Wu, C.A.; Squelch, A.; Jansen, S.; Sun, Z. Optimization of computed tomography angiography protocols for follow-up type B aortic dissection patients by using 3D printed model. *Appl. Sci.* **2021**, *11*, 6844. [CrossRef]

11. Lau, I.; Wong, Y.H.; Yeong, C.H.; Aziz, Y.F.A.; Sari, N.A.M.; Hashim, S.A.; Sun, Z. Quantitative and qualitative comparison of low-and high-cost 3D-printed heart models. *Quant. Imaging Med. Surg.* **2019**, *9*, 107. [CrossRef] [PubMed]
12. Paxton, N.C. Navigating the intersection of 3D printing, software regulation and quality control for point-of-care manufacturing of personalized anatomical models. *3D Print. Med.* **2023**, *9*, 9. [CrossRef]
13. Chen, F.-Q.; Leng, Y.-F.; Ge, J.-F.; Wang, D.-W.; Li, C.; Chen, B.; Sun, Z.-L. Effectiveness of virtual reality in nursing education: Meta-analysis. *J. Med. Internet Res.* **2020**, *22*, e18290. [CrossRef]
14. Tene, T.; Vique López, D.F.; Valverde Aguirre, P.E.; Orna Puente, L.M.; Vacacela Gomez, C. Virtual reality and augmented reality in medical education: An umbrella review. *Front. Digit. Health* **2024**, *6*, 1365345. [CrossRef]
15. Bruno, R.R.; Wolff, G.; Wernly, B.; Masyuk, M.; Piayda, K.; Leaver, S.; Erkens, R.; Oehler, R.; Afzal, S.; Heidari, H. Virtual and augmented reality in critical care medicine: The patient's, clinician's, and researcher's perspective. *Crit. Care* **2022**, *26*, 326. [CrossRef] [PubMed]
16. Lau, I.; Gupta, A.; Sun, Z. Clinical value of virtual reality versus 3D printing in congenital heart disease. *Biomolecules* **2021**, *11*, 884. [CrossRef]
17. Kieu, V.; Sumski, C.; Cohen, S.; Reinhardt, E.; Axelrod, D.M.; Handler, S.S. The Use of Virtual Reality Learning on Transition Education in Adolescents with Congenital Heart Disease. *Pediatr. Cardiol.* **2023**, *44*, 1856–1860. [CrossRef]
18. Awori, J.; Friedman, S.D.; Howard, C.; Kronmal, R.; Buddhe, S. Comparative effectiveness of virtual reality (VR) vs 3D printed models of congenital heart disease in resident and nurse practitioner educational experience. *3D Print. Med.* **2023**, *9*, 2. [CrossRef]
19. Galeczka, M.; Smerdzinski, S.; Tyc, F.; Fiszer, R. Virtual reality for transcatheter procedure planning in congenital heart disease. *Pol. Heart J.* **2023**, *81*, 1026–1027. [CrossRef]
20. Ong, C.S.; Krishnan, A.; Huang, C.Y.; Spevak, P.; Vricella, L.; Hibino, N.; Garcia, J.R.; Gaur, L. Role of virtual reality in congenital heart disease. *Congenit. Heart Dis.* **2018**, *13*, 357–361. [CrossRef]
21. Kim, B.; Loke, Y.-H.; Mass, P.; Irwin, M.R.; Capeland, C.; Olivieri, L.; Krieger, A. A novel virtual reality medical image display system for group discussions of congenital heart disease: Development and usability testing. *JMIR Cardio* **2020**, *4*, e20633. [CrossRef]
22. Priya, S.; La Russa, D.; Walling, A.; Goetz, S.; Hartig, T.; Khayat, A.; Gupta, P.; Nagpal, P.; Ashwath, R. From Vision to Reality: Virtual Reality's Impact on Baffle Planning in Congenital Heart Disease. *Pediatr. Cardiol.* **2024**, *45*, 165–174. [CrossRef]
23. Kiraly, L.; Shah, N.C.; Abdullah, O.; Al-Ketan, O.; Rowshan, R. Three-dimensional virtual and printed prototypes in complex congenital and pediatric cardiac surgery—A multidisciplinary team-learning experience. *Biomolecules* **2021**, *11*, 1703. [CrossRef]
24. Lau, I.; Gupta, A.; Ihdayhid, A.; Sun, Z. Clinical applications of mixed reality and 3D printing in congenital heart disease. *Biomolecules* **2022**, *12*, 1548. [CrossRef] [PubMed]
25. Lim, T.R.; Wilson, H.C.; Axelrod, D.M.; Werho, D.K.; Handler, S.S.; Yu, S.; Afton, K.; Lowery, R.; Mullan, P.B.; Cooke, J. Virtual reality curriculum increases paediatric residents' knowledge of CHDs. *Cardiol. Young* **2023**, *33*, 410–414. [CrossRef] [PubMed]
26. Eroğlu, F.S.; Erkan, B.; Koyuncu, S.B.; Komşal, Z.R.; Çiçek, F.E.; Ülker, M.; Toklu, M.; Atlan, M.; Kıyak, Y.S.; Kula, S. Effectiveness of using 2D atlas and 3D PDF as a teaching tool in anatomy lectures in initial learners: A randomized controlled trial in a medical school. *BMC Med. Educ.* **2023**, *23*, 962. [CrossRef] [PubMed]
27. Valverde, I.; Gomez-Ciriza, G.; Hussain, T.; Suarez-Mejias, C.; Velasco-Forte, M.N.; Byrne, N.; Ordoñez, A.; Gonzalez-Calle, A.; Anderson, D.; Hazekamp, M.G. Three-dimensional printed models for surgical planning of complex congenital heart defects: An international multicentre study. *Eur. J. Cardiothorac. Surg.* **2017**, *52*, 1139–1148. [CrossRef]
28. Sun, Z.; Wong, Y.H.; Yeong, C.H. Patient-specific 3D-printed low-cost models in medical education and clinical practice. *Micromachines* **2023**, *14*, 464. [CrossRef]
29. Traynor, G.; Shearn, A.I.; Milano, E.G.; Ordonez, M.V.; Velasco Forte, M.N.; Caputo, M.; Schievano, S.; Mustard, H.; Wray, J.; Biglino, G. The use of 3D-printed models in patient communication: A scoping review. *J. 3D Print. Med.* **2022**, *6*, 13–23. [CrossRef]
30. Castellanos, J.M.; Barbery, D.; Yefimov, A.; Dang, P.N. Preoperative planning using virtual reality for percutaneous transseptal valve-in-valve transcatheter mitral valve replacement: A case report. *Eur. Heart J. Case Rep.* **2022**, *6*, ytac384. [CrossRef]
31. Raimondi, F.; Vida, V.; Godard, C.; Bertelli, F.; Reffo, E.; Boddaert, N.; EI Beheiry, M.; Masson, J.B. Fast-track virtual reality for cardiac imaging in congenital heart disease. *J. Card. Surg.* **2021**, *36*, 2598–2602. [CrossRef]
32. Illmann, C.F.; Hosking, M.; Harris, K.C. Utility and access to 3-dimensional printing in the context of congenital heart disease: An international physician survey study. *CJC Open* **2020**, *2*, 207–213. [CrossRef]
33. Deng, X.; He, S.; Huang, P.; Luo, J.; Yang, G.; Zhou, B.; Xiao, Y. A three-dimensional printed model in preoperative consent for ventricular septal defect repair. *J. Cardiothorac. Surg.* **2021**, *16*, 229. [CrossRef]

Journal of
Cardiovascular
Development and Disease

MDPI

Review

The Role of Coronary Imaging in Chronic Total Occlusions: Applications and Future Possibilities

Giuseppe Panuccio [1,2,*,†], Youssef S. Abdelwahed [2,†], Nicole Carabetta [3], Ulf Landmesser [2], Salvatore De Rosa [3] and Daniele Torella [1]

1 Department of Experimental and Clinical Medicine, Magna Graecia University, 88100 Catanzaro, Italy; dtorella@unicz.it
2 Department of Cardiology, Angiology and Intensive Care Medicine, Deutsches Herzzentrum der Charité, 12200 Berlin, Germany; youssef.abdelwahed@dhzc-charite.de (Y.S.A.); ulf.landmesser@dhzc-charite.de (U.L.)
3 Department of Medical and Surgical Sciences, Magna Graecia University, 88100 Catanzaro, Italy; nicole.carabetta95@gmail.com (N.C.); saderosa@unicz.it (S.D.R.)
* Correspondence: panuccio@unicz.it
† These authors contributed equally to this work.

Abstract: Chronic total occlusions (CTOs) represent a challenging scenario in coronary artery disease (CAD). The prevalence of CTOS in patients undergoing coronary angiography underscores the need for effective diagnostic and therapeutic strategies. Coronary angiography, while essential, offers limited insights into lesion morphology, vessel course, and myocardial viability. In contrast, coronary imaging techniques—including optical coherence tomography (OCT), intravascular ultrasound (IVUS), and coronary computed tomography angiography (CCTA)—provide comprehensive insights for each stage of CTO percutaneous coronary intervention (PCI). OCT facilitates the assessment of plaque morphology and stent optimization, despite low evidence and several limitations in CTO-PCI. IVUS offers deeper penetration, allowing managing proximal cap scenarios and guiding subintimal navigation. CCTA provides a non-invasive, three-dimensional view of coronary anatomy, enabling the precise evaluation of myocardial mass at risk and detailed procedural planning. Despite their individual limitations, these imaging modalities have enhanced the success rates of CTO-PCI, thus reducing procedural and long-term complications and improving patient outcomes. The future of CTO management lies in further technological advancements, including hybrid imaging, artificial intelligence (AI) integration, and improved fusion imaging. These innovations promise to refine procedural precision and personalize interventions, ultimately improving the care of patients with complex coronary artery disease.

Keywords: chronic total occlusions; CTOs; coronary imaging; IVUS; OCT; computed tomography; precision medicine

1. Introduction

Chronic total occlusions (CTOs) represent a challenging scenario in coronary artery disease (CAD), characterized by increasing morbidity and adverse clinical outcomes [1]. The prevalence of CTOs among patients undergoing coronary angiography is about 16–18%, highlighting the importance of diagnostic and therapeutic strategies in this setting [2]. Coronary revascularization, including coronary artery bypass grafting (CABG) and percutaneous coronary intervention (PCI) represent a cornerstone treatment in CAD, including CTOs [3–5]. The clinical implications of CTOs are mainly a significant increase in angina symptoms and exercise tolerance, thus reducing quality of life [6]. However, despite the lack of randomized data, observational studies have shown a significant improvement in ejection fraction and in long-term survival in patients undergoing the successful recanalization of a CTO [7–9]. Coronary angiography has been the gold standard for the anatomical assessment of CTOs for years. However, it provides limited information about lesion's morphology, vessel course and myocardial viability, as well as about stent implantation and optimization. This limitation has been overcome by coronary imaging techniques, which provide useful information in every step of CTO-PCI, ranging from pre-procedural planning to enabling successful CTO crossing and achieving procedural success. Since its complexity, the management of CTOs often benefits from the support of coronary imaging in several phases, even before the CTO-PCI procedure. Non-invasive imaging modalities such as coronary computed tomography angiography (CCTA) offer comprehensive insights into CTO vessel and myocardial perfusion [10]. Invasive imaging techniques, including intravascular ultrasound (IVUS) and optical coherence tomography (OCT) provide detailed information of plaque composition, vessel size, and stent optimization. Moreover, IVUS can guide CTO crossing by extra-plaque techniques [11]. Since its many applications in CTO-PCI, coronary imaging has become an essential tool in this clinical scenario, especially in complex CTO lesions. Therefore, the aim of this work is to explore the current applications of coronary imaging techniques in the context of CTO-PCI, highlighting the strengths and limitations of each modality. Furthermore, we provide a discussion about emerging technologies related to coronary imaging and future perspective that may shape the field of CTO intervention.

Optical Coherence Tomography

OCT is a high-resolution intravascular imaging modality which uses near-infrared light to produce cross-sectional images of the coronary artery. Thanks to its high resolution (10–20 μm), OCT enables a detailed assessment of arterial wall and plaque morphology [12,13], as well as the optimization of stent deployment [8]. Although the evidence in the context of CTO-PCI is limited in respect to the other coronary imaging modalities, OCT has several applications. During CTO-PCI, the guidewire crossing of the lesions is a major challenge. OCT can help to confirm the intraluminal position of the guidewire, thereby decreasing the risk of subintimal course and potential perforation or dissection [14]. Moreover, in extra-plaque techniques used to cross the CTO lesion, case reports showed the feasibility of an antegrade dissection-and re-entry (ADR) approach through a novel OCT-guided CTO re-entry device, which provides real-time image guidance for true lumen re-entry [15]. After successful guidewire crossing, OCT can help to analyze the CTO-plaque, assessing its composition (fibrous, calcific, lipid-rich). In some CTOs, thanks to its high-resolution, OCT can identify microchannels within the context of the plaque, which sometimes may facilitate the progression of soft, low-profile guidewires [16]. Finally, OCT favors stent deployment and optimization (Figure 1A–C), which resulted in a significantly lower risk of target vessel failure (TVF) in a prespecified sub-study of the RENOVATE-COMPLEX-PCI trial [17]. However, despite its applications, OCT presents several limitations in CTO-PCI. First, its limited penetration depth (1–2 mm) could be a drawback in cases with large or heavily calcified plaques where a deeper visualization is required. Second, OCT imaging requires the clearance of blood from the vessel, typically achieved through contrast injection. This requirement can increase the risk of extending a dissection rim when it has been caused by guidewire crossing. Further studies will provide further data about OCT use in CTO-PCI.

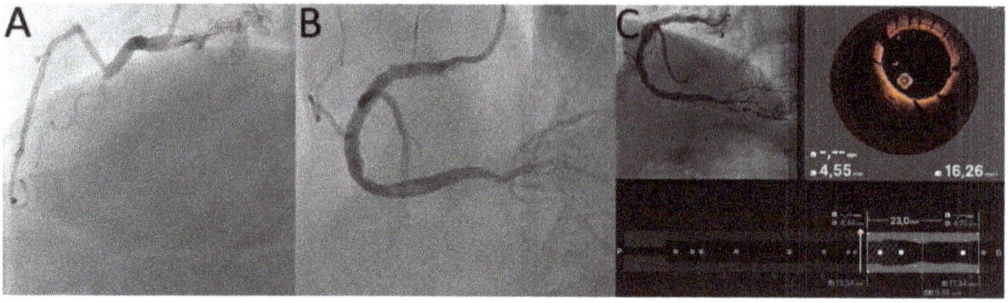

Figure 1. CTO-PCI of a right coronary artery (**A**,**B**) and OCT showing a good stent struts apposition and stent area (**C**).

2. Intravascular Ultrasound

IVUS is an imaging modality that uses high-frequency sound waves to create detailed cross-sectional images of the coronary arteries. IVUS catheters are equipped with ultrasound transducers that emit sound waves, which reflect off the vessel wall and the surrounding structures, and the reflected signals are then converted into images that provide the real-time visualization of the vessel lumen and wall [18,19]. IVUS catheters can be either phased array or mechanical. Phased array catheters present multiple transducers that electronically steer the ultrasound beam, while mechanical catheters have a single rotating transducer [20]. Thanks to its high penetration, IVUS has several applications in CTO-PCI (Figure 2A,B).

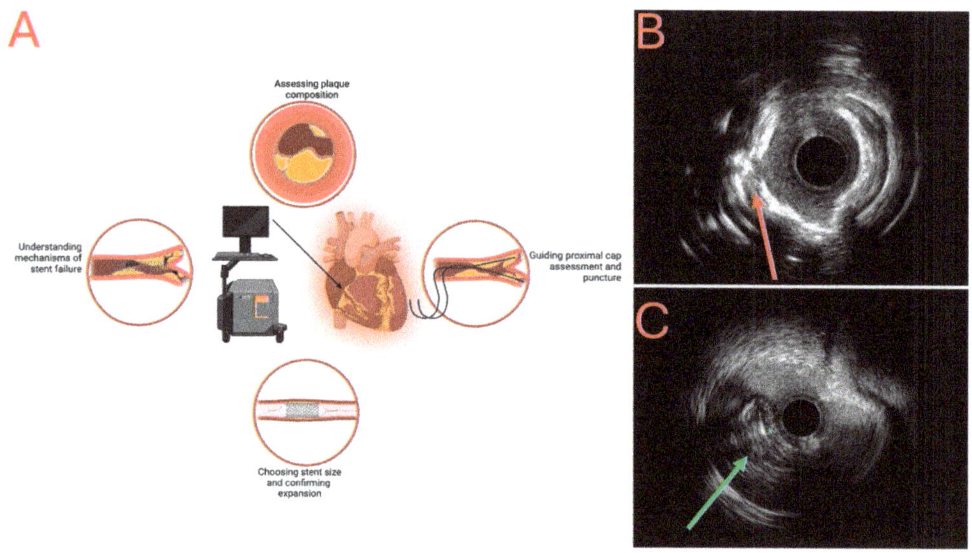

Figure 2. (**A**) IVUS applications in CTO-PCI. (**B**) Practical IVUS examples a heavily calcified CTO-plaque with evidence of calcium fracture after rotational atherectomy (red arrow). (**C**) Tip detection antegrade dissection and re-entry (TD-ADR) showing an IVUS catheter in the subintimal space guiding the penetration of the wire (green mark) in the true lumen (green arrow).

2.1. Proximal Cap Ambiguity

The proximal cap ambiguity is defined as the inability to clearly define the proximal entry point of the plaque, with a prevalence in approximately 30% of CTOs [21]. The presence of proximal cap ambiguity is also associated with higher rates of major adverse cardiac events (MACE) and retrograde crossing attempts [21]. In this scenario, an IVUS catheter can be advanced over a guidewire into a side branch adjacent to the proximal cap. Accordingly, subsequent IVUS pullback allows us to correctly assess the proximal cap and its composition, therefore, helps in making the choice between a high-penetration guidewire or a soft, polymer-jacketed guidewire [22].

2.2. Support in Antegrade Dissection and Re-Entry (ADR)

During CTO-PCI, the operators may direct the guidewire to the subintimal space in order to enable re-entry into the intimal space through different ways: (a) a dedicated device such as the Stingray™ (Boston Scientific, Marlborough, MA, USA) balloon or a dual lumen microcatheter; (b) redirecting the guidewire; (c) using another guidewire (parallel wire technique); or (d) using IVUS guidance in order to re-enter the intimal space with another guidewire. This last approach, called tip detection antegrade dissection and re-entry (TD-ADR) represents one of the most recent techniques in the CTO-PCI field and requires IVUS guidance to guide a stiff guidewire to re-enter the intimal space (Figure 2C) [23,24]; this approach shows higher procedural success rates and significantly lower procedural time in comparison to the conventional Stingray-assisted ADR [25].

2.3. Support in Reverse Controlled Antegrade and Retrograde Tracking (CART)

The retrograde approach allows us to cross the CTO distally through the collaterals, which could be septal, epicardial, or bypass collaterals. Thanks to this approach, the success rates of CTO-PCI significantly increased over years [26]. The indications for the use of the retrograde approach range from proximal cap ambiguity, long CTO lesions, bifurcation at the distal cap, and aorto-ostial lesions [27]. During this approach, the retrograde guidewire can be used: (a) as a marker for directing an antegrade wire which crosses the lesion; (b) for a retrograde true lumen puncture of the distal cap; or (c) for a retrograde dissection and re-entry approach, with the reverse CART being the most common strategy used in this setting. This consists of an antegrade knuckled guidewire delivered in the subintimal space, with a balloon sized 1:1 deflated on the antegrade wire which creates a connection between the subintimal and the intimal space. Subsequently, the retrograde wire advances from the distal to the proximal true lumen through the created space [28]. In this scenario, IVUS can help to define the position of both antegrade and retrograde guidewires and to identify plaque morphology and vessel size. This last phase is crucial for reversing the CART technique, because IVUS helps to identify the best segment of the vessel where a space connection between subintimal and intimal space can be created and can guide the selection of the appropriate guidewire to perform CTO crossing [29].

2.4. Stent Deployment and Optimization

After CTO crossing, IVUS allows the precise measurement of a vessel's dimension as well as the lesion's length to precisely identify stent's size and its landing zones. Since the geographical miss, stent under-sizing or malposition are the major predictors of stent thrombosis, IVUS acquires a significant impact in this scenario [30–32]. Although IVUS guidance in complex CAD is recommended since it significantly improves clinical outcomes, there is limited evidence regarding the clinical impact of IVUS in CTO-PCI [33]. Table 1 shows the studies reporting a comparison between IVUS- and angiography-guided CTO-PCI and shows a significant reduction in major adverse cardiac events (MACE), myocardial infarction, stent thrombosis, and in-stent late luminal loss [34–38]. Thanks to the appropriate vessel size and length estimation, summoning the evidence of recent trials showed that an IVUS-guided CTO-PCI is related to higher stent length and stent diameter, resulting in evidence of a significantly lower risk of stent thrombosis [39].

Table 1. Studies reporting a comparison between IVUS- and angiography-guided CTO-PCI.

Study	K-CTO	CTO-IVUS	Air-CTO	Progress-CTO	Kalogeropoulos et al. [38]
Year	2014	2015	2015	2020	2021
Study type	Observational	Randomized Controlled Trial	Randomized controlled trial	Observational	Observational
Sample Size	402 IG: 201 AG: 201	402 IG: 201 AG: 201	230 IG: 115 AG: 115	922 IG: 344 AG: 578	364 IG: 182 AG: 182
Follow Up (Years)	2	1	1	1	4
Primary Endpoint	Definite or probable stent thrombosis	Cardiac Death	in-stent late lumen loss (LLL)	CD, MI, TVR	All cause death, CD, MI, TVR
Procedural Success	**NR**	IG 99 AG 98	IG 91 AG 68	**NR**	NR
Retrograde Approach (%)	**NR**	IG: 7 AG 9.5	IG: 10.4 AG: 19.1	IG: 28.8 AG: 21.4	25.5 IG: 30.2 AG: 20.9
Anterograde Approach (%)	**NR**	IG: 93 AG: 90.5	IG: 89.6 AG: 80.9	IG: AWE 53.5 ADR:17.4 AG: AWE 57.1 ADR: 19.8	IG: AWE 60.4 ADR: 9.3 AG: AWE 69.2 ADR: 9.9
Second-Generation DES (%)	100	100	IG 27.8 AG 20.0	**NR**	100

CD: cardiac death; MI: myocardial infarction; TVR: target vessel revascularization; AWE: antegrade wire escalation; ADR: antegrade dissection re-entry; IG: intravascular ultrasound-guided group; AG: angiography-guided group.

2.5. IVUS Limitations

Despite its several applications, IVUS has some limitations that must be considered, including lower resolution compared to OCT, which may preclude the detailed visualization of microstructures within the plaque. IVUS also requires significant operator expertise for accurate image interpretation, especially in subintimal approaches, leading to a variability in outcomes.

3. Coronary Computed Tomography Angiography (CCTA)

CCTA is a non-invasive imaging modality which provides detailed three-dimensional images of the coronary arteries [40]. Utilizing CT technology, CCTA acquires high-resolution images that can be reconstructed to evaluate coronary anatomy, plaque characteristics and vessel course [41]. The extracted CCTA images of the coronary arteries are paired utilizing bifurcation points as markers to fluoroscopic diastolic images in order to balance breathing and cardiac rhythm. Co-registration between CCTA and fluoroscopic images facilitates the detection of angiographic projections that reduce vascular overlap and the foreshortening of the segment of interest. Through automatic softwares, it is feasible to reconstruct the centerline in the non-occluded segments of the vessel by identifying the contrast-filled lumen, while in the occluded segments, the difference in the Hounsfield Unit (HU) related to calcifications can aid in recognizing the vessel lumen of the CTO [42,43]. Thanks to its visualization modalities, CCTA allows for the multi-parametric evaluation of the CTO lesion. Slab maximum intensity projection (MIP) generates a projection image of a slab of tissue, highlighting the most intense structures. This method is effective in identifying calcified plaques and visualizing the overall vessel architecture [44] (Figure 3A). Curved multiplanar reconstruction (MPR) allows for the visualization of the coronary arteries along their natural course, providing a continuous view of the vessel, while stretched MPR visualizes the artery in a straightened format, making it easier to measure lesion length and identifying the occlusion site (Figure 3B). Finally, volume rendering creates a three-dimensional representation of the coronary arteries by combining data from multiple CT slices. This provides a comprehensive view of the vessel anatomy (Figure 3C). By providing a three-dimensional rendering of the coronary arteries, CCTA allows a precise identification of the occluding segments and their supply territories, enabling the quantification of the amount of myocardium at risk.

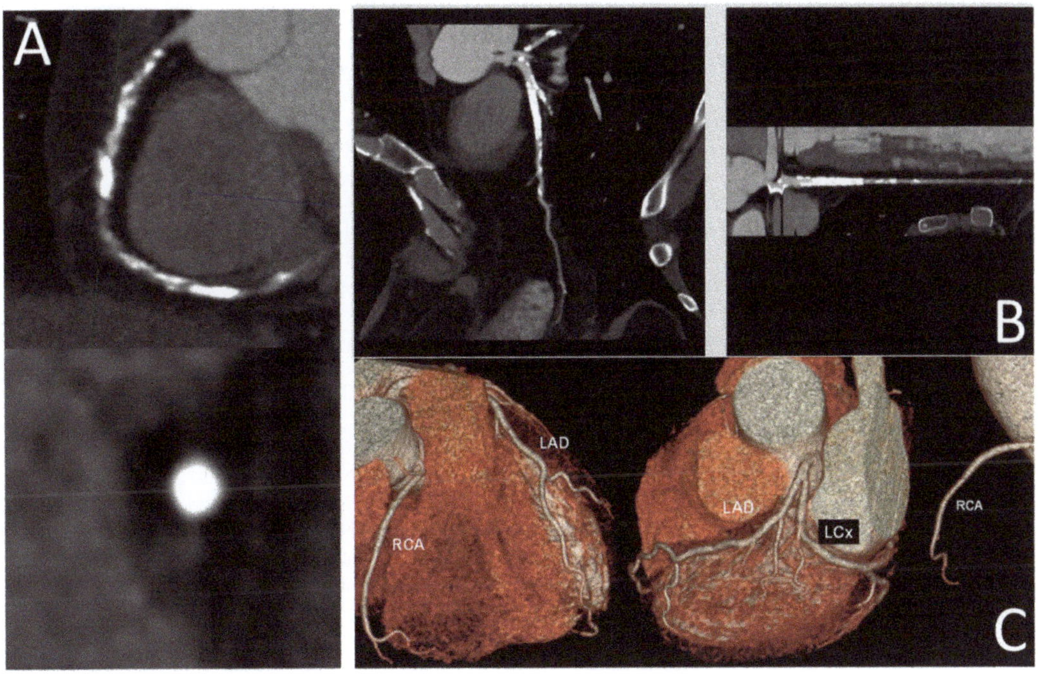

Figure 3. (**A**) visualization of a high-calcified CTO plaque of a right coronary artery with the slab maximum intensity projection (MIP) technique; (**B**) curved and stretched multi-planar reconstruction of a LAD-CTO; (**C**) three-dimensional reconstruction of coronary arteries through the volume rendering approach.

CCTA can be used to analyze the characteristics of the CTO segment before PCI. The non-invasive estimation of the proximal cap location and its features, the precise artery trajectory, and the calcium distribution are made possible by CCTA [45]. In fact, with traditional angiography, these data are less accurate. Thus, CCTA provides a better assessment of complex CTO, which may lead to shorter procedural time, less radiation and contrast injection, and consequently, the better planning of the procedure [46,47]. A functional assessment of wall motion and myocardial perfusion is also made possible by the ongoing advancement of scanner technologies [48]. Thanks to CCTA, several predictors of procedure's complexity have been identified, including the extent of calcification, lesion length, negative remodeling, blunt stump, vessel bending and the presence of side branches [49–51]. Among these risk factors of procedural complexity, calcification has several implications. Heavy calcifications within the CTO-plaque may impede device delivery, often forcing operators to adopt extra plaque approaches, burdened by higher periprocedural risks and worse outcomes [52]. Severe calcifications can compromise optimal stent expansion, which is a major risk factor for stent thrombosis [30]. CCTA allows us to adequately identify calcium burden, allowing an adequate planning of the procedure. Particularly, CCTA allows us to identify heavy calcification with a circular disposition of 360° and on the 100% of cross-sectional area (CSA), defined as "full-moon" calcifications, which have been shown to be independent predictors of an inability to cross the lesion or the need for intense debulking devices such as intravascular lithotripsy and rotational atherectomy, thus increasing the risk of procedural complications like coronary perforations [53,54]. In the evaluation of CTOs, several scores are useful tools to assess a lesion's complexity. The most used score is the J-CTO score, an angiographic score that identifies the probability of successful guidewire crossing within 30 min [55]. Recently, two CCTA-based scores (CT-RECTOR and KCCT) have been developed and have demonstrated a better predictive performance than the J-CTO angiographic score [56,57]. CT-RECTOR score predicts 30 min wire crossing by examining anatomical features such as stump morphology, multiple occlusions, the calcification extent of >50% of the vessel area, bending within the occlusion of greater than 45° and clinical characteristics as prior attempt, and the duration of CTO of >12 months [58]. In addition, the KCCT score considers other two features as the presence of an adjacent side branch and gives a supplementary point to central calcifications (360° and 100% CSA; Table 2). Recent evidence has examined the success rate of CTO-PCI after a pre-procedural CCTA, with higher success rates and fewer complications in the CCTA group compared to the angiography-only group [59]. According to these mentioned data, it seems feasible to apply CCTA in CTO-PCI procedures, especially for patients with high-score CTOs (e.g., J-CTO ≥ 2), in cases of prior failed procedures, in patients with previous CABG, and in situations with poor visualization of the vessel's course [60]. Further studies are ongoing (NCT05364827); these will examine patients randomly assigned to CCTA-guided CTO-PCI or only PCI. The primary endpoint will be the success rate, while the secondary endpoints will be the assessment of angina valued by the Seattle Angina Questionnaire, the need for a second CTO procedure, procedural complications, wire crossing time, and procedural time. The main limitation of the use of CCTA in this field is the additional use of radiation and contrast agents, although modern CT scanners have significantly decreased radiation and contrast while simultaneously enhancing picture quality. Likewise, we should expect further improvements in the fusion imaging of CCTA and fluoroscopy, and future research should identify the features of lesions that will benefit most from these new techniques.

Table 2. Overview of the CT-based CTO scores, along with the angiography-based J-CTO score.

	J-CTO Score	CT-RECTOR Score	KCCT Score
Morphology	☐ Tapered stump (0) ☐ Blunt stump (1)	☐ Blunt stump (1)	☐ Blunt stump (1)
Calcification	☐ Calcification within the CTO segment (1)	☐ Calcification extent>50% of the vessel CSA (1)	☐ Calcification with encircling <180° or CSA<50% (0) ☐ Peripheral calcification (≥180° or CSA≥50%) (1) ☐ Central calcification (360° and CSA 100%) (2)
Bending	☐ Bending ≥45 degrees (1)	☐ Bending ≥45 degrees (1)	☐ Bending > 45 degrees (1)
Length	☐ <20 mm (0) ☐ ≥20 mm (1)		☐ <15 mm (0) ☐ ≥15 mm (1)
Proximal Adjacent Side Branch			☐ No (0) ☐ Yes (1)
Re-Attempt	☐ Re-try lesion (1)	☐ Re-try lesion (1)	☐ Re-try lesion (1)
Occlusion		☐ Multiple occlusions (1)	

Table 2. *Cont.*

	J-CTO Score	CT-RECTOR Score	KCCT Score
Duration		☐ Duration of CTO ≥12 months or unknown (1)	☐ Duration of CTO ≥12 months or unknown (1)
Total Score	☐ 0 Easy ☐ 1 Intermediate ☐ 2 Difficult ☐ ≥3 Very Difficult	☐ 0 Easy ☐ 1 Intermediate ☐ 2 Difficult ☐ ≥3 Very Difficult	☐ 0 Easy ☐ 1 Intermediate ☐ 2 Difficult ☐ 3 Very Difficult ☐ ≥4 Extremely Difficult

4. Discussion

Coronary imaging techniques have revolutionized approaches to managing CTOs in CAD. Each modality offers unique advantages and plays a crucial role in different phases of CTO-PCI (Table 3). The importance of coronary imaging in this field has been widely recognized, not only for the increased technical success rates provided by these approaches. In fact, coronary imaging guidance has shown not only a significant improvement in quality of life [61,62] but also a significant reduction in procedural and long-term complications in respect to an angiography-only guidance, which is pivotal in the context of CTO-PCI. In more detail, in the recent OCCUPI trial, an OCT guidance led to a significant reduction in a composite endpoint of cardiac death, myocardial infarction, ischemia-driven target lesion revascularization, and stent thrombosis in complex CAD, including patients with CTOs [63]. Similarly, several studies showed a lower incidence of stent-thrombosis after IVUS guidance in CTO-PCI [39]. Finally, in patients undergoing CCTA before CTO-PCI, lower rates of intraprocedural complications like coronary perforations were observed [59]. Despite their individual strengths, these imaging modalities also present some limitations that should be carefully considered when planning and performing CTO-PCI. OCT, with its high-resolution, plays an important role in identifying microchannels and for stent optimization. However, its limited penetration depth restricts its utility in heavily calcified lesions and the requirement for blood clearance during imaging may increase procedural complications due to the enlargement of dissections. Therefore, while OCT plays a role in the later stages of CTO-PCI, its use during crossing phase remains limited. IVUS, with its deeper penetration, offers comprehensive insights into vessel's lumen and wall, which is particularly useful in ambiguous proximal cap scenarios and subintimal navigation during ADR or retrograde approach. IVUS-guided CTO-PCIs have also shown to reduce the short- and long-term complications of stent implantation [39]. However, operator-dependent interpretations may cause variability in outcomes, which may be mitigated by future technological developments and artificial intelligence (AI) algorithms, and its low resolution may miss microchannels or small dissections. CCTA serves as a useful non-invasive tool, providing the three-dimensional reconstructions of coronary anatomy, plaque characteristics, and vessel direction. The possibility of identifying myocardial mass at risk, combined with advance imaging techniques such as slab MIP, curved and stretched MPR, and volume rendering, allows for detailed procedural planning and risk stratification. Despite these advancements, several challenges persist, including cost, accessibility, and operator expertise. The high costs of imaging devices and limited availability can restrict their routine use, particularly in resource-limited settings. Additionally, the learning curve associated with coronary imaging can result in variability in outcomes, especially in less experienced operators. Further training protocols and the standardization of imaging protocols will help to reduce these issues, enabling more consistent results across centers, and aiding in the dissemination of these fundamental tools to achieve procedural success and increase safety.

Table 3. Basic principles, strengths and weaknesses of coronary imaging techniques in CTO-PCI.

Imaging Modality	Basic Principles	Strengths	Weaknesses
OCT (Optical coherence tomography)	Near-infrared light	-High-resolution (10-20 μm), allowing detailed assessment of plaque morphology -Detection of microchannels, thrombus, edge dissection -Useful for guiding stent deployment/optimization	-Limited penetration depth -Requires blood clearance with contrast, may enlarge dissections -Supplementary contrast use may impair renal function
IVUS (Intravascular ultrasound)	High-frequency sound waves	-Good penetration depth -Assessment of vessel size, plaque burden, calcification -Useful for guiding stent deployment/optimization -Helpful for solving proximal cap ambiguity -Support in retrograde and antegrade dissection and re-entry (ADR) approaches, including tip-detection ADR	-Lower resolution comparing to OCT -Interpretation is operator-dependent -Unable to detect thin fibrous caps or microcalcifications
CCTA (Coronary Computed Tomography Angiography)	X-rays	-Non-invasive modality -Slab maximum intensity projection (MIP) allows high-quality images. -Curved and stretched multi-planar (MPR) reconstructions allow easy measurement of occlusion length. -Volume rendering (VR) creates a three-dimensional view of the vessel. -Identification of calcium patterns around the CTO-lesion. -Simulation of angiographic views, friendly to interventional cardiologists. -CCTA based scores (KCCT and CT-rector) predict success rates.	-Lacking real-time imaging during PCI -Contrast and radiation exposure -Blooming effect due to heavy calcification may reduce diagnostic accuracy -Training needed to use CCTA programs -High costs

5. Future Possibilities

The future of coronary imaging in CTO intervention is poised for significant advancements, driven by technological innovation and interdisciplinary research. The integration of multiple imaging modalities with hybrid assessment holds promises to provide insights that leverage the strengths of each technique. Advancements in imaging technology, such as high-definition IVUS and ultra-high-resolution CCTA will offer more detailed images during CTO analyses. Further, AI and machine learning (ML) algorithms are set to reform the analysis and interpretation of coronary imaging, improving the reconstruction of the vessel, reducing postprocessing time and favoring the prediction of the successful percutaneous recanalization of CTO lesions [64–66]. Automated image segmentation and plaque characterization can reduce operator dependency and enhance diagnostic accuracy. The development of fusion imaging techniques that combine CCTA with real-time fluoroscopy can provide dynamic, real-time guidance during CTO-PCI. This approach can help reduce procedural time, minimize radiation exposure, and improve the accuracy of guidewire crossing and stent deployment. Continued innovation, research and collaboration across disciplines will be essential in unveiling the full potential of these advanced imaging techniques, ultimately improving the management of this complex scenario.

6. Conclusions

Advanced coronary imaging techniques have significantly improved the management of CTOs. OCT, IVUS, and CCTA provide irreplaceable support, from non-invasive anatomical evaluation and procedural planning detailed to plaque assessment and stent optimization. While each modality has its limitations, their integration into clinical practice has enhanced procedural success, safety, and patient outcomes. The development of AI and

ML algorithms, along with fusion imaging approaches, will overcome the limitations of these techniques, broadening their use and significantly increasing operators' expertise and confidence in performing CTO-PCI. Future advancement in these technologies promises greater precision and personalized approaches to CTO interventions.

Author Contributions: Conceptualization, G.P., S.D.R. and D.T.; methodology, G.P., N.C., S.D.R. and D.T.; software, G.P.; validation, G.P., Y.S.A., N.C., U.L., S.D.R. and D.T.; formal analysis, G.P., Y.S.A. and N.C.; investigation, G.P. and N.C.; resources, G.P., Y.S.A., U.L., S.D.R. and D.T.; data curation, G.P. and N.C.; writing—original draft preparation, G.P. and N.C.; writing—review and editing, G.P., Y.S.A., N.C., U.L., S.D.R. and D.T.; visualization, G.P., Y.S.A., N.C., U.L., S.D.R. and D.T.; supervision, G.P., S.D.R. and D.T.; project administration, G.P., S.D.R. and D.T.; funding acquisition, G.P., S.D.R. and D.T. All authors have read and agreed to the published version of the manuscript.

Funding: This work was in part supported by a grant from the Italian Ministry of Health: PSC SALUTE 2014–2020—POS4 "Cal-Hub-Ria" (T4-AN-09).

Institutional Review Board Statement: Not applicable.

Informed Consent Statement: Not applicable.

Data Availability Statement: No new data were created or analyzed in this study.

Conflicts of Interest: The authors declare no conflict of interest.

References

1. Råmunddal, T.; Hoebers, L.P.; Henriques, J.P.S.; Dworeck, C.; Angerås, O.; Odenstedt, J.; Ioanes, D.; Olivecrona, G.; Harnek, J.; Jensen, U.; et al. Prognostic Impact of Chronic Total Occlusions: A Report From SCAAR (Swedish Coronary Angiography and Angioplasty Registry). *JACC Cardiovasc. Interv.* **2016**, *9*, 1535–1544. [CrossRef] [PubMed]
2. Fefer, P.; Knudtson, M.L.; Cheema, A.N.; Galbraith, P.D.; Osherov, A.B.; Yalonetsky, S.; Gannot, S.; Samuel, M.; Weisbrod, M.; Bierstone, D.; et al. Current Perspectives on Coronary Chronic Total Occlusions: The Canadian Multicenter Chronic Total Occlusions Registry. *J. Am. Coll. Cardiol.* **2012**, *59*, 991–997. [CrossRef] [PubMed]
3. Panuccio, G.; Carabetta, N.; Torella, D.; De Rosa, S. Clinical Impact of Coronary Revascularization over Medical Treatment in Chronic Coronary Syndromes: A Systematic Review and Meta-Analysis. *Hell. J. Cardiol. HJC Hell. Kardiol. Ep.* **2024**, *78*, 60–71. [CrossRef] [PubMed]
4. Werner, G.S.; Hildick-Smith, D.; Martin Yuste, V.; Boudou, N.; Sianos, G.; Gelev, V.; Rumoroso, J.R.; Erglis, A.; Christiansen, E.H.; Escaned, J.; et al. Three-Year Outcomes of A Randomized Multicentre Trial Comparing Revascularization and Optimal Medical Therapy for Chronic Total Coronary Occlusions (EuroCTO). *EuroIntervention* **2023**, *19*, 571–579. [CrossRef] [PubMed]
5. Panuccio, G.; Carabetta, N.; Torella, D.; De Rosa, S. Percutaneous Coronary Revascularization versus Medical Therapy in Chronic Coronary Syndromes: An Updated Meta-Analysis of Randomized Controlled Trials. *Eur. J. Clin. Investig.* **2024**, e14303. [CrossRef] [PubMed]
6. Di Mario, C.; Mashayekhi, K.A.; Garbo, R.; Pyxaras, S.A.; Ciardetti, N.; Werner, G.S. Recanalisation of Coronary Chronic Total Occlusions. *EuroIntervention* **2022**, *18*, 535–561. [CrossRef] [PubMed]
7. Christakopoulos, G.E.; Christopoulos, G.; Carlino, M.; Jeroudi, O.M.; Roesle, M.; Rangan, B.V.; Abdullah, S.; Grodin, J.; Kumbhani, D.J.; Vo, M.; et al. Meta-Analysis of Clinical Outcomes of Patients Who Underwent Percutaneous Coronary Interventions for Chronic Total Occlusions. *Am. J. Cardiol.* **2015**, *115*, 1367–1375. [CrossRef]
8. Stojkovic, S.; Juricic, S.; Dobric, M.; Nedeljkovic, M.A.; Vukcevic, V.; Orlic, D.; Stankovic, G.; Tomasevic, M.; Aleksandric, S.; Dikic, M.; et al. Improved Propensity-Score Matched Long-Term Clinical Outcomes in Patients with Successful Percutaneous Coronary Interventions of Coronary Chronic Total Occlusion. *Int. Heart J.* **2018**, *59*, 719–726. [CrossRef]
9. Teramoto, T.; Tsuchikane, E.; Yamamoto, M.; Matsuo, H.; Kawase, Y.; Suzuki, Y.; Kanou, S.; Shimura, T.; Sato, H.; Habara, M.; et al. Successful Revascularization Improves Long-Term Clinical Outcome in Patients with Chronic Coronary Total Occlusion. *Int. J. Cardiol. Heart Vasc.* **2017**, *14*, 28–32. [CrossRef]
10. Melotti, E.; Belmonte, M.; Gigante, C.; Mallia, V.; Mushtaq, S.; Conte, E.; Neglia, D.; Pontone, G.; Collet, C.; Sonck, J.; et al. The Role of Multimodality Imaging for Percutaneous Coronary Intervention in Patients with Chronic Total Occlusions. *Front. Cardiovasc. Med.* **2022**, *9*, 823091. [CrossRef]
11. Xenogiannis, I.; Pavlidis, A.N.; Kaier, T.E.; Rigopoulos, A.G.; Karamasis, G.V.; Triantafyllis, A.S.; Vardas, P.; Brilakis, E.S.; Kalogeropoulos, A.S. The Role of Intravascular Imaging in Chronic Total Occlusion Percutaneous Coronary Intervention. *Front. Cardiovasc. Med.* **2023**, *10*, 1199067. [CrossRef] [PubMed]
12. Prati, F.; Jenkins, M.W.; Di Giorgio, A.; Rollins, A.M. Intracoronary Optical Coherence Tomography, Basic Theory and Image Acquisition Techniques. *Int. J. Cardiovasc. Imaging* **2011**, *27*, 251–258. [CrossRef] [PubMed]

13. Engel, L.-C.; Landmesser, U.; Abdelwahed, Y.S.; Jaguszewski, M.; Gigengack, K.; Wurster, T.-H.; Skurk, C.; Manes, C.; Schuster, A.; Noutsias, M.; et al. Comprehensive Multimodality Characterization of Hemodynamically Significant and Non-Significant Coronary Lesions Using Invasive and Noninvasive Measures. *PLoS ONE* **2020**, *15*, e0228292. [CrossRef] [PubMed]
14. Schultz, C.; van der Ent, M.; Serruys, P.W.; Regar, E. Optical Coherence Tomography to Guide Treatment of Chronic Occlusions? *JACC Cardiovasc. Interv.* **2009**, *2*, 366–367. [CrossRef]
15. Sandesara, P.B.; Robertson, G.C.; Chan, K.F.; Rowe, D.; Ebner, A.; Minarsch, L.; Lombardi, W.; Kandzari, D.E.; Hinohara, T.; Simpson, J.B. Clinical Experience of a Novel Optical Coherence Tomography-Guided Coronary Chronic Total Occlusion Re-Entry Device. *JACC Case Rep.* **2023**, *26*, 102041. [CrossRef]
16. Teijeiro Mestre, R.; Alegría-Barrero, E.; Di Mario, C. Microchannels in Recent Chronic Total Occlusions Assessed with Frequency-Domain Optical Coherence Tomography. *Rev. Esp. Cardiol. Engl. Ed.* **2013**, *66*, 907. [CrossRef]
17. Hong, D.; Kim, S.M.; Lee, S.Y.; Choi, K.H.; Song, Y.B.; Lee, J.-Y.; Lee, S.-J.; Yun, K.H.; Cho, J.Y.; Kim, C.J.; et al. Prognostic Impact of Intravascular Imaging-Guided Percutaneous Coronary Intervention in Chronic Total Occlusion. *Circulation* **2023**, *148*, 903–905. [CrossRef]
18. Koskinas, K.C. IVUS for Guidance of Coronary Interventions: Applying Optimisation Targets to Improve Clinical Outcomes. *EuroIntervention* **2020**, *16*, e448–e450. [CrossRef]
19. Panuccio, G.; De Rosa, S.; Landmesser, U.; Leistner, D.M.; Abdelwahed, Y.S. Role of Integrated Intracoronary Imaging to Identify Surgical Clip as a Trigger for ACS-NSTE. *JACC Case Rep.* **2024**, *29*, 102152. [CrossRef]
20. Bourantas, C.V.; Tenekecioglu, E.; Radu, M.; Räber, L.; Serruys, P.W. State of the Art: Role of Intravascular Imaging in the Evolution of Percutaneous Coronary Intervention—a 30-Year Review. *EuroIntervention* **2017**, *13*, 644–653. [CrossRef]
21. Karatasakis, A.; Danek, B.A.; Karmpaliotis, D.; Alaswad, K.; Jaffer, F.A.; Yeh, R.W.; Patel, M.P.; Bahadorani, J.N.; Wyman, R.M.; Lombardi, W.L.; et al. Impact of Proximal Cap Ambiguity on Outcomes of Chronic Total Occlusion Percutaneous Coronary Intervention: Insights From a Multicenter US Registry. *J. Invasive Cardiol.* **2016**, *28*, 391–396. [PubMed]
22. Galassi, A.R.; Sumitsuji, S.; Boukhris, M.; Brilakis, E.S.; Di Mario, C.; Garbo, R.; Spratt, J.C.; Christiansen, E.H.; Gagnor, A.; Avran, A.; et al. Utility of Intravascular Ultrasound in Percutaneous Revascularization of Chronic Total Occlusions: An Overview. *JACC Cardiovasc. Interv.* **2016**, *9*, 1979–1991. [CrossRef]
23. Tanaka, K.; Okamura, A.; Tsuchikane, E.; Matsuda, H.; Kawahira, M.; Sumiyoshi, A.; Watanabe, S.; Iwamoto, M.; Tanaka, N.; Koyama, Y.; et al. New Antegrade Dissection Re-Entry Technique with Tip Detection Method and New Puncture Wire in CTO-PCI. *JACC Cardiovasc. Interv.* **2023**, *16*, 1546–1548. [CrossRef] [PubMed]
24. Sakakura, K. Tip Detection-Antegrade Dissection and Re-Entry: Is This the Beginning of a New Era? *JACC Asia* **2024**, *4*, 373–374. [CrossRef]
25. Tanaka, K.; Okamura, A.; Yoshikawa, R.; Tsuchikane, E.; Ishikawa, M.; Suzuki, S.; Nagai, H.; Sumiyoshi, A.; Kawahira, M.; Yamasaki, T.; et al. Tip Detection-Antegrade Dissection and Re-Entry with New Puncture Wire in CTO Intervention: Revolution Through 3D-Wiring. *JACC Asia* **2024**, *4*, 359–372. [CrossRef] [PubMed]
26. Megaly, M.; Xenogiannis, I.; Abi Rafeh, N.; Karmpaliotis, D.; Rinfret, S.; Yamane, M.; Burke, M.N.; Brilakis, E.S. Retrograde Approach to Chronic Total Occlusion Percutaneous Coronary Intervention. *Circ. Cardiovasc. Interv.* **2020**, *13*, e008900. [CrossRef]
27. Brilakis, E.S.; Mashayekhi, K.; Tsuchikane, E.; Abi Rafeh, N.; Alaswad, K.; Araya, M.; Avran, A.; Azzalini, L.; Babunashvili, A.M.; Bayani, B.; et al. Guiding Principles for Chronic Total Occlusion Percutaneous Coronary Intervention. *Circulation* **2019**, *140*, 420–433. [CrossRef]
28. Matsuno, S.; Tsuchikane, E.; Harding, S.A.; Wu, E.B.; Kao, H.-L.; Brilakis, E.S.; Mashayekhi, K.; Werner, G.S. Overview and Proposed Terminology for the Reverse Controlled Antegrade and Retrograde Tracking (Reverse CART) Techniques. *EuroIntervention* **2018**, *14*, 94–101. [CrossRef]
29. Rathore, S.; Katoh, O.; Tuschikane, E.; Oida, A.; Suzuki, T.; Takase, S. A Novel Modification of the Retrograde Approach for the Recanalization of Chronic Total Occlusion of the Coronary Arteries Intravascular Ultrasound-Guided Reverse Controlled Antegrade and Retrograde Tracking. *JACC Cardiovasc. Interv.* **2010**, *3*, 155–164. [CrossRef]
30. Ullrich, H.; Münzel, T.; Gori, T. Coronary Stent Thrombosis—Predictors and Prevention. *Dtsch. Arztebl. Int.* **2020**, *117*, 320–326. [CrossRef]
31. Choi, S.-Y.; Witzenbichler, B.; Maehara, A.; Lansky, A.J.; Guagliumi, G.; Brodie, B.; Kellett, M.A.; Dressler, O.; Parise, H.; Mehran, R.; et al. Intravascular Ultrasound Findings of Early Stent Thrombosis after Primary Percutaneous Intervention in Acute Myocardial Infarction: A Harmonizing Outcomes with Revascularization and Stents in Acute Myocardial Infarction (HORIZONS-AMI) Substudy. *Circ. Cardiovasc. Interv.* **2011**, *4*, 239–247. [CrossRef] [PubMed]
32. Calvert, P.A.; Brown, A.J.; Hoole, S.P.; Obaid, D.R.; West, N.E.J.; Bennett, M.R. Geographical Miss Is Associated with Vulnerable Plaque and Increased Major Adverse Cardiovascular Events in Patients with Myocardial Infarction. *Catheter. Cardiovasc. Interv. Off. J. Soc. Card. Angiogr. Interv.* **2016**, *88*, 340–347. [CrossRef] [PubMed]
33. Räber, L.; Mintz, G.S.; Koskinas, K.C.; Johnson, T.W.; Holm, N.R.; Onuma, Y.; Radu, M.D.; Joner, M.; Yu, B.; Jia, H.; et al. Clinical Use of Intracoronary Imaging. Part 1: Guidance and Optimization of Coronary Interventions. An Expert Consensus Document of the European Association of Percutaneous Cardiovascular Interventions. *Eur. Heart J.* **2018**, *39*, 3281–3300. [CrossRef] [PubMed]
34. Hong, S.-J.; Kim, B.-K.; Shin, D.-H.; Kim, J.-S.; Hong, M.-K.; Gwon, H.-C.; Kim, H.-S.; Yu, C.W.; Park, H.S.; Chae, I.-H.; et al. Usefulness of Intravascular Ultrasound Guidance in Percutaneous Coronary Intervention with Second-Generation Drug-

Eluting Stents for Chronic Total Occlusions (from the Multicenter Korean-Chronic Total Occlusion Registry). *Am. J. Cardiol.* **2014**, *114*, 534–540. [CrossRef]
35. Kim, B.-K.; Shin, D.-H.; Hong, M.-K.; Park, H.S.; Rha, S.-W.; Mintz, G.S.; Kim, J.-S.; Kim, J.S.; Lee, S.-J.; Kim, H.-Y.; et al. Clinical Impact of Intravascular Ultrasound-Guided Chronic Total Occlusion Intervention with Zotarolimus-Eluting Versus Biolimus-Eluting Stent Implantation: Randomized Study. *Circ. Cardiovasc. Interv.* **2015**, *8*, e002592. [CrossRef]
36. Tian, N.-L.; Gami, S.-K.; Ye, F.; Zhang, J.-J.; Liu, Z.-Z.; Lin, S.; Ge, Z.; Shan, S.-J.; You, W.; Chen, L.; et al. Angiographic and Clinical Comparisons of Intravascular Ultrasound- versus Angiography-Guided Drug-Eluting Stent Implantation for Patients with Chronic Total Occlusion Lesions: Two-Year Results from a Randomised AIR-CTO Study. *EuroIntervention* **2015**, *10*, 1409–1417. [CrossRef]
37. Vemmou, E.; Khatri, J.; Doing, A.H.; Dattilo, P.; Toma, C.; Sheikh, A.; Alaswad, K.; Jefferson, B.K.; Patel, T.N.; Chandwaney, R.H.; et al. Impact of Intravascular Ultrasound Utilization for Stent Optimization on 1-Year Outcomes After Chronic Total Occlusion Percutaneous Coronary Intervention. *J. Invasive Cardiol.* **2020**, *32*, 392–399. [PubMed]
38. Kalogeropoulos, A.S.; Alsanjari, O.; Davies, J.R.; Keeble, T.R.; Tang, K.H.; Konstantinou, K.; Vardas, P.; Werner, G.S.; Kelly, P.A.; Karamasis, G.V. Impact of Intravascular Ultrasound on Chronic Total Occlusion Percutaneous Revascularization. *Cardiovasc. Revascularization Med. Mol. Interv.* **2021**, *33*, 32–40. [CrossRef]
39. Panuccio, G.; Abdelwahed, Y.S.; Carabetta, N.; Salerno, N.; Leistner, D.M.; Landmesser, U.; De Rosa, S.; Torella, D.; Werner, G.S. Clinical and Procedural Outcomes of IVUS-Guided vs. Angiography-Guided CTO-PCI: A Systematic Review and Meta-Analysis. *J. Clin. Med.* **2023**, *12*, 4947. [CrossRef]
40. Carabetta, N.; Siller-Matula, J.M.; Boccuto, F.; Panuccio, G.; Indolfi, C.; Torella, D.; De Rosa, S. Commissural Alignment during TAVR Reduces the Risk of Overlap to Coronary Ostia. *Int. J. Cardiol.* **2024**, *395*, 131572. [CrossRef]
41. El Merhi, F.; Bou-Fakhredin, R.; El Ashkar, B.; Ghieh, D.; Ghosn, Y.; Saade, C. State of the Art of Coronary Computed Tomography Angiography. *Radiography* **2020**, *26*, 174–182. [CrossRef] [PubMed]
42. Zheng, Y.; Tek, H.; Funka-Lea, G. Robust and Accurate Coronary Artery Centerline Extraction in CTA by Combining Model-Driven and Data-Driven Approaches. In Proceedings of the International Conference on Medical Image Computing and Computer Assisted Intervention, Nagoya, Japan, 22–26 September 2013; Volume 16, pp. 74–81. [CrossRef]
43. Rivest-Hénault, D.; Sundar, H.; Cheriet, M. Nonrigid 2D/3D Registration of Coronary Artery Models with Live Fluoroscopy for Guidance of Cardiac Interventions. *IEEE Trans. Med. Imaging* **2012**, *31*, 1557–1572. [CrossRef] [PubMed]
44. Napel, S.; Rubin, G.D.; Jeffrey, R.B. STS-MIP: A New Reconstruction Technique for CT of the Chest. *J. Comput. Assist. Tomogr.* **1993**, *17*, 832–838. [CrossRef]
45. Yamamoto, M.H.; Maehara, A.; Poon, M.; Guo, J.; Yamashita, K.; Yakushiji, T.; Saito, S.; Koyama, K.; Mintz, G.S.; Ochiai, M. Morphological Assessment of Chronic Total Occlusions by Combined Coronary Computed Tomographic Angiography and Intravascular Ultrasound Imaging. *Eur. Heart J. Cardiovasc. Imaging* **2017**, *18*, 315–322. [CrossRef]
46. La Scala, E.; Peyre, J.-P.; Maupas, E.; ReSurg; CT-CTO PCI Study Group. Effect of Preoperative Coronary CT for Planning of Percutaneous Coronary Intervention for Complex Chronic Total Occlusion (CTS-C-CTOPCI): Study Protocol for an Open-Label Randomised Controlled Trial. *Trials* **2023**, *24*, 560. [CrossRef] [PubMed]
47. Magro, M.; Schultz, C.; Simsek, C.; Garcia-Garcia, H.M.; Regar, E.; Nieman, K.; Mollet, N.; Serruys, P.W.; van Geuns, R.-J. Computed Tomography as a Tool for Percutaneous Coronary Intervention of Chronic Total Occlusions. *EuroIntervention* **2010**, *6* (Suppl. G), G123–G131.
48. Danad, I.; Szymonifka, J.; Schulman-Marcus, J.; Min, J.K. Static and Dynamic Assessment of Myocardial Perfusion by Computed Tomography. *Eur. Heart J. Cardiovasc. Imaging* **2016**, *17*, 836–844. [CrossRef]
49. Ehara, M.; Terashima, M.; Kawai, M.; Matsushita, S.; Tsuchikane, E.; Kinoshita, Y.; Kimura, M.; Nasu, K.; Tanaka, N.; Fujita, H.; et al. Impact of Multislice Computed Tomography to Estimate Difficulty in Wire Crossing in Percutaneous Coronary Intervention for Chronic Total Occlusion. *J. Invasive Cardiol.* **2009**, *21*, 575–582.
50. Mollet, N.R.; Hoye, A.; Lemos, P.A.; Cademartiri, F.; Sianos, G.; McFadden, E.P.; Krestin, G.P.; Serruys, P.W.; de Feyter, P.J. Value of Preprocedure Multislice Computed Tomographic Coronary Angiography to Predict the Outcome of Percutaneous Recanalization of Chronic Total Occlusions. *Am. J. Cardiol.* **2005**, *95*, 240–243. [CrossRef]
51. Soon, K.H.; Cox, N.; Wong, A.; Chaitowitz, I.; Macgregor, L.; Santos, P.T.; Selvanayagam, J.B.; Farouque, H.M.O.; Rametta, S.; Bell, K.W.; et al. CT Coronary Angiography Predicts the Outcome of Percutaneous Coronary Intervention of Chronic Total Occlusion. *J. Intervent. Cardiol.* **2007**, *20*, 359–366. [CrossRef]
52. Brilakis, E.S.; Banerjee, S. Dancing with the "STAR": The Role of Subintimal Dissection/Re-Entry Strategies in Coronary Chronic Total Occlusion Interventions. *Catheter. Cardiovasc. Interv. Off. J. Soc. Card. Angiogr. Interv.* **2012**, *79*, 28–29. [CrossRef] [PubMed]
53. Panuccio, G.; Werner, G.S.; De Rosa, S.; Torella, D.; Leistner, D.M.; Siegrist, P.T.; Haghikia, A.; Skurk, C.; Mashayekhi, K.; Landmesser, U.; et al. Full-Moon Coronary Calcification as Detected with Computed Tomography Angiography in Chronic Total Occlusion Percutaneous Coronary Intervention. *Am. J. Cardiol.* **2024**, *222*, 149–156. [CrossRef] [PubMed]
54. Panuccio, G.; Skurk, C.; Landmesser, U.; Abdelwahed, Y.S. Double "Full Moon" CTO Plaque Detected by Computed Tomography Could Predict High-Grade Debulking Techniques: A Case-Report. *Clin. Case Rep.* **2023**, *11*, e7325. [CrossRef] [PubMed]

55. Morino, Y.; Abe, M.; Morimoto, T.; Kimura, T.; Hayashi, Y.; Muramatsu, T.; Ochiai, M.; Noguchi, Y.; Kato, K.; Shibata, Y.; et al. Predicting Successful Guidewire Crossing through Chronic Total Occlusion of Native Coronary Lesions within 30 Minutes: The J-CTO (Multicenter CTO Registry in Japan) Score as a Difficulty Grading and Time Assessment Tool. *JACC Cardiovasc. Interv.* **2011**, *4*, 213–221. [CrossRef] [PubMed]
56. Tan, Y.; Zhou, J.; Zhang, W.; Zhou, Y.; Du, L.; Tian, F.; Guo, J.; Chen, L.; Cao, F.; Chen, Y. Comparison of CT-RECTOR and J-CTO Scores to Predict Chronic Total Occlusion Difficulty for Percutaneous Coronary Intervention. *Int. J. Cardiol.* **2017**, *235*, 169–175. [CrossRef] [PubMed]
57. Yu, C.-W.; Lee, H.-J.; Suh, J.; Lee, N.-H.; Park, S.-M.; Park, T.K.; Yang, J.H.; Song, Y.B.; Hahn, J.-Y.; Choi, S.H.; et al. Coronary Computed Tomography Angiography Predicts Guidewire Crossing and Success of Percutaneous Intervention for Chronic Total Occlusion: Korean Multicenter CTO CT Registry Score as a Tool for Assessing Difficulty in Chronic Total Occlusion Percutaneous Coronary Intervention. *Circ. Cardiovasc. Imaging* **2017**, *10*, e005800. [CrossRef]
58. Opolski, M.P.; Achenbach, S.; Schuhbäck, A.; Rolf, A.; Möllmann, H.; Nef, H.; Rixe, J.; Renker, M.; Witkowski, A.; Kepka, C.; et al. Coronary Computed Tomographic Prediction Rule for Time-Efficient Guidewire Crossing through Chronic Total Occlusion: Insights from the CT-RECTOR Multicenter Registry (Computed Tomography Registry of Chronic Total Occlusion Revascularization). *JACC Cardiovasc. Interv.* **2015**, *8*, 257–267. [CrossRef]
59. Hong, S.-J.; Kim, B.-K.; Cho, I.; Kim, H.-Y.; Rha, S.-W.; Lee, S.-H.; Park, S.M.; Kim, Y.H.; Chang, H.-J.; Ahn, C.-M.; et al. Effect of Coronary CTA on Chronic Total Occlusion Percutaneous Coronary Intervention: A Randomized Trial. *JACC Cardiovasc. Imaging* **2021**, *14*, 1993–2004. [CrossRef]
60. Werner, G.S. Use of Coronary Computed Tomographic Angiography to Facilitate Percutaneous Coronary Intervention of Chronic Total Occlusions. *Circ. Cardiovasc. Interv.* **2019**, *12*, e007387. [CrossRef]
61. Lee, S.-W.; Lee, P.H.; Ahn, J.-M.; Park, D.-W.; Yun, S.-C.; Han, S.; Kang, H.; Kang, S.-J.; Kim, Y.-H.; Lee, C.W.; et al. Randomized Trial Evaluating Percutaneous Coronary Intervention for the Treatment of Chronic Total Occlusion. *Circulation* **2019**, *139*, 1674–1683. [CrossRef]
62. Juricic, S.A.; Stojkovic, S.M.; Galassi, A.R.; Stankovic, G.R.; Orlic, D.N.; Vukcevic, V.D.; Milasinovic, D.G.; Aleksandric, S.B.; Tomasevic, M.V.; Dobric, M.R.; et al. Long-Term Follow-up of Patients with Chronic Total Coronary Artery Occlusion Previously Randomized to Treatment with Optimal Drug Therapy or Percutaneous Revascularization of Chronic Total Occlusion (COMET-CTO). *Front. Cardiovasc. Med.* **2022**, *9*, 1014664. [CrossRef] [PubMed]
63. Hong, S.-J.; Lee, S.-J.; Lee, S.-H.; Lee, J.-Y.; Cho, D.-K.; Kim, J.W.; Kim, S.M.; Hur, S.-H.; Heo, J.H.; Jang, J.-Y.; et al. Optical Coherence Tomography-Guided versus Angiography-Guided Percutaneous Coronary Intervention for Patients with Complex Lesions (OCCUPI): An Investigator-Initiated, Multicentre, Randomised, Open-Label, Superiority Trial in South Korea. *Lancet* **2024**, *404*, 1029–1039. [CrossRef] [PubMed]
64. Nakachi, T.; Yamane, M.; Kishi, K.; Muramatsu, T.; Okada, H.; Oikawa, Y.; Yoshikawa, R.; Kawasaki, T.; Tanaka, H.; Katoh, O. Machine Learning for Prediction of Technical Results of Percutaneous Coronary Intervention for Chronic Total Occlusion. *J. Clin. Med.* **2023**, *12*, 3354. [CrossRef] [PubMed]
65. Li, M.; Ling, R.; Yu, L.; Yang, W.; Chen, Z.; Wu, D.; Zhang, J. Deep Learning Segmentation and Reconstruction for CT of Chronic Total Coronary Occlusion. *Radiology* **2023**, *306*, e221393. [CrossRef]
66. Zhou, Z.; Gao, Y.; Zhang, W.; Zhang, N.; Wang, H.; Wang, R.; Gao, Z.; Huang, X.; Zhou, S.; Dai, X.; et al. Deep Learning-Based Prediction of Percutaneous Recanalization in Chronic Total Occlusion Using Coronary CT Angiography. *Radiology* **2023**, *309*, e231149. [CrossRef]

Journal of
*Cardiovascular
Development and Disease*

MDPI

Article

Association of Cardiovascular Risk Factors and Coronary Calcium Burden with Epicardial Adipose Tissue Volume Obtained from PET–CT Imaging in Oncological Patients

Carmela Nappi [1], Andrea Ponsiglione [1], Carlo Vallone [1], Roberto Lepre [1], Luigi Basile [1], Roberta Green [1], Valeria Cantoni [1], Ciro Gabriele Mainolfi [1], Massimo Imbriaco [1], Mario Petretta [2,*] and Alberto Cuocolo [1]

1 Department of Advanced Biomedical Sciences, University Federico II, 80131 Naples, Italy; c.nappi@unina.it (C.N.); andrea.ponsiglione@unina.it (A.P.); carlo.vallone@unina.it (C.V.); roberto.lepre@unina.it (R.L.); luigi.basile@unina.it (L.B.); roberta.green@unina.it (R.G.); valeria.cantoni@unina.it (V.C.); cirogabriele.mainolfi@unina.it (C.G.M.); massimo.imbriaco@unina.it (M.I.); cuocolo@unina.it (A.C.)
2 IRCCS Synlab SDN, 80143 Naples, Italy
* Correspondence: mariopetretta1@gmail.com

Abstract: Whole-body positron emission tomography (PET)–computed tomography (CT) imaging performed for oncological purposes may provide additional parameters such as the coronary artery calcium (CAC) and epicardial adipose tissue (EAT) volume with cost-effective prognostic information in asymptomatic people beyond traditional cardiovascular risk factors. We evaluated the feasibility of measuring the CAC score and EAT volume in cancer patients without known coronary artery disease (CAD) referred to whole-body ^{18}F-FDG PET–CT imaging, regardless of the main clinical problem. We also investigated the potential relationships between traditional cardiovascular risk factors and CAC with EAT volume. A total of 109 oncological patients without overt CAD underwent whole-body PET–CT imaging with ^{18}F-fluorodeoxyglucose (FDG). Unenhanced CT images were retrospectively viewed for CAC and EAT measurements on a dedicated platform. Overall, the mean EAT volume was 99 ± 49 cm^3. Patients with a CAC score ≥ 1 were older than those with a CAC = 0 (p < 0.001) and the prevalence of hypertension was higher in patients with detectable CAC as compared to those without (p < 0.005). The EAT volume was higher in patients with CAC than in those without (p < 0.001). For univariable age, body mass index (BMI), hypertension, and CAC were associated with increasing EAT values (all p < 0.005). However, the correlation between the CAC score and EAT volume was weak, and in multivariable analysis only age and BMI were independently associated with increased EAT (both p < 0.001), suggesting that potential prognostic information on CAC and EAT is not redundant. This study demonstrates the feasibility of a cost-effective assessment of CAC scores and EAT volumes in oncological patients undergoing whole-body ^{18}F-FDG PET–CT imaging, enabling staging cancer disease and atherosclerotic burden by a single test already included in the diagnostic work program, with optimization of the radiation dose and without additional costs.

Keywords: coronary artery disease; coronary artery calcium; epicardial adipose tissue; PET/CT imaging

1. Introduction

Since 1991, the risk of death from oncological reasons has declined continuously, with an overall drop of 32% when compared to up-to-date rates [1]. On the other hand, while we are assisting such a cancer-related death decline due to the refinement of both diagnostic capabilities and therapeutic armamentarium, cardiovascular diseases currently remain the main cause of death, and it is precisely oncological patients who are at a higher risk of developing coronary artery disease (CAD) compared to the general population. This finding is partially due to common CAD and cancer risk factors and partially related to specific oncological therapeutic approaches such as thoracic external beam radiotherapy and chemotherapy, including anthracycline treatments [2,3]. Hence, in cancer patients, especially in those with a high probability of long-term survival, it is important to assess cardiovascular risk. The role of standard modifiable cardiovascular risk factors in determining CAD has been widely investigated [4–6]. On the other hand, imaging data may contribute to improving CAD risk stratification. Coronary artery calcium (CAC) burden, obtained using different methods including unenhanced computed tomography (CT), has emerged as the most predictive single cardiovascular risk marker in asymptomatic persons, capable of adding predictive information beyond traditional cardiovascular risk factors, with cost effectiveness [7,8].

Available data from large population analysis studies are consistent with the concept that CAC testing represents a reasonable option to risk stratify cardiovascular impairment without increased costs [3,9]. On the other hand, a recent meta-analysis evaluated the incremental benefit of adding CAC scoring to standard cardiovascular disease risk calculators, considering six studies with a total of 1043 cardiovascular events among 17,961 participants [10]. Although the results indicated that CAC scoring provided some additional discrimination beyond traditional risk assessment equations, with this improvement being relatively consistent across the studies, the authors highlighted that this slight improvement is often counterbalanced by the associated costs, incidental findings, and radiation exposure, affirming that it is unclear which patients would truly benefit. There is also growing evidence that the quantification of epicardial adipose tissue (EAT) by cardiac imaging may play a significant role in CAD risk stratification in patients with suspected atherosclerosis [11–15].

With regard to the oncological population, Lee et al. [16] suggested that the EAT area on low-dose chest CT could be used to predict coronary atherosclerosis in an asymptomatic population considered for lung cancer screening. The potential role of EAT as a biomarker of cancer-related therapy cardiotoxicity has also been proposed [17]. A recent study evaluated changes in the EAT in patients with follicular lymphoma treated with two therapeutic approaches and with different potential cardiotoxicities and demonstrated that an EAT increase may be a marker for the early detection of myocardial damage [18].

The purpose of the present study was to evaluate the feasibility of measuring, in a cost-effective manner, CAC scores and EAT volumes in patients referred to whole-body ^{18}F-FDG PET–CT imaging, regardless of the main clinical question. We also assessed the association of cardiovascular risk factors and coronary calcium content with the EAT volume obtained from whole-body positron emission tomography (PET)–CT imaging in oncological patients without known CAD.

2. Materials and Methods

2.1. Study Population

From February 2022 to March 2023, 109 consecutive patients were enrolled. Only patients undergoing whole-body PET–CT imaging with ^{18}F-fluorodeoxyglucose (FDG), as part of their diagnostic or follow-up program, for oncological reasons were included. The following data were considered for exclusion criteria: previously diagnosed CAD including a history of myocardial infarction (chest pain or equivalent symptom complex, positive cardiac biomarkers, or typical electrocardiographic changes), of percutaneous coronary intervention, or of coronary artery bypass grafting; severe valvular or congenital heart disease; and the presence of implantable cardiac devices.

As part of the baseline examination, clinical information including traditional cardiovascular risk factors, current smoker status, hypercholesterolemia, diabetes mellitus, and hypertension was collected. Current smoking was defined if patients had regularly smoked ($\geq$1 cigarette per day) within the past month before imaging. Hypercholesterolemia was defined as having a previous diagnosis of the mentioned condition, previous or ongoing oral low-density lipoprotein cholesterol (LDL-C) lowering treatment, an LDL-C concentration of 3.5 mmol/L or higher, or a total cholesterol concentration of 5.5 mmol/L or higher at the time of imaging. Diabetes (type 1 and type 2) was identified when patients demonstrated a previous diagnosis of diabetes or current glucose lowering therapy [19]. Hypertension was defined as a blood pressure > 140/90 mm Hg or current anti-hypertensive therapy [20]. A familiar history of premature CAD was noted in the case of a diagnosis of CAD in a first degree relative prior to or at 55 years of age in men or 65 years in women [21]. Patients reporting anginal symptoms were defined as symptomatic. Chest pain was classified as non-anginal chest pain, atypical angina, or typical angina [22]. The review committee of our institution approved this study, and all patients gave informed consent.

2.2. PET/CT Imaging

All patients were required to fast for at least 6 h prior to unenhanced PET/CT imaging, and in all subjects included in this study blood glucose levels were <180 mg/dL at the time of the ^{18}F-FDG injection. ^{18}F-FDG PET/CT unenhanced images were acquired using a PET/CT Ingenuity TF (Philips Healthcare, Best, The Netherlands) 60 min after the tracer administration (activity range 200–300 MBq, according to body weight) [23,24].

All examinations were performed in a three-dimensional mode. An emission scan was completed, from the upper thigh to the base of the skull, in the caudocranial direction (4 min for each bed position). Iterative image reconstruction was finalized with an ordered subset expectation maximization algorithm (2 iterations, 28 subsets). A T 4-slice multi-detector helical CT scanner was used (detector row configuration, 4 × 5 mm; pitch, 1.5; gantry rotation speed, 0.8 s per revolution; table speed, 30 mm per gantry rotation; 140 kV and 80 mA). Using filtered back projection CT reconstructed images (Gaussian filter with 8 mm full width at half maximum) to match the PET resolution, attenuation-corrected emission data were attained. Transaxial, sagittal, and coronal images and co-registered images were evaluated using Philips IntelliSpace Portal, Image and information management software version 9.0 (Philips Medical Systems, Veenpluis, Best, The Netherlands). The co-registered CT images were recovered and estimated with a dedicated workstation for post-processing and analysis as previously illustrated [25].

The CT studies were analyzed by consensus from experienced nuclear medicine physicians and radiologists blinded to the PET results. Calcium was defined as the presence of at least 3 contiguous pixels with a density > 130 HU. The total calcium load in the coronary arteries was measured based on the scoring algorithm proposed by Agatston et al. [26]. CAC scores were estimated separately for left anterior descending, left circumflex, and right coronary arteries, and they were then summed to obtain a total CAC score. For quantification of the EAT volume, the image processing started at the level of the pulmonary trunk and ended at the level of the inferior diaphragmatic surface of the heart to manually trace pericardial borders. The area outside the traced pericardium was excluded. An attenuation range of between −30 and −190 HU was then set [27,28]. Lastly, the images were checked and revised by operators to correct potential mistakes, and the total EAT volume was provided [12,29].

2.3. Statistical Analysis

For statistical analysis purposes, categorical data are expressed as a percentage and continuous data as the mean ± standard deviation. The χ^2 test and two-sample t test were used to evaluate the differences in the categorical and continuous variables, respectively. The ln (CAC score +1) transformation was used to adjust for the rightward skew of the data and to reduce heteroscedasticity. Statistical significance was considered in the case of a p value < 0.05 (two-sided). In order to identify the variables associated with an increasing EAT volume and CAC, univariable and multivariable linear regression analyses were performed. Variables showing a p value < 0.05 in a univariable analysis were used to provide a multivariable model. All the analyses were performed using STATA version 18.

3. Results

The study population comprised 109 subjects with ages ranging from 18 to 74 years. Table 1 illustrates the main clinical indications for the PET/CT imaging test.

Table 1. Main clinical indications for PET–CT imaging.

Tumor	Patients (n = 109)
Hematological, n (%)	43 (39)
Urogenital, n (%)	22 (21)
Lung, n (%)	13 (12)
Breast, n (%)	8 (7)
Gastrointestinal, n (%)	7 (6)
Thyroid, n (%)	6 (6)
Melanoma, n (%)	3 (3)
Others, n (%)	7 (6)

The baseline demographic and clinical characteristics of the study population according to CAC are illustrated in Table 2. In 38 (35%) patients, CAC was not detectable, and in 71 (65%), the CAC score was ≥1 with a mean ln (CAC +1) of 2.7 ± 2.6. The mean CAC score in patients with a CAC score ≥ 1 was 358 ± 743. Patients with a CAC score ≥ 1 were older than those without CAC ($p < 0.001$) and the prevalence of hypertension was higher in patients with detectable CAC compared to those without ($p < 0.005$). Similarly, patients with relevant coronary calcification (CAC score ≥ 160) were older than those with non-relevant coronary calcification (68 ± 9 vs. 55 ± 16 years, $p < 0.005$), while the other clinical characteristics did not differ between the two groups.

Table 2. Demographic data and clinical characteristics according to CAC.

	All Patients (n = 109)	Without CAC (n = 38)	With CAC (n = 71)	p Value
Age (years)	58 ± 5	45 ± 17	64 ± 10	<0.001
Male gender, n (%)	53 (49)	19 (50)	37 (52)	0.83
Diabetes, n (%)	10 (9)	2 (5)	8 (11)	0.30
Hypertension, n (%)	47 (43)	9 (23)	38 (51)	<0.005
Hypercholesterolemia, n (%)	18 (17)	4 (11)	14 (20)	0.22
Smoking, n (%)	34 (31)	9 (23)	25 (35)	0.22
Family history of CAD, n (%)	18 (17)	6 (16)	15 (21)	0.50
Body mass index (kg/m^2)	26.0 ± 4.1	25.6 ± 4.5	25.6 ± 4.5	0.99

Values are expressed as mean value ± standard deviation, as number (percentage) of subjects; CAC, coronary artery calcium; CAD, coronary artery disease.

In the overall population, the mean EAT value was 99 ± 49 cm^3, and it was higher in patients with CAC than in those without (110 ± 48 cm^3 vs. 78 ± 43, $p < 0.005$). Within the limits of free breathing imaging, no focal tracer uptake on the EAT volume was observed.

Forty-five patients (41%) were treated with chemotherapy and/or radiotherapy before imaging. Of note, the ln (CAC +1) (2.8 ± 2.8 vs. 2.6 ± 2.5, $p = 0.4$) and EAT volume (102 ± 51 cm^3 vs. 97 ± 47 cm^3, $p = 0.6$) were not different between patients who underwent prior chemotherapy and/or radiotherapy and those who did not.

The findings of the univariable and multivariable linear regression analyses are depicted in Table 3. Age, body mass index (BMI), hypertension, and ln (CAC +1) were significantly associated with increasing EAT values in the univariable analysis. In the overall population, a significant relationship ($R^2 = 0.347$, $p < 0.001$) between the ln (CAC +1) and EAT volume was observed (Figure 1). However, when including clinical variables and CAC in the multivariable model, only age and BMI were independently associated with increasing EAT ($R^2 = 0.571$, $p < 0.001$).

Table 3. Linear regression analysis for prediction of increasing EAT volume in overall population.

	Univariable Analysis			Multivariable Analysis		
	SE	**ß Coefficient**	***p* Value**	**SE**	**ß Coefficient**	***p* Value**
Age	0.27	0.47	<0.001	0.32	0.45	<0.001
Male gender	9.3	−0.12	0.21			
Body mass index	0.99	0.31	<0.001	0.9	0.06	<0.001
Diabetes	16.1	0.13	0.18			
Hypertension	9.1	0.28	0.003	8.7	0.30	0.61
Hypercholesterolemia	12.4	0.17	0.70			
Smoking	10	0.14	0.14			
Family history of CAD	11.8	0.11	0.24			
Ln(CAC +1)	1.67	0.35	<0.001	1.83	0.12	0.25

EAT, epicardial adipose tissue, CAD, coronary artery disease, CAC, coronary artery calcium.

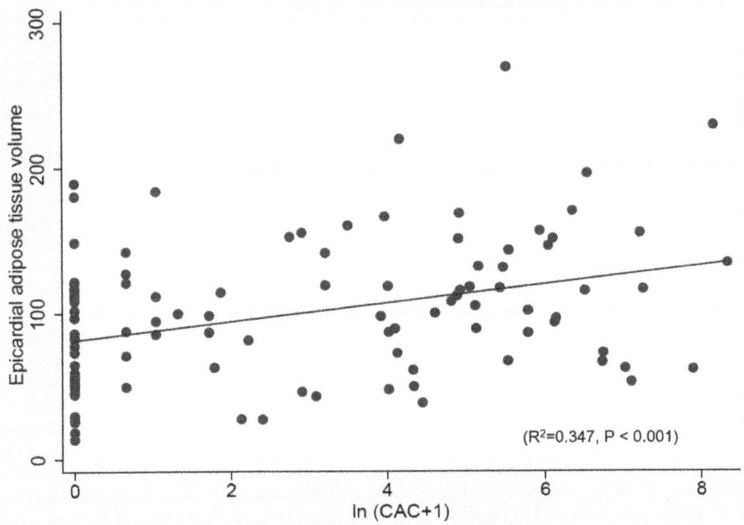

Figure 1. Correlation between epicardial adipose tissue (EAT) volume and coronary artery calcium (CAC) score.

In the univariable analysis, age ($p < 0.001$) and hypertension ($p < 0.005$) were associated with an increasing CAC score. In the multivariable model, only age was independently associated with increasing CAC ($p < 0.001$).

The examples of a 20-year-old man with a diagnosis of Hodgkin's lymphoma, with a BMI of 21.8 and without risk factors, and an 80-year-old man with a diagnosis of colorectal cancer, with a BMI of 30 and hypertension, are presented in Figures 2 and 3, respectively. As shown, in the old obese patient with hypertension, high values in the CAC score and EAT volume were measured, while in the young patient without risk factors, CAC was not detectable and the EAT volume values were negligible.

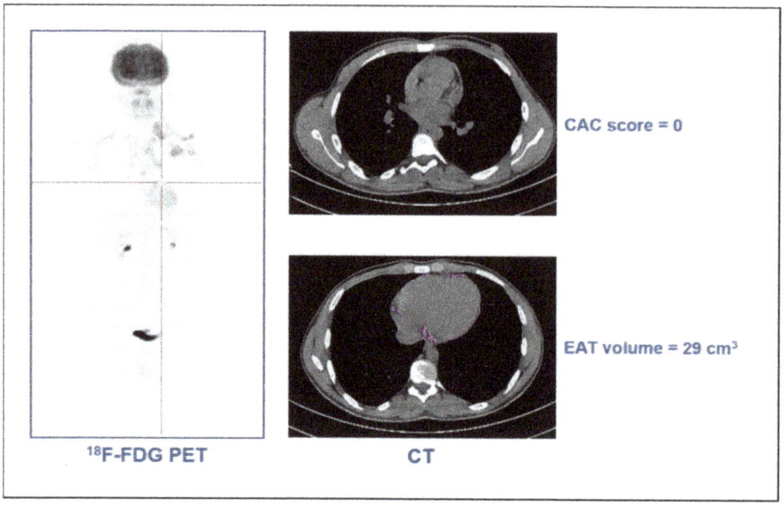

Figure 2. Case example of a 20-year-old man with Hodgkin's lymphoma.

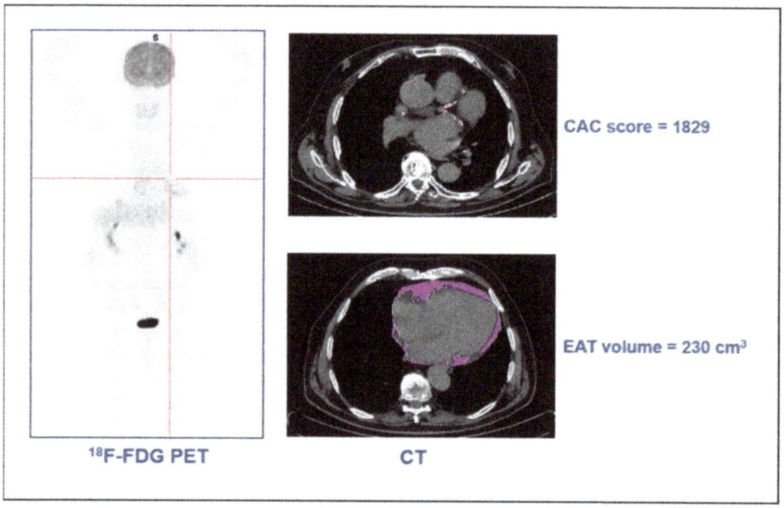

Figure 3. Case example of an 80-year-old man with colorectal cancer.

4. Discussion

The present study demonstrates for the first time the feasibility of the cost-effective evaluation of established markers of CAD, such as CAC scores and EAT, in patients without overt CAD undergoing whole-body PET–CT imaging for oncological reasons while also exploring the association of EAT volume with traditional cardiac risk factors. From an overall population of 109 patients, the majority (65%) demonstrated detectable coronary calcium. The role of CAC score measurements over cardiovascular risk factors has been established [30–32]. As expected, patients with detectable calcium burden were older than those without calcium. Starting from 50 years, age became the main cardiovascular risk factor due to the progressive accretion of atherosclerotic plaques over time [32,33]. The role of ageing in CAD development has been so widely demonstrated that novel concepts related to coronary calcium accumulation have been considered. In particular, coronary vascular age may be used as a surrogate for atherosclerotic burden [34]. Also, the higher prevalence of hypertension in patients with detectable CAC has been demonstrated [35–37]. Hence, the incorporation of CAC measurements into all non-contrast chest examinations may contribute to a significant jump forward in the early detection and treatment of CAD [29]. In our study population, age, BMI, hypertension, and CAC were associated with increasing EAT values. A significant but moderate relationship between EAT volume and CAC has been observed, with a large scattering. It is likely that a significantly larger patient cohort would have resulted in higher correlation. However, when the clinical variables and CAC were tested in a multivariable model, only age and BMI were independently associated with increasing EAT, suggesting that if on one hand there is a strong interplay between calcium burden and cardiac fat depot, on the other hand fat accumulation may have a direct link with other cardiovascular risk factors regardless of calcium load development. Therefore, even in cancer patients, the measurement of EAT volume does not seem redundant with respect to the evaluation of the CAC score for the purpose of estimating cardiovascular risk. Accordingly, our findings seem more relevant considering that EAT may contribute to the development of coronary vascular dysfunction before CAC accumulation [12]. The interplay between EAT and micro- and macro-vessel dysfunction has been demonstrated [38,39]. A recent cross-sectional study demonstrated that EAT volume was independently associated with CAC in a population of 409 patients with diabetes [40]. These latter findings are consistent with a previous investigation conducted on 127 patients that showed a significant relationship between EAT volume and diabetes, BMI, waist circumference, cholesterol, HDL-cholesterol, triglyceride levels, and the presence of metabolic syndrome [41]. On the other hand, EAT is at present attracting interest on the research ground as an early biomarker of atherosclerosis [11,40]. With regard to cancer populations, increasing EAT has recently been observed in breast cancer patients undergoing neoadjuvant chemotherapy [42]. The potential to expand cardiovascular assessment through whole-body unenhanced imaging using CT by evaluating both EAT volume and CAC scores can lead to a significant enhancement in clinical practice. This assumption should be read in light of the change in the natural history of oncological pathologies [43–45]. According to United States National Institute of Health [46], the amount of cancer survivors is expected to upsurge by 24.4%, to 22.5 million, by 2032. This trend, coupled with evidence indicating that cancer patients across all sites face an increased risk of cardiovascular death compared to the general population [3,47–53], underscores the imperative for establishing more streamlined cardiovascular care for cancer patients. This involves not only enhancing multidisciplinary collaboration among specialists including oncologists, cardiologists, and primary care physicians but also integrating diverse categories of information obtained from comprehensive imaging examinations.

The potential utility of CAC and EAT evaluation should be taken into consideration to stratify oncological patients referred to chemotherapy and/or radiotherapy at risk not only of adverse cardiovascular events for atherosclerotic development but also for cardiotoxicity [54,55]. This is even more relevant in the case of both occurrences. Furthermore, the potential to integrate CT with PET findings offers the possibility to look at metabolic data also for cardiovascular evaluation. Indeed, it has been demonstrated that an increased splenic ^{18}F-FDG uptake is associated with cardiovascular events and the proinflammatory remodeling of circulating leukocytes, suggesting the presence of a cardio-splenic axis [56].

Although different studies have proposed EAT and CAC as markers of cardiac toxicity related to oncological therapy, in our population, these parameters were not different between patients who underwent prior chemotherapy and/or radiotherapy and those who did not. However, to deeply investigate the role of chemotherapy in the onset of cardiovascular disease, EAT and CAC scores should both be tested using serial imaging in a more homogeneous population.

Certain limitations of the present study should be acknowledged. Firstly, the retrospective nature of this single-center investigation contributes to the heterogeneous enrolled population, compounded by a small sample size. Therefore, a study in a homogeneous category of patients would have strengthened the value of the investigation. It should also be considered that 41% of our patients already received chemotherapy and/or radiotherapy before the imaging test. In spite of this, when patients were tested regarding the differences in CAC and EAT volumes according to previous chemotherapy, no statistical differences were found between the groups. Patients were tested under fasting conditions that lead to fatty acid metabolism activation, and ketosis was not measured. However, to our knowledge, there are no studies testing potential EAT characteristics changes in CT images under a fasting state. In addition, the CT imaging was performed without electrocardiographic gating or triggering, and cardiac motion artifacts might have affected the evaluation of the pericardium. The occurrence of cardiovascular events has not been considered in the analysis. The inclusion of patients without documented cardiovascular diseases and the absence of prognostic data and cardiac imaging results may also impact patient management. Furthermore, a control group of patients without cancer would have provided additional data and empowered the value of the reported findings. There is clear evidence on the prognostic role of EAT and CAC in patients with cardiovascular diseases [57,58]. However, further studies linking EAT volume and CAC to cardiovascular outcomes in cancer patients are needed. Finally, other risk factors should be considered as possible explanations for increased BMIs and EAT and consequently CAC in older oncological patients. In particular, sedentary lifestyles and a lack of physical activity, which are associated with unhealthy habits and hypercaloric diets, are additional influencing factors, leading to an increase in several chronic diseases such as high blood pressure, diabetes, obesity, and cholesterol, among others.

There is still an open debate regarding the choice of the best parameter that may indicate pathological adiposity [59]. Further studies are warranted to correlate the prevalence of sedentary behavior with pathological obesity parameters including not only BMI but also waist-to-hip ratio, EAT, and CAC in oncological patients with long life expectancies. Moreover, even if age and BMI are easier to measure than EAT, patients' assessments may benefit from available data to provide a more holistic approach that looks at cancer and cardiovascular disease at a single time.

5. Conclusions

This study shows the feasibility of assessing, in a cost-effective manner, CAC scores and EAT volumes in patients referred to whole-body ^{18}F-FDG PET–CT imaging, regardless of the main clinical question. This approach may allow the evaluation, at the same time, of cancer disease and atherosclerotic burden in a single test already included in the diagnostic program of oncological patients with radiation dose optimization and without additional costs. In the present investigation, increased age, hypertension, BMIs, and CAC scores are associated with EAT in oncological patients without known CAD.

Author Contributions: Conceptualization, C.N., A.P., M.P. and A.C.; methodology, C.N. and M.P.; software, C.V. and R.L.; validation, R.G. and V.C.; formal analysis, C.G.M., R.G. and V.C.; investigation, C.N. and M.P.; resources, L.B., R.L. and C.V.; data curation, C.N., A.P., M.P., R.G. and V.C.; writing—original draft preparation, C.N., M.P. and A.C.; writing—review and editing, C.N., A.P., M.P., A.C. and M.I.; visualization, C.N., M.P. and A.C.; supervision, M.P., M.I. and A.C.; project administration, A.C. All authors have read and agreed to the published version of the manuscript.

Funding: This research received no external funding.

Institutional Review Board Statement: This study was conducted in accordance with the Declaration of Helsinki and approved by the Institutional Review Board of Federico II University (31012022).

Informed Consent Statement: Informed consent was obtained from all subjects involved in this study.

Data Availability Statement: The data presented in this study are available on request from the corresponding author. The data are not publicly available due to privacy restrictions.

Conflicts of Interest: All authors declare that the research was conducted in the absence of any commercial or financial relationships that could be construed as a potential conflict of interest.

References

1. Siegel, R.L.; Miller, K.D.; Fuchs, H.E.; Jemal, A. Cancer statistics, 2022. *CA Cancer J. Clin.* **2022**, *72*, 7–33. [CrossRef]
2. Martin, S.S.; Aday, A.W.; Almarzooq, Z.I.; Anderson, C.A.M.; Arora, P.; Avery, C.L.; Baker-Smith, C.M.; Barone Gibbs, B.; Beaton, A.Z.; Boehme, A.K.; et al. 2024 Heart Disease and Stroke Statistics: A Report of US and Global Data From the American Heart Association. *Circulation* **2024**, *149*, 8. [CrossRef]
3. Velusamy, R.; Nolan, M.; Murphy, A.; Thavendiranathan, P.; Marwick, T.H. Screening for Coronary Artery Disease in Cancer Survivors. *JACC CardioOncology* **2023**, *5*, 22–38. [CrossRef]
4. Megna, R.; Petretta, M.; Nappi, C.; Assante, R.; Zampella, E.; Gaudieri, V.; Mannarino, T.; D'Antonio, A.; Green, R.; Cantoni, V.; et al. Age-Specific Cardiovascular Risk Factors for Major Adverse Cardiac Events in Patients Undergoing Myocardial Perfusion Imaging. *J. Cardiovasc. Dev. Dis.* **2023**, *10*, 395. [CrossRef]
5. O'Sullivan, J.W.; Ashley, E.A.; Elliott, P.M. Polygenic risk scores for the prediction of cardiometabolic disease. *Eur. Heart J.* **2023**, *44*, 89–99. [CrossRef]
6. Mensah, G.A.; Brown, D.W.; Croft, J.B.; Greenlund, K.J. Major Coronary Risk Factors and Death from Coronary Heart Disease. *Am. J. Prev. Med.* **2005**, *29*, 68–74. [CrossRef]
7. Budoff, M.J.; Young, R.; Burke, G.; Jeffrey Carr, J.; Detrano, R.C.; Folsom, A.R.; Kronmal, R.; Lima, J.A.C.; Liu, K.J.; McClelland, R.L.; et al. Ten-year association of coronary artery calcium with atherosclerotic cardiovascular disease (ASCVD) events: The multi-ethnic study of atherosclerosis (MESA). *Eur. Heart J.* **2018**, *39*, 2401–2408. [CrossRef]
8. Arad, Y.; Goodman, K.J.; Roth, M.; Newstein, D.; Guerci, A.D. Coronary calcification, coronary disease risk factors, C-reactive protein, and atherosclerotic cardiovascular disease events: The St. Francis Heart Study. *J. Am. Coll. Cardiol.* **2005**, *46*, 158–165. [CrossRef]
9. Lyon, A.R.; López-Fernández, T.; Couch, L.S.; Asteggiano, R.; Aznar, M.C.; Bergler-Klein, J.; Boriani, G.; Cardinale, D.; Cordoba, R.; Cosyns, B.; et al. 2022 ESC Guidelines on cardio-oncology developed in collaboration with the European Hematology Association (EHA), the European Society for Therapeutic Radiology and Oncology (ESTRO) and the International Cardio-Oncology Society (IC-OS). *Eur. Heart J.* **2022**, *43*, 4229–4361. [CrossRef]
10. Bell, K.J.L.; White, S.; Hassan, O.; Zhu, L.; Scott, A.M.; Clark, J.; Glasziou, P. Evaluation of the Incremental Value of a Coronary Artery Calcium Score Beyond Traditional Cardiovascular Risk Assessment: A Systematic Review and Meta-analysis. *JAMA Intern Med.* **2022**, *182*, 634–642. [CrossRef]
11. Iacobellis, G. Epicardial adipose tissue in contemporary cardiology. *Nat. Rev. Cardiol.* **2022**, *19*, 593–606. [CrossRef]
12. Nappi, C.; Ponsiglione, A.; Acampa, W.; Gaudieri, V.; Zampella, E.; Assante, R.; Cuocolo, R.; Mannarino, T.; Dell'Aversana, S.; Petretta, M.; et al. Relationship between epicardial adipose tissue and coronary vascular function in patients with suspected coronary artery disease and normal myocardial perfusion imaging. *Eur. Heart J. Cardiovasc. Imaging* **2019**, *20*, 1379–1387. [CrossRef]
13. Miller, R.J.H.; Shanbhag, A.; Killekar, A.; Lemley, M.; Bednarski, B.; Van Kriekinge, S.D.; Kavanagh, P.B.; Feher, A.; Miller, E.J.; Einstein, A.J.; et al. AI-derived epicardial fat measurements improve cardiovascular risk prediction from myocardial perfusion imaging. *NPJ Digit. Med.* **2024**, *7*, 24. [CrossRef]
14. Nappi, C.; Megna, R.; Volpe, F.; Ponsiglione, A.; Caiazzo, E.; Piscopo, L.; Mainolfi, C.G.; Vergara, E.; Imbriaco, M.; Klain, M.; et al. Quantification of Coronary Artery Atherosclerotic Burden and Muscle Mass: Exploratory Comparison of Two Freely Available Software Programs. *Appl. Sci.* **2022**, *12*, 5468. [CrossRef]
15. Si, N.; Shi, K.; Li, N.; Dong, X.; Zhu, C.; Guo, Y.; Hu, J.; Cui, J.; Yang, F.; Zhang, T. Identification of patients with acute myocardial infarction based on coronary CT angiography: The value of pericoronary adipose tissue radiomics. *Eur. Radiol.* **2022**, *32*, 6868–6877. [CrossRef]
16. Lee, K.C.; Yong, H.S.; Lee, J.; Kang, E.Y.; Na, J.O. Is the epicardial adipose tissue area on non-ECG gated low-dose chest CT useful for predicting coronary atherosclerosis in an asymptomatic population considered for lung cancer screening? *Eur. Radiol.* **2019**, *29*, 932–940. [CrossRef]
17. Monti, C.B.; Schiaffino, S.; Galimberti Ortiz, M.D.M.; Capra, D.; Zanardo, M.; De Benedictis, E.; Luporini, A.G.; Spagnolo, P.; Secchi, F.; Sardanelli, F. Potential role of epicardial adipose tissue as a biomarker of anthracycline cardiotoxicity. *Insights Imaging* **2021**, *12*, 161. [CrossRef]
18. Esposito, F.; Mezzanotte, V.; Tesei, C.; Luciano, A.; Gigliotti, P.E.; Nunzi, A.; Secchi, R.; Angeloni, C.; Pitaro, M.; Meconi, F.; et al. CT Images in Follicular Lymphoma: Changes after Treatment Are Predictive of Cardiac Toxicity in Patients Treated with Anthracycline-Based or R-B Regimens. *Cancers* **2024**, *16*, 563. [CrossRef]
19. Figtree, G.A.; Vernon, S.T.; Hadziosmanovic, N.; Sundström, J.; Alfredsson, J.; Arnott, C.; Delatour, V.; Leósdóttir, M.; Hagström, E. Mortality in STEMI patients without standard modifiable risk factors: A sex-disaggregated analysis of SWEDEHEART registry data. *Lancet* **2021**, *397*, 1085–1094. [CrossRef]
20. Williams, B.; Mancia, G.; Spiering, W.; Agabiti Rosei, E.; Azizi, M.; Burnier, M.; Clement, D.L.; Coca, A.; de Simone, G.; Dominiczak, A.; et al. 2018 ESC/ESH Guidelines for the management of arterial hypertension. *Eur. Heart J.* **2018**, *39*, 3021–3104. [CrossRef]
21. Scheuner, M.T.; Whitworth, W.C.; McGruder, H.; Yoon, P.W.; Khoury, M.J. Expanding the definition of a positive family history for early-onset coronary heart disease. *Genet. Med.* **2006**, *8*, 491–501. [CrossRef]

22. Gibbons, R.J.; Balady, G.J.; Bricker, J.T.; Chaitman, B.R.; Fletcher, G.F.; Froelicher, V.F.; Mark, D.B.; McCallister, B.D.; Mooss, A.N.; O'Reilly, M.G.; et al. ACC/AHA 2002 guideline update for exercise testing: Summary article. *J. Am. Coll. Cardiol.* **2002**, *40*, 1531–1540. [CrossRef]
23. Boellaard, R.; Delgado-Bolton, R.; Oyen, W.J.; Giammarile, F.; Tatsch, K.; Eschner, W.; Verzijlbergen, F.J.; Barrington, S.F.; Pike, L.C.; Weber, W.A.; et al. FDG PET/CT: EANM procedure guidelines for tumour imaging: Version 2.0. *Eur. J. Nucl. Med. Mol. Imaging* **2015**, *42*, 328–354. [CrossRef]
24. Petranović Ovčariček, P.; Giovanella, L.; Carrió Gasset, I.; Hindié, E.; Huellner, M.W.; Luster, M.; Piccardo, A.; Weber, T.; Talbot, J.N.; Verburg, F.A. The EANM practice guidelines for parathyroid imaging. *Eur. J. Nucl. Med. Mol. Imaging* **2021**, *48*, 2801–2822. [CrossRef]
25. Megna, R.; Petretta, M.; Assante, R.; Zampella, E.; Nappi, C.; Gaudieri, V.; Mannarino, T.; D'Antonio, A.; Green, R.; Cantoni, V.; et al. A Comparison among Different Machine Learning Pretest Approaches to Predict Stress-Induced Ischemia at PET/CT Myocardial Perfusion Imaging. *Comput. Math. Methods Med.* **2021**, *2021*, 3551756. [CrossRef]
26. Agatston, A.S.; Janowitz, W.R.; Hildner, F.J.; Zusmer, N.R.; Viamonte, M.; Detrano, R. Quantification of coronary artery calcium using ultrafast computed tomography. *J. Am. Coll. Cardiol.* **1990**, *15*, 827–832. [CrossRef]
27. Yoshizumi, T.; Nakamura, T.; Yamane, M.; Islam, A.H.; Menju, M.; Yamasaki, K.; Arai, T.; Kotani, K.; Funahashi, T.; Yamashita, S.; et al. Abdominal Fat: Standardized Technique for Measurement at CT. *Radiology* **1999**, *211*, 283–286. [CrossRef]
28. Nardone, O.M.; Ponsiglione, A.; de Sire, R.; Calabrese, G.; Liuzzi, R.; Testa, A.; Guarino, A.D.; Olmo, O.; Rispo, A.; Camera, L.; et al. Impact of Sarcopenia on Clinical Outcomes in a Cohort of Caucasian Active Crohn's Disease Patients Undergoing Multidetector CT-Enterography. *Nutrients* **2022**, *14*, 3460. [CrossRef]
29. Wang, T.D.; Lee, W.J.; Shih, F.Y.; Huang, C.H.; Chang, Y.C.; Chen, W.J.; Lee, Y.T.; Chen, M.F. Relations of Epicardial Adipose Tissue Measured by Multidetector Computed Tomography to Components of the Metabolic Syndrome Are Region-Specific and Independent of Anthropometric Indexes and Intraabdominal Visceral Fat. *J. Clin. Endocrinol. Metab.* **2009**, *94*, 662–669. [CrossRef]
30. Boccalini, S.; Teulade, M.; Paquet, E.; Si-Mohamed, S.; Rapallo, F.; Moreau-Triby, C.; Charrière, S.; Mewton, N.; Boussel, L.; Bergerot, C.; et al. Silent myocardial infarction fatty scars detected by coronary calcium score CT scan in diabetic patients without history of coronary heart disease. *Eur. Radiol.* **2024**, *34*, 214–225. [CrossRef]
31. Greenland, P.; LaBree, L.; Azen, S.P.; Doherty, T.M.; Detrano, R.C. Coronary Artery Calcium Score Combined With Framingham Score for Risk Prediction in Asymptomatic Individuals. *JAMA* **2004**, *291*, 210–215. [CrossRef]
32. Acquah, I.; Cainzos-Achirica, M.; Taha, M.B.; Lahan, S.; Blaha, M.J.; Al-Kindi, S.G.; Khan, S.U.; Sharma, G.; Budoff, M.J.; Nasir, K. Social disadvantage, coronary artery calcium, and their interplay in the prediction of atherosclerotic cardiovascular disease events. *Atherosclerosis* **2024**, *388*, 117355. [CrossRef]
33. McClelland, R.L.; Nasir, K.; Budoff, M.; Blumenthal, R.S.; Kronmal, R.A. Arterial Age as a Function of Coronary Artery Calcium (from the Multi-Ethnic Study of Atherosclerosis [MESA]). *Am. J. Cardiol.* **2009**, *103*, 59–63. [CrossRef]
34. Nappi, C.; Gaudieri, V.; Acampa, W.; Arumugam, P.; Assante, R.; Zampella, E.; Mannarino, T.; Mainolfi, C.G.; Imbriaco, M.; Petretta, M.; et al. Coronary vascular age: An alternate means for predicting stress-induced myocardial ischemia in patients with suspected coronary artery disease. *J. Nucl. Cardiol.* **2019**, *26*, 1348–1355. [CrossRef]
35. Jensen, S.M.; Prescott, E.I.B.; Abdulla, J. The prognostic value of coronary flow reserve in patients with non-obstructive coronary artery disease and microvascular dysfunction: A systematic review and meta-analysis with focus on imaging modality and sex difference. *Int. J. Cardiovasc. Imaging* **2023**, *39*, 2545–2556. [CrossRef]
36. Ahmed, A.I.; Saad, J.M.; Han, Y.; Malahfji, M.; Al-Mallah, M.H. Incremental prognostic value of positron emission tomography derived left ventricular mass. *J. Nucl. Cardiol.* **2023**, *30*, 254–263. [CrossRef]
37. Akşit, E.; Kırılmaz, B.; Özdemir, S. The importance of myocardial perfusion imaging in patients with ischemia and nonobstructive coronary arteries. *J. Nucl. Cardiol.* **2023**, *33*, 101791. [CrossRef]
38. Bakkum, M.J.; Danad, I.; Romijn, M.A.; Stuijfzand, W.J.; Leonora, R.M.; Tulevski, I.I.; Somsen, G.A.; Lammertsma, A.A.; van Kuijk, C.; van Rossum, A.C.; et al. The impact of obesity on the relationship between epicardial adipose tissue, left ventricular mass and coronary microvascular function. *Eur. J. Nucl. Med. Mol. Imaging* **2015**, *42*, 1562–1573. [CrossRef]
39. Nerlekar, N.; Muthalaly, R.G.; Wong, N.; Thakur, U.; Wong, D.T.L.; Brown, A.J.; Marwick, T.H. Association of Volumetric Epicardial Adipose Tissue Quantification and Cardiac Structure and Function. *J. Am. Heart Assoc.* **2018**, *7*, e009975. [CrossRef]
40. Cosson, E.; Nguyen, M.T.; Rezgani, I.; Berkane, N.; Pinto, S.; Bihan, H.; Tatulashvili, S.; Taher, M.; Sal, M.; Soussan, M.; et al. Epicardial adipose tissue volume and myocardial ischemia in asymptomatic people living with diabetes: A cross-sectional study. *Cardiovasc. Diabetol.* **2021**, *20*, 224. [CrossRef]
41. Wang, C.P.; Hsu, H.L.; Hung, W.C.; Yu, T.H.; Chen, Y.H.; Chiu, C.A.; Lu, L.F.; Chung, F.M.; Shin, S.J.; Lee, Y.J. Increased epicardial adipose tissue (EAT) volume in type 2 diabetes mellitus and association with metabolic syndrome and severity of coronary atherosclerosis. *Clin. Endocrinol.* **2009**, *70*, 876–882. [CrossRef]
42. Wang, X.; Tan, Y.; Liu, D.; Shen, H.; Deng, Y.; Tan, Y.; Wang, L.; Zhang, Y.; Ma, X.; Zeng, X.; et al. Chemotherapy-associated steatohepatitis was concomitant with epicardial adipose tissue volume increasing in breast cancer patients who received neoadjuvant chemotherapy. *Eur. Radiol.* **2022**, *32*, 4898–4908. [CrossRef]
43. Verdecchia, A.; Guzzinati, S.; Francisci, S.; De Angelis, R.; Bray, F.; Allemani, C.; Tavilla, A.; Santaquilani, M.; Sant, M. Survival trends in European cancer patients diagnosed from 1988 to 1999. *Eur. J. Cancer* **2009**, *45*, 1042–1066. [CrossRef]

44. Herrmann, J.; Lerman, A.; Sandhu, N.P.; Villarraga, H.R.; Mulvagh, S.L.; Kohli, M. Evaluation and Management of Patients With Heart Disease and Cancer: Cardio-Oncology. *Mayo Clin. Proc.* **2014**, *89*, 1287–1306. [CrossRef]
45. Abbema, D.V.; Vissers, P.; de Vos-Geelen, J.; Lemmens, V.; Janssen-Heijnen, M.; Tjan-Heijnen, V. Trends in Overall Survival and Treatment Patterns in Two Large Population-Based Cohorts of Patients with Breast and Colorectal Cancer. *Cancers* **2019**, *11*, 1239. [CrossRef]
46. Available online: https://cancercontrol.cancer.gov/ocs/statistics (accessed on 15 February 2024).
47. Choi, D.; Choi, S.; Kim, K.H.; Kim, K.; Chang, J.; Kim, S.M.; Kim, S.R.; Cho, Y.; Lee, G.; Son, J.S.; et al. Combined Associations of Physical Activity and Particulate Matter With Subsequent Cardiovascular Disease Risk Among 5-Year Cancer Survivors. *J. Am. Heart Assoc.* **2022**, *11*, e022806. [CrossRef]
48. Yang, L.; Zhang, N.; Yue, Q.; Song, W.; Zheng, Y.; Huang, S.; Qiu, J.; Tse, G.; Li, G.; Wu, S.; et al. Long-Term Atherosclerotic Cardiovascular Disease Risk in Patients With Cancer: A Population-Based Study. *Curr. Probl. Cardiol.* **2023**, *48*, 101693. [CrossRef]
49. Raisi-Estabragh, Z.; Kobo, O.; Freeman, P.; Petersen, S.E.; Kolman, L.; Miller, R.J.H.; Roguin, A.; Van Spall, H.G.C.; Vuong, J.; Yang, E.H.; et al. Temporal trends in disease-specific causes of cardiovascular mortality amongst patients with cancer in the USA between 1999 and 2019. *Eur. Heart J. Qual. Care Clin. Outcomes* **2022**, *9*, 54–63. [CrossRef]
50. Sturgeon, K.M.; Deng, L.; Bluethmann, S.M.; Zhou, S.; Trifiletti, D.M.; Jiang, C.; Kelly, S.P.; Zaorsky, N.G. A population-based study of cardiovascular disease mortality risk in US cancer patients. *Eur. Heart J.* **2019**, *40*, 3889–3897. [CrossRef]
51. Zhang, S.; Liu, L.; Shi, S.; He, H.; Shen, Q.; Wang, H.; Qin, S.; Chang, J.; Zhong, R. Bidirectional Association Between Cardiovascular Disease and Lung Cancer in a Prospective Cohort Study. *J. Thorac. Oncol.* **2024**, *19*, 80–93. [CrossRef]
52. Barish, R.; Lynce, F.; Unger, K.; Barac, A. Management of Cardiovascular Disease in Women With Breast Cancer. *Circulation* **2019**, *139*, 1110–1120. [CrossRef]
53. Melson, J.W.; Koethe, B.; Mohanty, S.; Babroudi, S.; Bao, C.; Chunduru, A.; Dwaah, H.; Finn, M.; Jain, A.; Lalla, M.; et al. Atherosclerotic Cardiovascular Disease Risk and Longitudinal Risk Factor Management Among Patients With Breast Cancer. *Clin. Breast Cancer* **2024**, *24*, e71–e79.e4. [CrossRef]
54. El-Sabbagh, A.; Osman, M.M.; Fesler, M.; Helmy, T.; Parker, N.; Muzaffar, R. Chemotherapy-induced coronary arteries calcium score deterioration as detected with unenhanced CT portion of FDG PET/CT. *Am. J. Nucl. Med. Mol. Imaging* **2018**, *8*, 303–310.
55. Shen, H.; Lian, Y.; Yin, J.; Zhu, M.; Yang, C.; Tu, C.; Peng, Y.; Li, X.; Zhang, J. Cardiovascular Risk Stratification by Automatic Coronary Artery Calcium Scoring on Pretreatment Chest Computed Tomography in Diffuse Large B-Cell Lymphoma Receiving Anthracycline-Based Chemotherapy: A Multicenter Study. *Circ. Cardiovasc. Imaging* **2023**, *16*, e014829. [CrossRef]
56. Emami, H.; Singh, P.; MacNabb, M.; Vucic, E.; Lavender, Z.; Rudd, J.H.; Fayad, Z.A.; Lehrer-Graiwer, J.; Korsgren, M.; Figueroa, A.L.; et al. Splenic metabolic activity predicts risk of future cardiovascular events: Demonstration of a cardiosplenic axis in humans. *JACC Cardiovasc. Imaging* **2015**, *8*, 121–130. [CrossRef]
57. Rämö, J.T.; Kany, S.; Hou, C.R.; Friedman, S.F.; Roselli, C.; Nauffal, V.; Koyama, S.; Karjalainen, J.; Maddah, M.; Palotie, A.; et al. Cardiovascular Significance and Genetics of Epicardial and Pericardial Adiposity. *JAMA Cardiol.* **2024**, *9*, 418–427. [CrossRef]
58. Sarwar, A.; Shaw, L.J.; Shapiro, M.D.; Blankstein, R.; Hoffman, U.; Cury, R.C.; Abbara, S.; Brady, T.J.; Budoff, M.J.; Blumenthal, R.S.; et al. Diagnostic and prognostic value of absence of coronary artery calcification. *JACC Cardiovasc. Imaging* **2009**, *2*, 675–688. [CrossRef]
59. Hashemy, H.; Nguyen, A.; Khafagy, R.; Roshandel, D.; Paterson, A.D.; Dash, S. Analyses of potential causal contributors to increased waist/hip ratio-associated cardiometabolic disease: A combined and sex-stratified Mendelian randomization study. *Diabetes Obes. Metab.* **2024**, *26*, 2284–2291. [CrossRef]

Journal of
Cardiovascular Development and Disease

MDPI

Communication

Mixed Reality (Holography)-Guided Minimally Invasive Cardiac Surgery—A Novel Comparative Feasibility Study †

Winn Maung Maung Aye [1,2,3,*], Laszlo Kiraly [1,2,3,4], Senthil S. Kumar [1], Ayyadarshan Kasivishvanaath [2], Yujia Gao [3] and Theodoros Kofidis [1,2,3]

1 Department of Cardiac, Thoracic and Vascular Surgery, Division of Congenital Cardiac Surgery, National University Hospital, National University Health System, Singapore 119228, Singapore; kiraly_laszlo@nuhs.edu.sg (L.K.); senthil_kumar_subbian@nuhs.edu.sg (S.S.K.); surtk@nus.edu.sg (T.K.)
2 Yong Loo Lin School of Medicine, National University of Singapore, Singapore 117597, Singapore; ayyadarshan.kasivishvanaath@mohh.com.sg
3 Department of Surgery, National University Hospital, National University Health System, Singapore 119228, Singapore; yujiagao@nuhs.edu.sg
4 Department of Public Health, Semmelweis University, 1085 Budapest, Hungary
* Correspondence: surwmma@nus.edu.sg; Tel.: +65-96550490
† This abstract was presented at the Virtual Meeting—The 30th Annual Meeting of the Asian Society for Cardiovascular and Thoracic Surgery (ASCVTS 2022)—Plenary 2, C-PL2-7, Nara, Japan, 25 March 2022.

Abstract: The operative field and exposure in minimally invasive cardiac surgery (MICS) are limited. Meticulous preoperative planning and intraoperative visualization are crucial. We present our initial experience with HoloLens® 2 as an intraoperative guide during MICS procedures: aortic valve replacement (AVR) via right anterior small thoracotomy, coronary artery bypass graft surgery (CABG) via left anterior small thoracotomy (LAST), and pulmonary valve replacement (PVR) via LAST. Three-dimensional (3D) segmentations were performed using the patient's computer tomography (CT) data subsequently rendered into a 3D hologram on the HoloLens® 2. The holographic image was then superimposed on the patient lying on the operating table, using the xiphoid and the clavicle as landmarks, and was used as a real-time anatomical image guide for the surgery. The incision site marking made using HoloLens® 2 differed by one intercostal space from the marking made using a conventional surgeon's mental reconstructed image from the patient's preoperative imaging and was found to be a more appropriate site of entry into the chest for the structure of interest. The transparent visor of the HoloLens® 2 provided unobstructed views of the operating field. A mixed reality (MR) device could contribute to preoperative surgical planning and intraoperative real-time image guidance, which facilitates the understanding of anatomical relationships. MR has the potential to improve surgical precision, decrease risk, and enhance patient safety.

Keywords: minimally invasive cardiac surgery; mixed reality; virtual reality; augmented reality; 3-dimensional holographic image; HoloLens® 2

1. Introduction

Unlike the abdominal wall, the chest wall is rigid and does not allow changes in the visual angle. The path of access to the three-dimensional (3D) target structures is deep, and the angle is fixed and restricted [1]. Appropriate incision and exposure to allow adequate visibility and access are of paramount importance in MICS [1,2]. Meticulous preoperative planning, especially determining the site of entry into the chest, and real-time intraoperative image guidance are necessary for successful surgery [3,4]. The main aim of the minimal invasive surgery (MIS) approach is to reduce collateral tissue damage and morbidity without risking the completeness of the intended surgical repair [1,2]. Possible advantages of MIS include faster and better postoperative mobilization, independence, fewer infections, less blood loss and need for transfusion, less trauma, less re-exploration, less postoperative lactate, and fewer arrhythmias [2]. Current preoperative imaging, e.g., 2/3D echocardiography, computer tomography angiography (CTA), and magnetic resonance imaging (MRI), display 2D or reconstructed 3D images, typically on a flat 2D screen, requiring the surgeon to create a mental model and apply it onto the patient's real anatomy during surgical planning and/or in surgery [1,5]. As spatial intelligence is variable, it may be difficult for individual surgeons to establish the 3D spatial relationship and correct depth perception of the patient's anatomy using preoperative imaging and their mental model [3].

This cognitive problem can be overcome by using HoloLens® 2 (Microsoft Corporation, Redmond, WA, USA), a head-mounted mixed-reality (MR) holographic device [6–8] (Figure 1a,b). It provides an immersive experience by superimposing a holographic 3D-rendered model onto the patient's anatomy [3,9] (Figure 2). Furthermore, the surgeon's line-in-sight is maintained throughout the procedure so that the operator is not distracted by another screen [9,10].

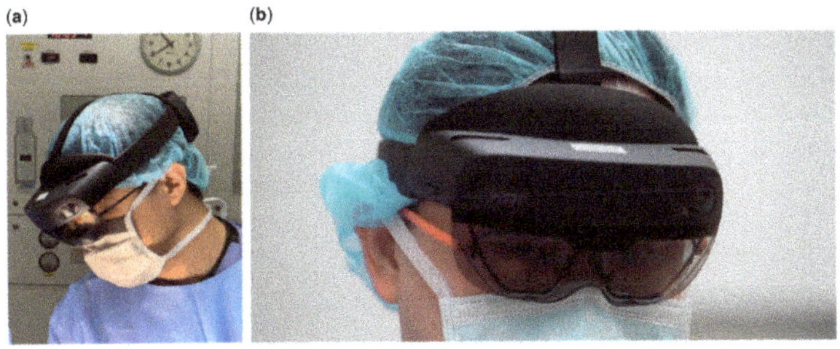

Figure 1. Surgeon wearing HoloLens® 2: (**a**) Looking at the patient on operating table; (**b**) looking through the clear visor onto the hologram.

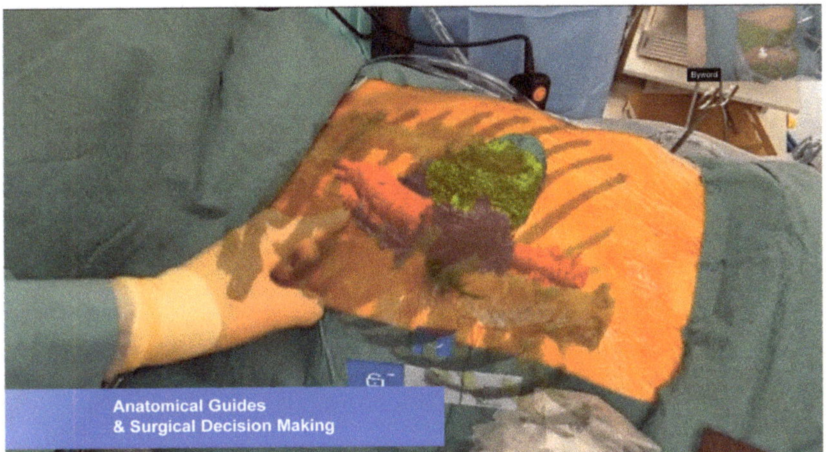

Figure 2. HoloLens® 2-guided minimally invasive surgery for aortic valve replacement.

In virtual reality (VR), the real environment is replaced by a virtual one, whereas augmented reality (AR) overlays virtual objects in the real, physical environment without the user being able to interact with them. Pokémon Go is a prime example of AR [4]. Mixed reality (MR) combines VR and AR [3,4,10,11], allowing surgeons to have simultaneous interactions with the virtual and physical world by superimposing holographic 3D images onto the operative field; thus, MR increases the user's experience of depth and perception [4,10].

Using HoloLens® 2, the patient's own virtual holographic model of the heart is anchored by selected landmarks on the thoracic wall, and the model is projected inside the chest cavity [4]. The main advantage of holograms placed inside the operative field is that surgeons have a better appreciation of the vector and magnitude of movement required [9]. HoloLens® 2 guides the surgeon to locate the most appropriate site of incision and auxiliary ports so that optimal visibility of and access to the operative field can be achieved [3].

To date, there are no reports in the MICS literature describing the use of HoloLens® 2 for improving surgical access. We present—to the best of our knowledge—a novel comparative study of three MICS procedures using HoloLens® 2 for preoperative planning and for real-time intraoperative guidance [9].

2. Materials and Methods

2.1. Computed Tomography Angiography (CTA)

A third-generation dual-source 2 × 192-slice scanner (SOMATOM Force, Siemens Healthcare, Forchheim, Germany), and the images are obtained using a prospectively ECG-triggered high-pitch spiral mode (Turbo Flash, 2 × 192 × 0.6 mm detector collimation, Siemens Healthcare) [9]. The slice thickness is based on detector collimation, which is 0.6 mm. The CT protocol was designed by radiologists and radiographers in consultation with the equipment vendor.

The images were then uploaded onto the HoloLens® 2 system to be rendered into a 3D holographic model [6].

2.2. Hologram Creation

Consent for photography or videography was obtained from each patient in accordance with institutional guidelines. CTA DICOM data were extracted from CT scans. Segmentation and alignment of the images were performed. These images were exported as a DICOM standard dataset, which was then uploaded onto HoloLens® 2 via Virtual Surgery Intelligence software version 1.5 (apoQlar GmbH, Hamburg, Germany) that generated the reference cardiothoracic hologram [9]. Additionally, segmentation of individual structures within the raw scan images was performed using 3D Slicer (The Slicer Community, www.slicer.org, v4.11.20210226) via manual segmentation to identify the individual cardiac chambers, valves, coronary arteries, and internal mammary arteries. The segmented images were exported as standard tessellation language (STL) files onto virtual surgery intelligence (VSI) and used for image superimposition and visualization [9]. The entire process of hologram creation took approximately 3 h. It was reviewed by the surgical team preoperatively.

2.3. Surgical Procedures

The patient was positioned on the operating table, and the surgeon marked the preferred site of entry employing conventional anatomical landmarks and their mental model. Then, they superimposed the reconstructed patient's cardiac hologram onto the chest using the xiphoid and the clavicle as reference landmarks for a real-time anatomical assessment. This enabled the surgeon to look "into" the chest organ topography in their line-in-sight [10]. The best incision site was again marked. In addition, insertion points of surgical instruments and accessories were chosen in reference to the intended incision site marked using HoloLens® 2. Assessment with the hologram also enabled anticipation of difficulties and to foresee any possible spatial confinement.

The technicalities of superimposing the 3D-rendered image on the operative field were initially challenging. They required the surgeon to virtually hold the holographic image in mid-air and place it onto the patient's chest using the landmarks as accurately as possible [3,10]. Surgeons had preoperative training sessions of approximately 20 min and quickly familiarized themselves with the movements of the holographic imagery [10].

The first procedure was an MIS aortic valve replacement (AVR) via right anterior small thoracotomy using a totally endoscopic technique (Figure 2). Using HoloLens® 2, a holographic image was superimposed onto the actual patient's chest. The position of the aorta and aortic valve annulus were visualized. With this guidance, the incision was made, and the chest was entered via the second intercostal space. The AVR was performed in the usual manner.

The second procedure was an MIS off-pump coronary artery bypass graft surgery (CABG) via left anterior small thoracotomy (LAST). A similar process was performed. The fixed holographic 3D image guided the best way for the surgeon to access the most appropriate intercostal space and to plan the entry into the chest cavity. It also facilitated decision-making over the placement of bypass grafts and projected the degree of difficulties of exposure.

The 3rd case was an MIS pulmonary valve replacement (PVR) (Figure 3). PVR following repair of Tetralogy of Fallot in childhood is conventionally carried out via redo-median sternotomy. In order to avoid redo-median sternotomy, PVR was planned via LAST. Three-dimensional superimposed holographic visualization adequately projected the position of the main pulmonary artery (MPA) and pulmonary valve annulus (PVA) and guided the most appropriate intercostal space to enter the chest.

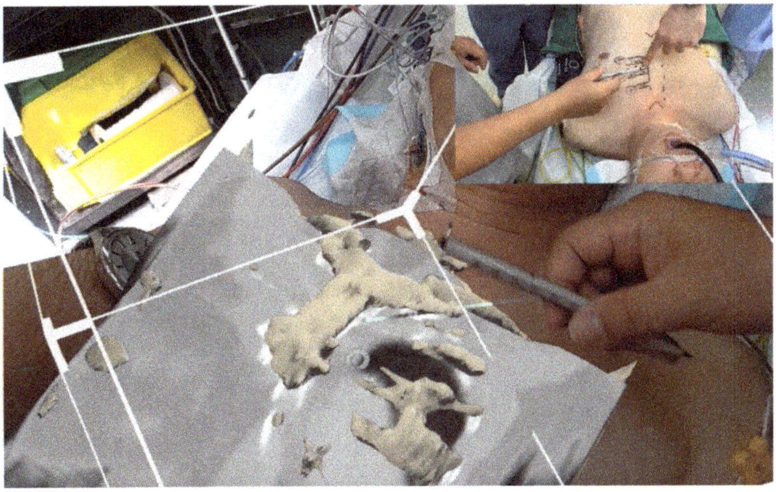

Figure 3. HoloLens® 2 guided minimally invasive surgery for pulmonary valve replacement.

3. Results

Approximately 3 hours of preoperative worktime was required to create a 3D holographic image to be viewed on the device. Production was performed by a different in-house team.

The xiphoid process and the clavicle provided consistent reference points to lock the hologram on the patient's chest, ensuring accurate placement. Hologram superimposition and fine adjustments were straightforward as surgeons had had prior training and were familiar with the technicalities. The OR time taken for the process was less than 10 min from mounting the device on the surgeon's head to marking the incision site. Dictated by the structures of interest, the most accurate and smallest, incision site could be selected.

In all three cases, the incision site marked with and without the HoloLens® 2 differed by one intercostal space. HoloLens® 2 provided more appropriate access to the operating field: one intercostal space cranial in MIS AVR and MIS PVR and one intercostal space caudal in MIS CABG. The endoscopic tool distribution (camera insertion, left ventricular vent, and their relation to the structures of interest/chest wall) could be better appreciated and/or planned. HoloLens® 2 references were found to be more suitable than the markings based on the surgeon's interpretation of the structures of interest from preoperative imaging. The transparent visor of the HoloLens® 2 allowed unobstructed views of the operating field. The operative time in 3 MIS cardiac surgical procedures described, with the use of HoloLens 2, was reduced by a mean duration of 34.3 ± 3.2 min. This could be attributed to the entry site being the most accurate without requiring change during the procedure, which can be time-consuming. A survey was also conducted to determine the level of user acceptability for MR devices in surgery. This survey was conducted in 2022, with 30 surgeons who had trialed the solution. Survey feedback was collected using a validated User Evaluation Questionnaire (UEQ), that uses a 26 point matrix to compare the new solution with existing devices. The survey results showed overwhelming positive response to the use of MR in surgery, as shown in Suppelementary File S2.

In this work, the study presented in [12] is expanded upon.

4. Discussion

The concept of holographic visualization and the necessary technology have existed for many decades [13,14]. The use of this technology in the medical field has been delayed by the bulky nature of the devices [3,13] and the inability to view high-quality images [3]. Microsoft HoloLens® 2, a head-mounted MR holographic device, was first made commercially available in 2016 [3] and is currently widely used in various medical and surgical subspecialties. MR technology, interconnected with both VR and AR, allows the user to interact with virtual reality in reality. MR has been applied in numerous medical [15–20] and surgical specialties, e.g., orthopedic surgery [21], neurosurgery [22], urology [23], general surgery [24], etc. Advantages have been demonstrated in both educational and clinical settings to help medical professionals better understand complex anatomical structures, so the modality is available for preoperative surgical planning and intraoperative guidance [25–27]. VR and 3D-printed heart models were also found to be superior for diagnostic assessment, medical education, and preoperative planning in comparison with conventional visualization techniques [28].

4.1. Benefits

MR devices offer multiple presumed benefits in MICS intraoperative visualization [10,29,30]. The patient's own 3D holographic model superimposed on the actual anatomy ascertains spatial anatomy. The hologram can be adjusted and rendered to anatomical landmarks in real time [9]. All this contributes to incisional precision and accuracy of access to the target structures [31,32]. In fact, in each of our presented cases, HoloLens® 2's superimposed model recommended a different intercostal space for chest entry from the one assumed by the surgeon's mental model. Modification of chest entry by one intercostal space can achieve a significantly better visualization of the structures of interest in a confined operating space in minimally invasive cardiac surgery. The superiority of HoloLens® 2 can be attributed to the fact that holograms not only revealed the appropriate depth and relationships but also the angulation and vector orientation of optimal access.

Furthermore, holographic models propose an optimal distribution and orientation of auxiliary ports for manipulation and visualization. Intrathoracic spatial anatomical findings proved the holographic recommendations and no need for interspace and/or port adjustment occurred. We propose that intraoperative MR technology is the ultimate step in the meticulous preoperative planning process that is required for MICS.

HoloLens® 2's superimposed model, in line with the surgeon's vision, optimizes ergonomics, i.e., the surgeon can focus on the progress of the procedure without any interruption to consult with an external 2D flat screen [10] and/or disturbance of the visual–motor axis or hand–eye coordination [7,33]. Assumed benefits include improved surgical performance, reduced procedural length, more accurate visualization, and identification of anatomical structures leading to decreased risk of iatrogenic injuries [5,10,30]. The operator's integrated perception of virtual and real structures and their spatial relationship contributes to cognitive coherence [11], reduced operator stress and fatigue, and less risk of complications; all this potentially translates into improved patient safety. Intraoperative holography, not involving physical contact with any material structure, is a non-invasive, aseptic modality [29].

MR offers a competitive advantage in avoiding median resternotomy in selected cases. Redo-sternotomy carries inherent risks of potentially fatal injury of the mediastinal structures upon chest entry [34,35]. CT angiography has been advocated as part of the preoperative work-up [36]. CT datasets converted into holographic models open an avenue for an alternative approach, e.g., LAST for PVR [37]. Holographic incisional guidance provides direct access to the target structures and significantly reduces operative risks while increasing precision [38]. The general acceptance and initial user experience were positive throughout our study.

4.2. Limitations

The alignment of 3D holographic images onto a patient's chest was carried out manually using only two anatomic landmarks, namely the xiphoid and clavicles. More alignment points on exposed landmarks might be required for better precision [4]. Manual alignment needs to be mastered and is time-consuming [10]. Similarly, accommodation to HoloLens® 2 headgear requires some habituation. Co-application of regular head-mounted surgical equipment, such as surgical loupes and headlights typically worn by cardiac surgeons during surgery might be difficult or even impossible with HoloLens® 2 [4]. The holographic images are static [4], and no magnification has yet been integrated into the models [10]. HoloLens® 2 was only applied in the initial phases of the operations, i.e., during chest entry and intrathoracic orientation; the surgical procedures did not require additional spatial guidance. Our study of three surgical procedures only represents our initial experience with MR and HoloLens® 2. The modality requires more exposure with a wider spectrum of anatomies and complexities in order to identify clinical applicability, accuracy, user comfort, and the device's place in the MICS armamentarium.

5. Conclusions

The use of an MR device in MICS could improve our understanding of anatomical spatial relationships. As an intraoperative form of real-time image guidance, it may be regarded as an important last step in pre- and intraoperative planning that offers improved precision of access and better intrathoracic orientation. In-line 3D visibility conjoining the patient's intrathoracic anatomy with the superimposed in-line reconstructed holographic model optimizes the surgeon's ergonomics and potentially enhances patient safety. The real value and place of the modality need further evaluation in an extended cohort of patients with a wider surgical spectrum and more degrees of complexity.

Supplementary Materials: The following supporting information can be downloaded at https://www.mdpi.com/article/10.3390/jcdd12020049/s1, File S1: HoloLens 2 Video; (https://youtu.be/rlC2IilA4i8, accessed on 11 September 2024); File S2: Survey for use of HoloLens 2 in MIS Cardiac Surgery; File S3: Manual Segmentation Protocol.

Author Contributions: Conceptualization, T.K. and L.K.; methodology, T.K.; writing—original draft preparation, W.M.M.A., S.S.K., A.K. and L.K.; writing—review and editing, L.K.; visualization, Y.G.; supervision: L.K. and T.K. All authors have read and agreed to the published version of the manuscript.

Funding: This study received no external funding.

Institutional Review Board Statement: This study was conducted in accordance with the Declaration of Helsinki and approved by the NHG Domain Specific Review Board (DSRB) Approval of Exemption (NHG DSRB Reference Number: 2020/01044) on 8 October 2020.

Informed Consent Statement: Informed consent was obtained from all subjects involved in the study in accordance with institutional guidelines.

Data Availability Statement: The original contributions presented in this study are included in the article/Supplementary Materials. Further inquiries can be directed to the corresponding author.

Acknowledgments: The authors would like thank Ilias Skaltsiotis, Jai Sule, and Guohao Chang for surgical assistance and providing the patients to be involved in this manuscript; Yujia Gao, Ng Kian Wai and Ngiam Kee Yuan for technical assistance and guidance using HoloLens® 2 during the surgeries.

Conflicts of Interest: The authors declare no competing interests. The authors have no financial interest in any of the products or devices that are described in this article.

References

1. Kofidis, T. *Minimally Invasive Cardiac Surgery. A Practical Guide*; CRC Press: Boca Raton, FL, USA, 2021.
2. Kiraly, L.; Aye, W.M.; Subbian, S.K.; Kofidis, T.; Al Hakami, A. Minimal incision and less invasive techniques in congenital cardiac surgery: A narrative review. *Pediatr. Med.* **2024**, *7*, 14. [CrossRef]
3. Ye, W.; Zhang, X.; Li, T.; Luo, C.; Yang, L. Mixed-reality hologram for diagnosis and surgical planning of double outlet right ventricle: A pilot study. *Clin. Radiol.* **2021**, *76*, 237. [CrossRef] [PubMed]
4. Brun, H.; Bugge, R.A.; Suther, L.K.; Birkeland, S.; Kumar, R.; Pelanis, E.; Elle, O.J. Mixed reality holograms for heart surgery planning: First user experience in congenital heart disease. *Eur. Heart J. Cardiovasc. Imaging* **2019**, *20*, 883–888. [CrossRef]
5. Liu, S.; Xie, M.; Zhang, Z.; Wu, X.; Gao, F.; Lu, L.; Zhang, J.; Xie, Y.; Yang, F.; Ye, Z. A 3 D Hologram with Mixed Reality Technique to improve Understanding of Pulmonary Lesions Caused by COVID-19; Randomised Control Trial. *Med. Internet Res.* **2021**, *23*, e24081. [CrossRef]
6. Karmonik, C.; Boone, T.B.; Khavari, R. Workflow for visualization of neuroimaging data with an augmented reality device. *J. Digit. Imaging* **2018**, *31*, 26–31. [CrossRef] [PubMed]
7. Tepper, O.M.; Rudy, H.L.; Lefkowitz, A.; Weimer, K.A.; Marks, S.M.; Stern, C.S.; Garfein, E.S. Mixed reality with HoloLens: Where virtual reality meets augmented reality in the operating room. *Plast. Reconstr. Surg.* **2017**, *140*, 1066–1070. [CrossRef] [PubMed]
8. Taylor, A.G. *What Is the Microsoft HoloLens? Develop Microsoft HoloLens Apps Now*; Springer: Berlin/Heidelberg, Germany, 2016; pp. 3–7.
9. Cai, E.Z.; Gao, Y.; Ngiam, K.Y.; Lim, T.C. Mixed Reality Intraoperative Navigation in Craniomaxillofacial Surgery. *Plast. Reconstr. Surg.* **2021**, *148*, 686e–688e. [CrossRef] [PubMed]
10. Scherl, C.; Stratemeier, J.; Rotter, N.; Hesser, J.; Schönberg, S.O.; Servais, J.J.; Männle, D.; Lammert, A. Augmented Reality with HoloLens in Parotid Tumour Surgery: A Prospective Feasibility Study. *ORL J. Otorhinolaryngol. Relat. Spec.* **2021**, *83*, 439–448. [CrossRef]

11. Deib, G.; Johnson, A.; Unberath, M.; Yu, K.; Andress, S.; Qian, L.; Osgood, G.; Navab, N.; Hui, F.; Gailloud, P. Image guided percutaneous spine procedures using an optical see-through head mounted display: Proof of concept and rational. *J. Neurointerv. Surg.* **2018**, *10*, 1187–1191. [CrossRef] [PubMed]
12. Aye, W.M.M.; Kiraly, L.; Kumar, S.S.; Kasivishvanaath, A.; Gao, Y.; Kofidis, T. Mixed Reality (Holography)-Guided Minimally Invasive Cardiac Surgery—A First-in-Man Comparative Feasibility Study. In Proceedings of the 30th Annual Meeting of the Asian Society for Cardiovascular and Thoracic Surgery (ASCVTS 2022)—Plenary 2, C-PL2-7, Nara, Japan, 25 March 2022.
13. Redman, J.D.; Wolton, W.P.; Shuttleworth, E. Use of holography to make truly three-dimensional X-ray images. *Nature* **1968**, *220*, 58–60. [CrossRef]
14. Carbone, M.; Piazza, R.; Condino, S. Commercially Available Head- Mounted Displays Are Unsuitable for Augmented Reality Surgical Guidance: A Call for Focused Research for Surgical Applications. *Surg. Innov.* **2020**, *27*, 254–255. [CrossRef] [PubMed]
15. Huber, T.; Hadzijusufovic, E.; Hansen, C.; Paschold, M.; Lang, H.; Kneist, W. Head-mounted mixed-reality technology during robotic-assisted transanal total mesorectal excision. *Dis. Colon. Rectum.* **2019**, *62*, 258–261. [CrossRef] [PubMed]
16. Ameri, G.; Baxter, J.S.; Bainbridge, D.; Peters, T.M.; Chen, E.C. Mixed reality ultrasound guidance system: A case study in system development and cautionary tale. *Int. J. Comput. Assist. Radiol. Surg.* **2018**, *13*, 495–505. [CrossRef] [PubMed]
17. Coelho, G.; Figueiredo, E.G.; Rabelo, N.N.; Teixeira, M.J.; Zanon, N. Development and evaluation of a new pediatric mixed-reality model for neurosurgical training. *J. Neurosurg. Pediatr.* **2019**, *2*, 423–432. [CrossRef]
18. Li, Y.; Chen, X.; Wang, N.; Zhang, W.; Li, D.; Zhang, L.; Qu, X.; Cheng, W.; Xu, Y.; Chen, W.; et al. A wearable mixed-reality holographic computer for guiding external ventricular draining insertion at the bedside. *J. Neurosurg.* **2018**, *10*, 1599–1606.
19. Sauer, I.M.; Queisner, M.; Tang, P.; Moosburner, S.; Hoepfner, O.; Horner, R.; Lohmann, R.; Pratschke, J. Mixed reality in visceral surgery development of a suitable workflow and evaluation of intraoperative use-cases. *Ann. Surg.* **2017**, *266*, 706–712. [CrossRef]
20. Pratt, P.; Ives, M.; Lawton, G. Through the HoloLens looking glass: Augmented reality for extremity reconstruction surgery using 3D vascular models with perforating vessels. *Eur. Radiol. Exp.* **2018**, *2*, 2. [CrossRef]
21. Elmi-Terander, A.; Nachabe, R.; Skulason, H.; Pedersen, K.; Söderman, M.; Racadio, J.; Babic, D.; Gerdhem, P.; Edström, E. Feasibility and accuracy of thoracolumbar minimally invasive pedicle screw placement with augmented reality navigation technology. *Spine* **2018**, *43*, 1018–1023. [CrossRef] [PubMed]
22. Li, Z.; Butler, E.; Li, K.; Lu, A.; Ji, S.; Zhang, S. Large-scale exploration of neuronal morphologies using deep learning and augmented reality. *Neuroinformatics* **2018**, *16*, 339–349. [CrossRef] [PubMed]
23. Porpiglia, F.; Fiori, C.; Checcucci, E.; Amparore, D.; Bertolo, R. Augmented reality robot-assist- ed radical prostatectomy: Preliminary experience. *Urology* **2018**, *115*, 184. [CrossRef]
24. Bong, J.H.; Song, H.J.; Oh, Y.; Park, N.; Kim, H.; Park, S. Endoscopic navigation system with extended field of view using augmented reality technology. *Int. J. Med. Robot.* **2018**, *14*, e1886. [CrossRef] [PubMed]
25. Hu, H.Z.; Feng, X.B.; Shao, Z.W.; Xie, M.; Xu, S.; Wu, X.H.; Ye, Z.W. Application and Prospect of Mixed Reality Technology in Medical Field. *Curr. Med. Sci.* **2019**, *39*, 1–6. [CrossRef] [PubMed]
26. Wainman, B.; Pukas, G.; Wolak, L.; Mohanraj, S.; Lamb, J.; Norman, G.R. The Critical Role of Stereopsis in Virtual and Mixed Reality Learning Environments. *Anat. Sci. Educ.* **2020**, *13*, 401–412. [CrossRef]
27. Hilt, A.D.; Kapllani, K.M.; Hierck, B.P.; Kemp, A.C.; Albayrak, A.; Melles, M.; Schalij, M.J.; Scherptong, R.W. Perspectives of Patients and Professionals on Information and Education After Myocardial Infarction With Insight for Mixed Reality Implementation: Cross-Sectional Interview Study. *JMIR Hum. Factors* **2020**, *7*, e17147. [CrossRef] [PubMed]
28. Lau, I.; Gupta, A.; Sun, Z. Clinical Valve of Virtual Reality versus 3D Printing in Congenital Heart Disease. *Biomolecules* **2021**, *11*, 884. [CrossRef]
29. Jang, J.; Tschabrunn, C.M.; Barkagan, M.; Anter, E.; Menze, B.; Nezafat, R. Three-dimensional holographic visualization of high-resolution myocardial scar on HoloLens. *PLoS ONE* **2018**, *13*, e0205188. [CrossRef] [PubMed]
30. Incekara, F.; Smits, M.; Dirven, C.; Vincent, A. Clinical feasibility of a wearable mixed-reality device in neurosurgery. *World Neurosurg.* **2018**, *118*, e422–e427. [CrossRef] [PubMed]
31. Kersten-Oertel, M.; Jannin, P.; Collins, D.L. The State of the Art of Visualization in Mixed Reality Image Guided Surgery. *Comput. Med. Imaging Graph.* **2013**, *37*, 98–112. [CrossRef] [PubMed]
32. Wu, X.; Liu, R.; Yu, J.; Xu, S.; Yang, C.; Yang, S.; Shao, Z.; Ye, Z. Mixed Reality Technology Launches in Orthopedic Surgery for Comprehensive Preoperative Management of Complicated Cervical Fractures. *Surg. Innov.* **2018**, *25*, 421–422. [CrossRef]
33. El Shallaly, G.; Cuschieri, A. Optimum view distance for laparoscopic surgery. *Surg. Endosc.* **2006**, *20*, 1879–1882. [CrossRef]
34. Kirshbom, P.M.; Myung, R.J.; Simsic, J.M.; Kramer, Z.B.; Leong, T.; Kogon, B.E.; Kanter, K.R. One Thousand repeat sternotomies for congenital cardiac surgery: Risk factors for re-entry injury. *Ann. Thorac. Surg.* **2009**, *88*, 158–161. [CrossRef] [PubMed]
35. Pahwa, S.; Stephens, E.H.; Dearani, J.A. High-Risk Reoperative Sternotomy-How We Do It, How We Teach It. *World J. Pediatr. Congenit. Heart Surg.* **2020**, *11*, 459–465. [CrossRef] [PubMed]

36. Valente, T.; Bocchini, G.; Rossi, G.; Sica, G.; Davison, H.; Scaglione, M. MDCT prior to median re-sternotomy in cardiovascular surgery: Our experiences, infrequent findings and the crucial role of radiological report. *Br. J. Radiol.* **2019**, *92*, 20170980. [CrossRef] [PubMed]
37. Henaine, R.; Yoshimura, N.; Di Filippo, S.; Ninet, J. Pulmonary valve replacement in repaired tetralogy of Fallot by left thoracotomy avoid ascending aorta injury. *J. Thorac. Cardiovasc. Surg.* **2011**, *141*, 590–592. [CrossRef] [PubMed]
38. Kumar, R.P.; Pelanis, E.; Bugge, R.; Brun, H.; Palomar, R.; Aghayan, D.L.; Fretland, Å.A.; Edwin, B.; Elle, O.J. Use of Mixed Reality for Surgery Planning: Assessment and Development Workflow. *J. Biomed. Inform.* **2020**, *112*, 100077. [CrossRef]

Journal of
Cardiovascular Development and Disease

MDPI

Review

Fractional Flow Reserve from Coronary CT: Evidence, Applications, and Future Directions

Arta Kasaeian [1], Mohadese Ahmadzade [2], Taylor Hoffman [1], Mohammad Ghasemi-Rad [2,*] and Anoop Padoor Ayyappan [3,*]

[1] Baylor College of Medicine, Houston, TX 77030, USA; arta.kasaeian@bcm.edu (A.K.); taylor.hoffman@bcm.edu (T.H.)
[2] Department of Radiology, Division of Vascular and Interventional Radiology, Baylor College of Medicine, Houston, TX 77030, USA; mohadese.ahmadzade@bcm.edu
[3] Department of Radiology, Division of Cardiothoracic Imaging, Baylor College of Medicine, Houston, TX 77030, USA
* Correspondence: mohammad.ghasemirad@bcm.edu (M.G.-R.); anoop.ayyappan@bcm.edu (A.P.A.)

Abstract: Coronary computed tomography angiography (CCTA) has emerged as the leading noninvasive imaging modality for the assessment of coronary artery disease (CAD), offering high-resolution visualization of the coronary anatomy and plaque characterization. The development of fractional flow reserve derived from CCTA (FFR-CT) has further transformed the diagnostic landscape by enabling the simultaneous evaluation of both anatomical stenosis and lesion-specific ischemia. FFR-CT has demonstrated diagnostic accuracy comparable to invasive FFR. The combined use of CCTA and FFR-CT is now pivotal in a broad range of clinical scenarios, including the evaluation of stable and acute chest pain, assessment of high-risk and complex plaque features, and preoperative planning. As evidence continues to mount, CCTA and FFR-CT are positioned to become the primary gatekeepers to the cardiac catheterization laboratory, potentially reducing the number of unnecessary invasive procedures. This review highlights the growing clinical utility of FFR-CT, its integration with advanced plaque imaging, and the future potential of these technologies in redefining the management of CAD, while also acknowledging current limitations, including image quality requirements, cost, and access.

Keywords: fractional flow reserve; coronary CT angiography; computational fluid dynamics; coronary artery disease; FFR-CT

1. Introduction

Coronary artery disease (CAD) is the leading cause of morbidity and mortality globally, accounting for approximately 17.8 million deaths each year and affecting about 1 in 20 adults in the United States alone [1]. As the prevalence of CAD continues to rise, there is a growing need for accurate and personalized ways to diagnose it as early as possible. Traditional methods for evaluating CAD, including clinical risk scoring, functional stress testing, and invasive coronary angiography (ICA), have long been the standard of care. However, each comes with notable limitations. ICA, while considered the gold standard, is invasive, expensive, and subject to interobserver variability. More importantly, it often fails to capture the true hemodynamic impact of coronary lesions. Visual assessment of stenosis severity can overlook pathophysiologic elements like collateral circulation or plaque morphology, potentially leading to overtreatment or underestimation of risk [2]. As the precision of CAD diagnostics has improved, the focus has shifted beyond simply identifying luminal stenosis. There is now greater emphasis on understanding the specific lesion site, the extent of luminal narrowing, composition of arterial plaques, and the presence of downstream ischemia and impaired myocardial perfusion [3]. This comprehensive approach is helping to improve risk stratification and guide more personalized treatment strategies.

Against this backdrop, coronary computed tomography angiography (CCTA) has emerged as a powerful, non-invasive tool for assessing CAD. Recent technological innovations have significantly enhanced the spatial and temporal resolution of CCTA while reducing radiation exposure. CCTA has a sensitivity of up to 99% and a negative predictive value of 97%, making it highly effective for excluding significant coronary artery disease in low- to intermediate-risk patients [4]. Current evidence supports a Class I, Level A recommendation for cardiac CT in both stable and acute chest pain, as outlined in the 2021 AHA–ACC Chest Pain Guidelines [5]. Specifically, CCTA is recommended (Class I) for intermediate-risk patients, while FFR-CT carries a Class IIa recommendation for evaluating 40–90% stenosis in proximal or mid-coronary arteries. In the SCOT-HEART trial, 23% of patients who received cardiac CT had their treatment changed within 6 weeks, compared to only 5% with standard care, showing that cardiac CT results can significantly impact individual treatment decisions [6]. The DISCHARGE trial, involving patients with stable chest pain and intermediate CAD risk, found that cardiac CT and invasive angiography had similar outcomes over 3.5 years, but cardiac CT led to fewer major procedural complications [7].

While CCTA has proven valuable for visualizing coronary anatomy, its limitation to anatomical assessment alone has driven the development of CT-derived fractional flow reserve (FFR-CT), an innovation that integrates both anatomical and functional insights. This advancement enhances the ability to evaluate the physiological significance of coronary lesions, improving diagnostic accuracy and guiding more effective treatment strategies. This review explores the role of FFR-CT and its potential to impact prognosis and reshape clinical practice in CAD.

2. Fractional Flow Reserve

Fractional flow reserve (FFR) is a physiological index developed in the early 1990s to assess the hemodynamic significance of coronary artery stenoses. In 1993, Dr. Nico H. J. Pijls and Dr. Bernard De Bruyne introduced FFR as a method to quantify the pressure gradient across a coronary lesion during conditions of maximal hyperemia [8,9]. This metric, defined as the ratio of distal coronary pressure to aortic pressure under maximal blood flow, enables a functional assessment of coronary stenoses that complements traditional anatomical imaging. The introduction of FFR marked a significant advancement in interventional cardiology by enhancing the precision of percutaneous coronary intervention (PCI), improving clinical decision-making, and leading to better patient outcomes.

3. Clinical Validation of Invasive FFR

3.1. The FAME Study: FFR-Guided PCI in Multivessel Disease

The FAME (Fractional Flow Reserve Versus Angiography for Multivessel Evaluation) study evaluated the clinical benefit of FFR-guided PCI in patients with multivessel CAD [10]. In this randomized trial involving 1005 patients, participants were assigned to PCI guided either by angiography alone or by FFR measurements. Lesions with FFR ≤ 0.80 were treated in the FFR group, whereas all angiographically significant lesions were stented in the other group. Although both groups had a similar number of target lesions, fewer stents were implanted in the FFR-guided group (1.9 vs. 2.7; $p < 0.001$). After two years, the FFR group had significantly lower rates of death or myocardial infarction (8.4% vs. 12.9%;

$p = 0.02$). Lesions deferred based on an FFR > 0.80 showed very low adverse-event rates. These findings support FFR's critical role in safely guiding PCI and improving long-term outcomes in multivessel CAD.

3.2. The FAME 2 Trial: FFR-Guided PCI vs. Medical Therapy

The FAME 2 study demonstrated that in patients with stable CAD and reduced fractional flow reserve (FFR $\leq$ 0.80), percutaneous coronary intervention (PCI) plus medical therapy (MT) significantly improved clinical outcomes, compared to MT alone [11]. Over three years, PCI reduced major adverse cardiac events (10.1% vs. 22.0%), primarily by lowering urgent revascularization rates. Death and myocardial infarction rates were also lower, though this decline was not statistically significant. Patients undergoing PCI experienced less severe angina and sustained quality-of-life improvements throughout follow-up. While initial costs were higher for PCI, long-term expenses were comparable to MT alone. The study supports FFR-guided PCI as a superior strategy over MT in stable coronary disease, enhancing survival, reducing cardiac events, and improving patient quality of life without increased long-term costs.

4. Emergence of Non-Invasive Coronary Physiology Assessment

Despite the advantages of invasive FFR, the need for pressure wires and pharmacologic agents such as adenosine introduces patient discomfort, procedural risk, and cost. These limitations spurred the development of non-invasive alternatives, particularly leveraging advancements in CCTA and computational modeling.

FFR-CT integrates the anatomical detail provided by CCTA with the physiological insights of traditional FFR, offering a comprehensive, non-invasive assessment of CAD. This approach eliminates the need for pharmacologic stress agents, such as adenosine, and obviates the use of invasive pressure wires. As a result, FFR-CT enhances patient comfort and streamlines the diagnostic process without compromising clinical accuracy.

5. Principles and Technology Behind FFR-CT

FFR-CT uses standard CCTA datasets combined with computational fluid dynamics to model coronary blood flow and evaluate the hemodynamic significance of coronary lesions. Traditionally, FFR is measured invasively using pressure wire and pharmacologic agents like adenosine. In contrast, FFR-CT estimates this value non-invasively by modeling blood flow as a Newtonian fluid governed by the Navier–Stokes equations [12]. FFR-CT estimates blood flow and pressure in coronary arteries non-invasively by applying computational fluid dynamics to CCTA images. Total coronary flow at rest is first estimated using heart size and mass as key parameters. Microvascular resistance is then assumed to be inversely related to the size of the epicardial arteries. Because the coronary response to vasodilators is predictable, maximal blood flow can be simulated using resting images. Finally, blood flow and pressure are modeled by solving the 3D Navier–Stokes equations.

5.1. HeartFlow® FFR-CT: A Pioneering Non-Invasive Solution

HeartFlow® FFR-CT is the non-invasive technology for assessing the physiological significance of CAD most widely adopted in the United States. It remains the only solution with FDA clearance, CE marking, and NICE endorsement for the functional evaluation of coronary lesions. This innovative approach leverages CCTA and applies advanced computational fluid dynamics (CFD) to simulate blood flow and pressure within the coronary arteries. To perform the analysis, CCTA data is securely transferred to HeartFlow®'s centralized core laboratory, where powerful off-site supercomputers process the information. The CFD model reconstructs a patient-specific 3D model of coronary anatomy, calculates pressure gradients, and generates an FFR-CT map that identifies flow-limiting stenoses (Figure 1). The entire process typically takes between one and four hours, providing clinicians with a detailed, non-invasive assessment of coronary physiology.

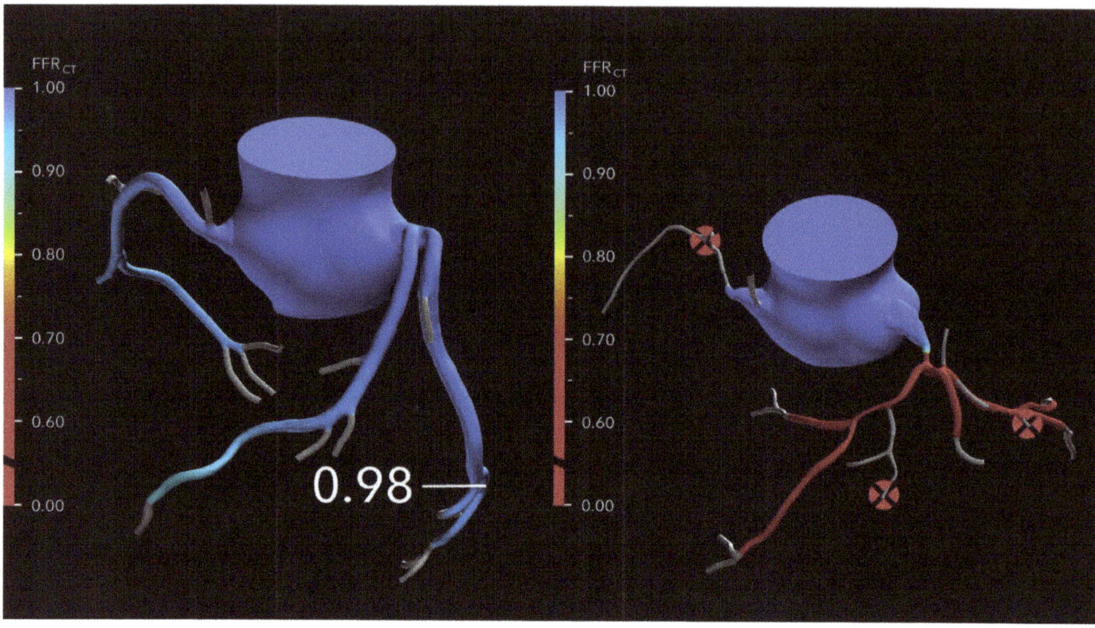

Figure 1. FFR-CT results are displayed using 3D-modeled representations of coronary arteries. (**Left**): A value above 0.80 is considered normal and is shown in blue. Borderline values ranging from 0.76 to 0.80 are depicted in orange and yellow. (**Right**): Values of 0.75 or below are classified as abnormal and marked in red. Areas of complete occlusion are indicated with an "X" symbol.

5.2. The Evolving Role of On-Site Machine Learning-Based FFR-CT in Clinical Practice

On-site machine learning-based FFR-CT (FFR-$CT_{ML)}$ represents a major advancement in the noninvasive physiologic assessment of coronary artery disease. Traditional FFR-CT solutions, such as HeartFlow®'s CFD-based platform, require an off-site supercomputing infrastructure. This approach poses limitations related to processing time, cost, and scalability, making it less accessible in time-sensitive or resource-limited settings. Recent developments in artificial intelligence have enabled on-site FFR-CT computation using deep learning models trained on synthetic coronary anatomies and corresponding hemodynamic data. These models rapidly approximate the complex nonlinear relationship between coronary anatomy and blood flow, bypassing the need for computational fluid dynamics. By operating on standard workstations, FFR-CT_{ML} enables faster reporting with a lower computational burden.

A recent meta-analysis evaluated the diagnostic performance of FFR-CT_{ML} [13]. A total of 23 studies on FFR-CT_{CFD} and 18 studies on FFR-CT_{ML} were included. The data encompassed 2501 patients and 3764 vessels in the CFD group, and 1323 patients and 4194 vessels in the ML group. The results demonstrated that FFR-CT_{ML} and FFR-CT_{CFD} had comparable specificity and AUC at both the patient (Z = 0.59, p = 0.55; AUC p = 0.5) and vessel (Z = 0.94, p = 0.34; AUC p = 0.74) levels. The diagnostic odds ratio was also similar at the vessel level (Z = 0.7, p = 0.48). However, FFR-CT_{ML} showed significantly lower sensitivity than FFR-CT_{CFD} at both the patient (Z = 3.85, p = 0.0001) and vessel

(Z = 2.05, $p = 0.04$) levels. While the sensitivity of CFD-based FFR-CT may be superior, the specificity and area under the receiver operating curve, more relevant for clinical decision-making, are largely equivalent in the ML and CFD models. Importantly, on-site FFR-CT_{ML} can optimize workflow, reduce turnaround time, and improve cost-effectiveness, which may be particularly impactful in high-volume or under-resourced healthcare systems. Given its favorable diagnostic profile, operational advantages, and potential to enhance equitable access to CAD diagnostics, on-site FFR-CT_{ML} is poised to become an integral component of contemporary cardiac imaging strategies. Cleerly ISCHEMIA is an FDA-cleared automated machine learning-based decision-support tool used for interpreting CCTA images to estimate the likelihood of ischemia in individual vessels.

6. Real-World Evidence and Clinical Validation of FFR-CT

FFR_{CT} has been evaluated in several large-scale multicenter trials. The DISCOVER-FLOW study was the first to evaluate the diagnostic performance of FFR-CT, using a first-generation algorithm in patients with suspected or known CAD [14]. Involving 103 patients and 159 vessels, the study compared non-invasive FFR-CT with traditional coronary CTA, using invasive FFR as the gold standard. An FFR threshold of $\leq$0.80 and a CTA stenosis threshold of $\geq$50% were applied to define ischemia-causing lesions. FFR-CT demonstrated superior diagnostic accuracy (84% vs. 59%) and specificity (82% vs. 40%) compared to CTA, with similar sensitivity (88% vs. 91%). The area under the receiver operating characteristic (ROC) curve was significantly higher for FFR-CT (0.90) than for CTA (0.75, $p = 0.001$), indicating better overall diagnostic discrimination. FFR-CT also showed strong correlation with invasive FFR (r = 0.717, $p < 0.001$), with only a minor systematic underestimation. These findings established FFR-CT as a highly accurate, non-invasive alternative for the identification of functionally significant coronary stenoses.

The DeFACTO study evaluated the diagnostic performance of FFR-CT combined with CCTA in 252 stable patients with suspected or known CAD [15]. Conducted across 17 centers in five countries, the study compared non-invasive FFR-CT against invasive FFR as the gold standard. While the study narrowly missed its pre-specified accuracy target, FFR-CT plus CCTA demonstrated improved diagnostic accuracy (73%) compared to CCTA alone (64%). Sensitivity for detecting ischemia was significantly higher with FFR-CT (90% vs. 84%), while specificity remained modest (54%). Importantly, overall diagnostic discrimination improved, with an area under the receiver operating characteristic curve (AUC) of 0.81 for FFR-CT compared to 0.68 for CCTA alone ($p < 0.001$). In patients with intermediate stenosis (30–70%), FFR-CT also showed markedly improved sensitivity (82% vs. 37%). These findings highlight FFR-CT's potential to enhance the physiological assessment of CAD beyond anatomical imaging alone.

The NXT study evaluated 254 patients with suspected stable coronary artery disease to assess the diagnostic performance of noninvasive FFR-CT [16]. Using invasive FFR $\leq$ 0.80 as the reference standard, FFR-CT demonstrated significantly improved diagnostic accuracy and discrimination compared to coronary CTA alone. The area under the curve (AUC) was 0.90 for FFR-CT versus 0.81 for CTA ($p = 0.0008$). While sensitivity was similar (86% for FFR-CT vs. 94% for CTA), specificity improved markedly (79% vs. 34%). These findings support FFR-CT as a superior noninvasive method for identifying ischemia-causing lesions.

A sub-analysis of the PACIFIC trial assessed 208 patients with suspected coronary artery disease, comparing the diagnostic performance of FFR-CT, coronary CTA, 99mTc-tetrofosmin SPECT, and $^{15}O\text{-}H_2O$ PET against invasive FFR as the reference [17]. On a per-vessel basis, FFR-CT demonstrated the highest AUC (0.94), outperforming CTA (0.83), SPECT (0.70), and PET (0.87). On a per-patient level, FFR-CT and PET had similar AUCs (0.92 vs. 0.91), both higher than CTA (0.81) and SPECT (0.75). However, on an intention-to-diagnose analysis, PET had superior performance due to FFR-CT's limited evaluability—17% of vessels and 25% of patients were not analyzable. This limitation of FFR-CT, the requirement of high-quality image data, is also evident in prior studies, where 11% and 13% of examinations were non-evaluable, due to artifacts, in the DeFACTO and NXT trials, respectively. These findings underscore PET's high diagnostic accuracy and suggest that while FFR-CT offers excellent functional assessment, its image quality dependency can affect real-world diagnostic utility compared to PET.

The PLATFORM trial was a multicenter study enrolling 584 patients with new-onset chest pain, comparing the usual care to a diagnostic strategy incorporating CCTA and selective fractional flow reserve derived from CTA (FFR-CT) [18]. Patients were assigned, based on the initial planned strategy, noninvasive testing or invasive coronary angiography (ICA), and then randomized to usual care or CTA plus FFR-CT. Among those for whom the initial plan was ICA, the CTA/FFR-CT strategy significantly reduced the number of patients undergoing ICA with no obstructive CAD, from 73% in usual care to 12% in the CTA/FFR-CT group. Additionally, 61% of invasive angiographies were avoided after CTA/FFR-CT results. Clinical event rates, including those for death and myocardial infarction, were low and similar between groups at one year. Moreover, the CTA/FFR-CT approach reduced costs by 33% in patients planned for invasive angiography, demonstrating that FFR-CT effectively acts as a gatekeeper to ICA, reducing the number of unnecessary invasive procedures without compromising patient outcomes.

The ADVANCE registry was a large prospective study of 5083 patients with suspected CAD, across 38 international centers [19]. It evaluated the real-world impact of incorporating FFR-CT into clinical decision-making. The study found that adding FFR-CT to standard CCTA led to changes in treatment strategy in nearly 67% of patients. Among those undergoing ICA, patients with an FFR-CT $\leq$ 0.80 had a significantly lower incidence of non-obstructive CAD (14.4%) compared to those with an FFR-CT > 0.80 (43.8%). Furthermore, 72.3% of patients with FFRCT $\leq$ 0.80 who underwent ICA proceeded to revascularization. At the 1-year follow-up, revascularization rates were substantially higher in the FFR-CT $\leq$ 0.80 group (38.4%) than in those with higher FFRCT values (5.6%). The findings highlight that FFR-CT effectively guides treatment by identifying patients likely to benefit from revascularization while reducing the number of unnecessary invasive procedures.

The SYNTAX III Revolution trial investigated how incorporating FFR-CT influences treatment decisions in patients with complex coronary artery disease, specifically those with left main or three-vessel disease [20]. The study randomized 223 patients to two heart teams, each comprising an interventional cardiologist, cardiac surgeon, and radiologist, who initially assessed patients using either coronary CTA or ICA. Each team calculated the anatomic SYNTAX score and recommended treatment strategies including coronary artery bypass grafting (CABG), percutaneous coronary intervention (PCI), and equipoise coronary artery bypass grafting–percutaneous coronary intervention. After reviewing the initial decisions, teams integrated FFR-CT data to reassess treatment plans. The addition of FFR-CT led to a change in overall treatment strategy in 7% of cases and altered vessel selection for revascularization in 12%. Furthermore, FFR-CT reclassified 14–16% of patients to a lower SYNTAX score category. These findings underscore the value of FFR-CT as a noninvasive functional tool that refines clinical decision-making and procedural planning in complex coronary disease.

A recent study evaluated the impact of FFR-CT on postprocedural myocardial injury (PMI) and long-term outcomes in revascularized OCAD patients, using data from a 2013–2021 tertiary hospital registry [21]. Among 559 revascularized patients (386 PCI, 166 CABG), FFR-CT was performed in 45.1%. Over 4.4 $\pm$ 2.2 years of follow-up, major adverse cardiovascular events (MACE) occurred in 24.5% of patients. FFR-

CT use was associated with significantly lower all-cause mortality (HR 0.476, 95% CI 0.230–0.985, $p = 0.046$) and a non-significant trend toward reduced MACE (HR 0.736, 95% CI 0.513–1.055, $p = 0.095$). Subgroup analysis in PCI and CABG cohorts showed no significant MACE reduction individually. Among 477 patients with cardiac troponin data, 42.5% had PMI, with a lower PMI incidence in CABG patients undergoing FFR-CT (5.3% vs. 15.6%, $p = 0.044$), though this was not significant in adjusted models. These findings suggest that FFR-CT may improve long-term outcomes, particularly survival, independent of procedural myocardial injury.

One meta-analysis, encompassing 43 studies and over 7000 vessels from 5236 patients, provides the most extensive evaluation to date of the diagnostic performance and clinical applicability of FFR-CT compared to invasive FFR [22]. This analysis found a moderate correlation between FFR-CT and invasive FFR (Spearman coefficient 0.67), with the level of agreement increasing in vessels with higher FFR values, particularly those with an FFR-CT > 0.90. Overall, FFR-CT demonstrated robust diagnostic accuracy, sensitivity, and specificity (82.2%, 80.9%, and 83.1%, respectively). The diagnostic performance of FFR-CT varied by value range: values > 0.90 had a 93% likelihood of ruling out hemodynamically significant CAD, while an FFR-CT < 0.49 had nearly 100% accuracy in identifying physiologically significant lesions. This suggests that at either end of the FFR-CT spectrum, the modality performs exceptionally well and can guide confident clinical decision-making. In contrast, diagnostic uncertainty increases within the intermediate range or "gray zone" of 0.75–0.80, in which the accuracy drops significantly, potentially requiring additional testing before deciding on revascularization or deferral. Notably, FFR-CT readings on average were only 0.01 lower than invasive FFR, indicating minimal systematic bias. This highlights the utility of raw FFR-CT values for guiding decisions, rather than relying solely on dichotomous classification (i.e., ≤0.80 vs. >0.80). The clinical implications of these findings are significant. When the FFR-CT is >0.90, ICA may be safely deferred in most patients, helping to reduce unnecessary procedures, associated complications, and healthcare costs. Conversely, lesions with an FFR-CT < 0.49 are highly likely to benefit from revascularization. As a result, FFR-CT may serve as an effective gatekeeper for ICA, offering a valuable adjunct to anatomical imaging from CTA by adding a functional dimension. This aligns with growing interest in noninvasive "one-stop shop" approaches for evaluating chest pain and suspected CAD.

7. When and How to Use FFR-CT: Guidance for Coronary CTA Interpretation and Reporting

FFR-CT is particularly valuable in evaluating patients with intermediate-risk coronary anatomy, typically characterized by one or more lesions causing 30–69% stenosis, or ≥70% stenosis in vessels other than the left main or proximal left anterior descending (LAD) artery. In these cases, FFR-CT helps determine the need for ICA versus optimal medical therapy (OMT). If the FFR-CT is >0.80, the likelihood of hemodynamically significant CAD is low, and patients can generally be managed safely with OMT alone, potentially avoiding unnecessary ICA or revascularization (Figures 2 and 3).

FFR-CT is generally not indicated in low-risk anatomy, such as patients with normal CCTA or stenosis < 30%, for whom OMT is the standard approach. In high-risk anatomy, including ≥50% left main stenosis, ≥70% proximal LAD stenosis, or three-vessel disease, patients are typically referred directly to ICA due to the high pre-test probability of significant disease. In the "gray zone" (0.75–0.80) management should be individualized based on lesion characteristics such as location (e.g., LAD vs. non-LAD vessels), lesion segment (proximal vs. distal), number of affected vessels, total plaque burden, and high-risk plaque features (e.g., low-attenuation plaque, napkin-ring sign, and positive remodeling). In the absence of high-risk features or symptoms, many patients in this range may be safely managed with OMT and close clinical follow-up. One commonly used approach includes a 3-month trial of OMT, with ICA reserved for persistent or worsening symptoms.

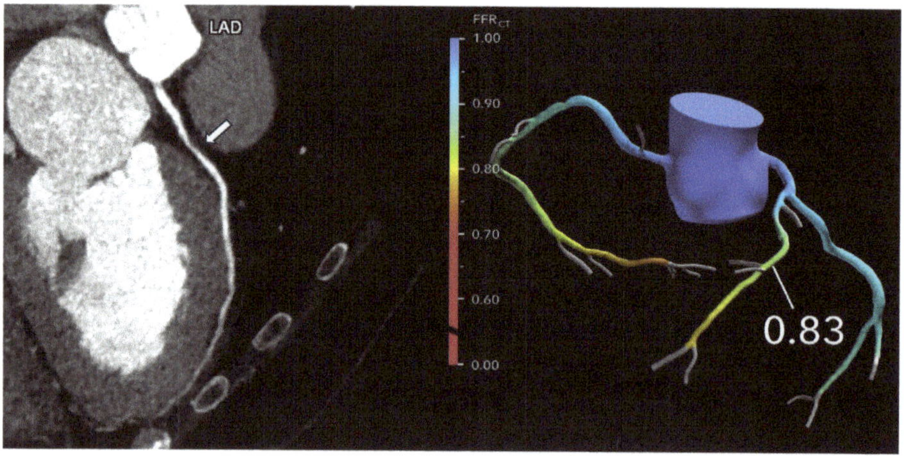

Figure 2. Optimizing treatment decisions with FFR-CT: (**Left**): A curved MPR coronary CTA image of the LAD in a 62-year-old man with atypical chest pain reveals severe stenosis (>70% diameter reduction) in the proximal LAD (arrow). (**Right**): The FFR-CT image demonstrates a value of 0.83 measured 2 cm distal to the lesion, indicating normal flow. As a result, invasive coronary angiography was deferred, and the patient was managed with medical therapy.

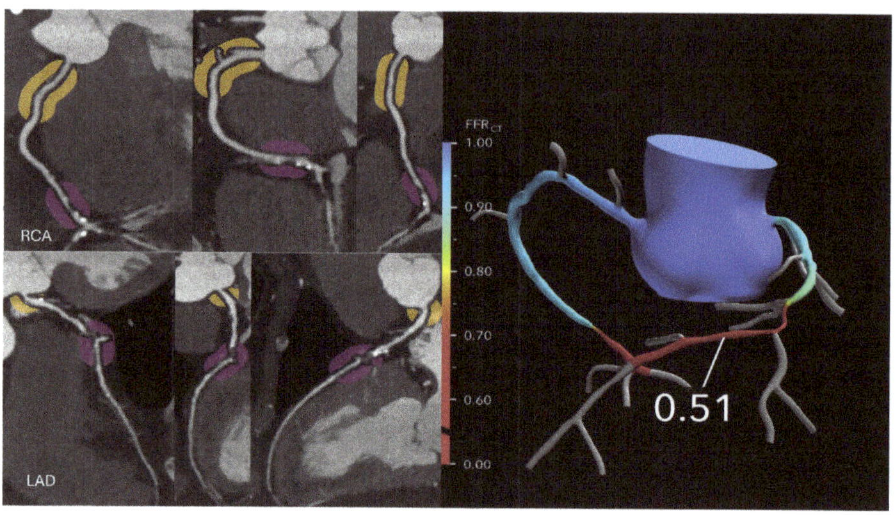

Figure 3. Optimizing treatment decisions with FFR-CT: (**Left**): A curved MPR coronary CTA image in a 64-year-old man with stable chest pain reveals severe stenoses in the mid left anterior descending (LAD) artery and distal right coronary artery. (**Right**): The corresponding FFRCT image shows a value of 0.51 measured 2 cm distal to the lesion, indicating severely reduced flow. Based on these findings, the patient proceeded to invasive coronary angiography followed by intervention.

A metric to enhance physiologic interpretation of FFR-CT is the ΔFFR-CT, defined as the difference in FFR-CT values proximal and distal to a coronary lesion. In a study involving 73 vessels from 50 patients who underwent CCTA, FFR-CT, and invasive FFR, a ΔFFR-CT ≥ 0.12 strongly predicted ischemia (invasive FFR ≤ 0.80), with an odds ratio of 10.2 [23] (Figure 4). ΔFFR-CT demonstrated superior diagnostic accuracy (AUC 0.86) compared to diameter stenosis (AUC 0.66) and other FFR-CT metrics. Its integration significantly improved ischemia classification and reclassification, suggesting ΔFFR-CT may serve as a valuable adjunct, particularly in intermediate lesions or diagnostic uncertainty.

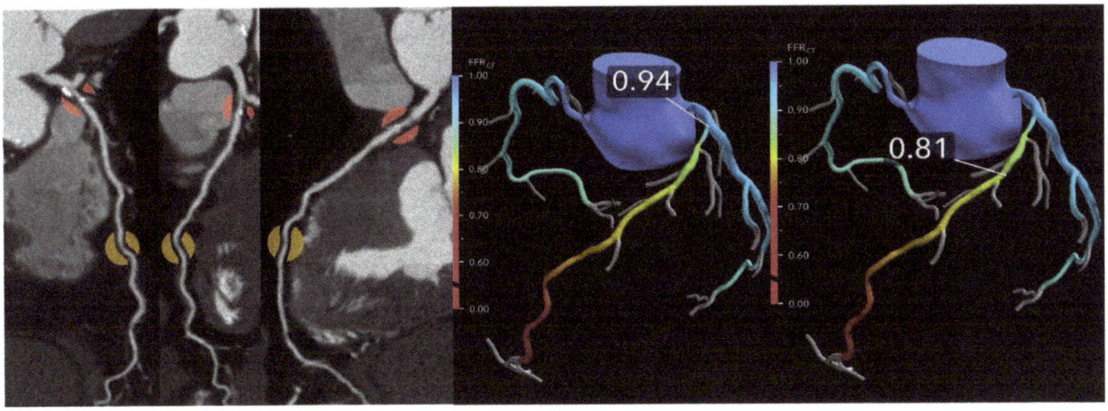

Figure 4. Lesion-specific ischemia: (**Left**): A curved multiplanar reformatted coronary CTA image in a 60-year-old man reveals moderate stenosis in the anterior left anterior descending (LAD) artery. (**Right**): The corresponding FFR-CT image shows an FFRCT value of 0.81 measured 2 cm distal to the lesion. The difference between the proximal and distal FFR-CT values across the lesion is 0.13, which exceeds the abnormal threshold of 0.12, confirming hemodynamically significant ischemia.

The location of FFR-CT measurement critically impacts diagnostic accuracy. Lesion-specific ischemia is best evaluated 1–2 cm distal to the stenosis rather than at the terminal vessel, where physiologic pressure naturally declines, even in the absence of disease, potentially leading to the overestimation of ischemia [24]. Thus, terminal-vessel measurements should be avoided. Distal-to-lesion FFR-CT measurement improves concordance with invasive FFR, enhances diagnostic precision, and may reduce unnecessary invasive testing.

The "gray zone" of FFR-CT values between 0.75 and 0.80 remains diagnostically challenging, as lesions in this range are ischemic on invasive FFR in approximately 50–60% of cases. To address this, a structured clinical algorithm is recommended:

7.1. Symptom Assessment

Prioritize patient-reported symptoms (frequency, exertional pattern, and response to anti-anginal therapy). Persistent angina or functional limitation may justify more aggressive investigation.

7.2. Anatomic Context

Evaluate lesion location (e.g., LAD vs. non-LAD), segment (proximal vs. distal), and number of affected vessels. Proximal LAD lesions in particular warrant lower thresholds for further testing or ICA.

7.3. Plaque Morphology

Use high-risk plaque features on CCTA, such as low-attenuation plaque, positive remodeling, napkin-ring sign, and spotty calcification, to stratify risk. The presence of ≥2 high-risk features favors early invasive evaluation.

7.4. Physiologic Adjuncts

Consider using ΔFFR-CT, defined as the difference in FFR-CT values proximal and distal to a coronary lesion. ΔFFR-CT may thus refine decision-making, especially when standard FFR-CT values are indeterminate.

7.5. Trial of Medical Therapy and Follow-Up

In the absence of high-risk features or disabling symptoms, initiate a 12-week trial of OMT with close outpatient follow-up. Repeated non-invasive testing (e.g., perfusion imaging or stress echo) or ICA should be reserved for symptom progression or diagnostic uncertainty.

This structured approach reinforces the utility of FFR-CT in intermediate-risk CAD while acknowledging its limitations as a standalone tool in borderline cases. It enables clinicians to combine physiologic, anatomic, and clinical factors in making safe and individualized decisions, thereby preserving the core benefit of FFR-CT, namely, reducing the incidence of unnecessary invasive testing without compromising diagnostic rigor.

8. Understanding the Limitations of the FFR-CT Technology

Accurate FFR-CT analysis relies on high-quality coronary CTA, requiring precise lumen segmentation and myocardial mass estimation; both are dependent on optimal spatial resolution and complete myocardial coverage. Image-degrading factors such as motion artifacts, calcium blooming, misalignment, noise, and poor contrast can obscure lumen boundaries or exclude sections of the myocardium from the field of view. Due to these limitations, 10–25% of studies are rejected and deemed unsuitable for FFR-CT analysis [16,18]. In approximately 80% of disqualified cases, motion artifacts were the main reason for inadequate image quality [25]. Additionally, FFR-CT is currently not feasible in patients who have undergone coronary stenting or coronary artery bypass grafting (CABG).

Coronary artery calcification (CAC) significantly affects the diagnostic accuracy of both CCTA FFR-CT. A recent meta-analysis evaluated ten studies comparing FFR-CT and CCTA performance across different coronary artery calcium score categories, using invasive FFR as the reference standard [26]. The results showed that FFR-CT consistently outperformed CCTA in detecting hemodynamically significant stenoses at low to moderate calcium levels (CACS < 400), with notably higher area under the curve (AUC) values, both per-patient and per-vessel. For example, in patients with a CACS < 100, FFR-CT AUC reached 0.9 versus 0.32 for CCTA, while in CACS 100–399, FFR-CT maintained superior accuracy. The superiority of FFR-CT at lower calcium burdens is attributed to its computational fluid dynamics (CFD) approach, which integrates global coronary anatomy and physiological flow models, reducing the impact of the calcification-related artifacts that limit CCTA's lumen assessment. However, in patients with severe calcification (CACS ≥ 400), FFR-CT's diagnostic advantage diminishes, with specificity decreasing and AUC values declining. Further research is needed to establish a clear CACS threshold guiding its clinical application.

Despite its diagnostic potential, the dependency of FFR-CT on high-quality image acquisition remains a critical limitation. In real-world practice, non-diagnostic scan rates ranging from 10–25% raise valid concerns about reproducibility, especially in high-volume centers managing patients with common comorbidities or suboptimal scan conditions. These failure rates can undermine diagnostic confidence, delay clinical decision-making, and reduce overall workflow efficiency. Until improvements in scanner technology, acquisition protocols, and motion correction algorithms become more widely adopted, the integration of FFR-CT into routine clinical workflows will need to be approached cautiously, with a realistic understanding of its current technical constraints. Overall, FFR-CT shows promise in improving non-invasive evaluation of CAD, but optimizing its robustness across diverse clinical scenarios remains an important area for future innovation.

9. The Cost-Effectiveness and Economic Impact of FFR-CT in Clinical Practice

The cost of FFR-CT also presents a barrier to its routine use, especially in non-invasive diagnostic pathways. The Centers for Medicare & Medicaid Services (CMS) have set national payment rates for the HeartFlow® FFR-CT at $1017 for hospital outpatient settings and $839 for physician office settings. These rates are established under the Hospital Outpatient Prospective Payment System (OPPS) and the Physician Fee Schedule (PFS), respectively.

The PLATFORM study showed that using FFR-CT in evaluating stable patients with chest pain reduced healthcare costs [27]. The study evaluated 584 patients and found that using FFR-CT reduced costs by 32% in the invasive testing group ($7343 vs. $10,734; $p < 0.0001$) and improved quality of life in the noninvasive group (Seattle Angina Questionnaire score increase: 19.5 vs. 11.4; $p = 0.003$), compared to usual care. In the FORECAST trial ($n = 1400$), an FFR-CT-guided strategy showed no significant difference in total cardiac costs compared to standard care (£114 higher; $p = 0.10$) but significantly reduced invasive coronary angiography rates (19% vs. 25%; $p = 0.01$), suggesting potential economic efficiency attained by avoiding unnecessary invasive procedures [28].

However, while early trials suggest the potential for cost containment, these findings have limited generalizability to broader, real-world populations. The upfront cost of FFR-CT, over $1000 per analysis, remains financially prohibitive for many institutions, especially those in low- and middle-income countries or under tight budgetary constraints. Furthermore, reimbursement pathways for FFR-CT vary widely across health systems, often lacking clarity or consistency, which can deter adoption. Economic modeling studies have attempted to project long-term cost-effectiveness based on reduced downstream testing and improved care triage, but real-world validation of these models is still lacking. To facilitate broader implementation, future studies must evaluate FFR-CT's value in diverse clinical settings, incorporating heterogeneous populations and real-world cost data. Additionally, health economic strategies, such as bundled payments, value-based reimbursement models, or integration into clinical decision-support tools, may help align FFR-CT adoption with sustainable cost structures. Without such considerations, the widespread integration of FFR-CT into routine practice may remain limited despite its clinical promise.

10. Looking Ahead: Unlocking the Future Potential of FFR-CT

10.1. Evaluation of Coronary Artery Anomalies

Anomalous aortic origin of a coronary artery (AAOCA), particularly with an interarterial course, is a known risk factor for sudden cardiac death, especially among young individuals. Traditional imaging often struggles to determine the functional significance of such anomalies. FFR-CT has emerged as a promising tool that provides both anatomical and physiological insight in a non-invasive manner. In the ANOCOR registry, 62 patients with AAOCA underwent FFR-CT analysis, revealing that FFR-CT values were significantly lower in those with key morphological markers of an intramural course, including a takeoff angle $< 30°$, luminal narrowing $>50\%$, and eccentricity > 1.5. A proximal FFR-CT cutoff of ≤ 0.83 demonstrated high sensitivity (96%) and specificity (100%) for identifying intramural pathways [29]. These findings are notable, as the diagnostic threshold for AAOCA appears to be higher than the conventional ≤ 0.80 used in atherosclerotic disease. While FFR-CT reflects only the fixed anatomical component of AAOCA at rest, it may still aid in risk stratification, especially when considering dynamic changes during exertion. Complementing this, a separate study involving 94 patients with an interarterial anomalous right coronary artery from the left coronary sinus found that anatomical features such as slit-like ostium, low takeoff level, and presence of an intramural course were significantly associated with abnormal FFR-CT values (≤0.80) [30] (Figure 5). These anatomical predictors also correlated with a higher prevalence of both typical and atypical angina, highlighting FFR-CT's potential to gauge clinical relevance and symptom burden in AAOCA.

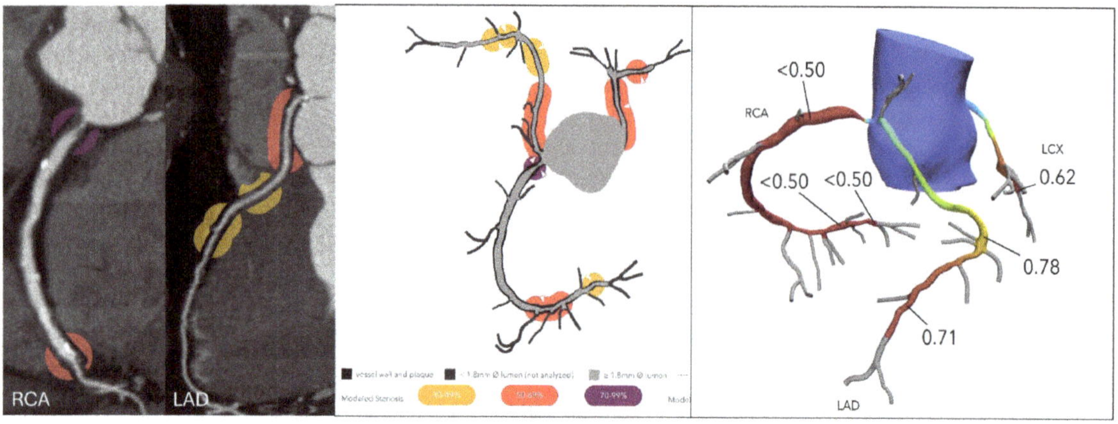

Figure 5. Anomalous aortic origin of the left coronary artery. (**Left**): Curved multiplanar reformatted coronary CT angiography (CTA) images in a 65-year-old male patient demonstrate severe stenosis at the ostium of the right coronary artery (RCA) and moderate stenosis at the ostium of the left anterior descending (LAD) artery, both originating from the right coronary cusp. (**Right**): Corresponding fractional flow reserve computed tomography (FFRCT) images show a value of 0.50 at 2 cm distal to the RCA ostial lesion, indicating significantly reduced flow. The mid LAD displays a value of 0.78, and the distal LAD shows a value of 0.71, suggesting a high likelihood of hemodynamic significance. Based on these findings, the patient proceeded to invasive coronary angiography and subsequent intervention for both lesions.

10.2. Plaque Characterization

Coronary computed tomography angiography has become the leading noninvasive tool for evaluating both calcified and high-risk coronary plaque features. Beyond identifying luminal narrowing, CCTA provides critical insight into plaque composition, including low-attenuation plaque (LAP), positive remodeling, and the overall plaque burden features collectively termed high-risk plaque (HRP) [31]. These advanced markers not only help refine risk assessment for CAD but also enhance the ability to predict ischemia and acute coronary syndromes.

Recent studies have demonstrated that total plaque volume and the presence of HRP features are more closely associated with ischemia, as measured by fractional flow reserve, whether invasive FFR or computed tomography-derived (FFR-CT), than stenosis severity alone. Specifically, LAP has emerged as a strong and independent predictor of ischemia. In fact, patients with two or more HRP features on CCTA have more than a threefold increased likelihood of ischemia on FFR-CT compared to those with only one HRP marker [32]. Together, plaque characterization with CCTA and physiological assessment with FFR-CT offer a comprehensive, noninvasive approach to understanding coronary disease and guiding patient management.

11. Myocardial Infarction and Ischemia in the Absence of Obstructive Coronary Artery Disease

Myocardial infarction with non-obstructive coronary arteries (MINOCA) and ischemia with non-obstructive coronary arteries (INOCA) represent distinct clinical conditions within the spectrum of ischemic heart disease, occurring in patients without significant coronary artery obstruction. MINOCA is characterized by elevated cardiac biomarkers indicative of myocardial infarction, despite angiographic evidence of minimal or no coronary stenosis. Its potential causes are diverse and include plaque disruption, spontaneous coronary artery dissection (SCAD), Takotsubo syndrome, myocarditis, coronary vasospasm, microvascular dysfunction, and supply–demand mismatch [33]. In a recent study, females aged 70 years or younger with myocardial infarction with MINOCA experienced a significantly higher incidence of major adverse events compared to both their male counterparts and females with myocardial infarction with obstructive coronary arteries (MIOCA). This difference is likely attributable to the distinct underlying pathophysiological mechanisms of ischemia in MINOCA, which may include coronary microvascular dysfunction, vasospasm, or spontaneous coronary artery dissection, rather than the atherosclerotic plaque rupture typically seen in MIOCA. These findings highlight the need for tailored diagnostic and therapeutic strategies in younger women presenting with MINOCA [34].

In such cases, ICA and intravascular imaging may be necessary, yet CCTA and FFR-CT can serve as valuable tools to exclude obstructive disease and detect alternative etiologies such as SCAD. INOCA, on the other hand, is defined by ischemic symptoms without biomarker elevation and is frequently underdiagnosed or misattributed to non-cardiac conditions. Common underlying mechanisms include coronary vasospasm and microvascular dysfunction [35].

Beyond FFR-CT, the HeartFlow® platform can compute the coronary volume-to-myocardial mass (V/M) ratio, offering additional insights into coronary flow capacity [36]. A low V/M ratio may suggest microvascular angina or myocardial supply–demand mismatch, helping to identify physiologic causes of ischemia in the absence of significant luminal narrowing [37,38]. Thus, in patients with MINOCA or INOCA, CCTA and FFR-CT, augmented by V/M analysis, offer a comprehensive, noninvasive approach to diagnosis and risk stratification.

In a prospective study of 153 patients with angina and nonobstructive coronary artery disease (ANOCA), 68 were found to have coronary microvascular dysfunction (CMD), and 22 of those exhibited high minimal microvascular resistance (>470 Wood units) [39]. Patients with CMD had a significantly lower coronary flow reserve compared to controls (1.9 ± 0.38 vs. 3.2 ± 0.81; $p < 0.001$). A strong inverse correlation was observed between lumen volume and microvascular resistance ($r = -0.59$; 95% CI: -0.45 to -0.71; $p < 0.001$). Those with CMD and high microvascular resistance had 40% smaller lumen volumes than controls (512.8 ± 130.3 mm^3 vs. 853.2 ± 341.2 mm^3; $p < 0.001$). Epicardial lumen volume, assessed by CCTA, was independently associated with microvascular resistance ($p < 0.001$). The ability of the CTA-derived lumen volume to predict high microvascular resistance demonstrated an area under the curve of 0.79 (95% CI: 0.69–0.88). These findings suggest CCTA may be valuable in the diagnostic workup of patients with CMD and ANOCA.

12. PCI and CABG Planning

One of the most promising advancements is the integration of FFR-CT into pre-procedural planning for PCI and coronary artery bypass grafting (CABG). The HeartFlow® Planner tool enables cardiologists to simulate revascularization strategies by assessing lesion-specific ischemia, determining optimal stent size and placement, and performing virtual remodeling of the coronary lumen. This allows for a functional evaluation of how PCI might impact coronary flow, before any intervention is performed.

Early feasibility studies have shown that FFR-CT values obtained after virtual stenting closely correlate with post-PCI invasive FFR, highlighting the potential of the technique to predict procedural success [40,41]. In a prospective, multicenter observational study involving 120 patients, the HeartFlow® Planner demonstrated high accuracy in matching both FFRINV and minimal stent area assessed via optical coherence tomography (OCT), even in complex scenarios involving diffuse disease and significant calcification [42]. In patients with tandem stenoses, the FFR-CT planner helps assess the added benefit of stenting each individual lesion. In cases of diffuse coronary disease, it supports optimizing the overall impact of the procedure while minimizing complications and limiting the total stent length used [43].

A recent patient-level meta-analysis of nine studies including 3336 coronary vessels (2760 patients) evaluated the prognostic value of post-PCI FFR across different coronary arteries [44]. The overall mean post-PCI FFR was 0.89 (95% CI: 0.87–0.90), with significantly lower values observed in left anterior descending (LAD) arteries compared to non-LAD vessels (0.86 vs. 0.93; $p < 0.001$). Lower post-PCI FFR was independently associated with increased risk of target vessel failure (TVF), primarily driven by target vessel revascularization. For every 0.10-unit decrease in FFR, the risk of TVF increased by 52%. However, predictive accuracy varied: post-PCI FFR had poor discrimination for TVF in the LAD (AUC: 0.52; 95% CI: 0.47–0.58) and moderate in non-LAD vessels (AUC: 0.66; 95% CI: 0.59–0.73; $p = 0.005$). These findings underscore the need for vessel-specific interpretation of post-PCI FFR and caution against applying uniform thresholds across all coronary territories.

Invasive coronary angiography has traditionally been the cornerstone for surgical planning in patients with complex multivessel CAD undergoing CABG. However, studies have shown that ICA alone may not reliably identify functionally significant stenoses, potentially leading to suboptimal graft targeting [45,46]. A major contributor to graft failure is competitive flow, particularly when grafts are placed to lesions that do not cause ischemia. This mechanism accounts for the failure of over 75% of internal thoracic artery (ITA) grafts in such cases [47]. Moreover, up to 25% of grafts do not result in improved regional myocardial perfusion post-CABG [48]. These findings underscore the importance of incorporating functional assessment into the preoperative evaluation to guide more effective and durable surgical revascularization strategies.

The role of FFR-CT as a non-invasive tool for identifying suitable CABG candidates and guiding surgical planning is increasingly recognized and supported by current clinical guidelines, based on evidence from multiple studies [49–52]. The first successful CABG procedure guided exclusively by FFR-CT has been recently documented [49], where post-operative FFR-CT assessments were also used to confirm functional improvement. Furthermore, the ongoing FASTTRACK CABG trial aims to evaluate the feasibility and reliability of planning CABG primarily using CCTA and FFR-CT, independent of invasive coronary angiography, potentially establishing a new paradigm in surgical decision-making [53]. These findings support the growing role of FFR-CT not only in diagnosis but also in guiding and optimizing therapeutic strategies, offering a noninvasive, patient-specific approach to coronary revascularization planning.

13. Filtering the Flow: FFR-CT as the New Gatekeeper to the Cath Lab

The main benefit of FFR-CT, demonstrated across multiple studies, is its ability to reduce unnecessary ICA [18,19,28]. In the PLATFORM trial, researchers found that an FFRCT-guided approach led to fewer referrals for cardiac catheterization, and patients who did undergo invasive coronary angiography were more likely to have obstructive CAD [18]. The ADVANCE study results demonstrated that FFR-CT led to a change in patient classification and influenced treatment plans in 66.9% of cases [19]. Additionally, among patients with an FFR-CT value of $\leq$0.80, subsequent invasive coronary angiography revealed a significantly higher likelihood of the identification of obstructive disease requiring revascularization [19].

The FORECAST trial was the first randomized study to evaluate the effectiveness of using CCTA combined with selective FFR-CT in patients with stable chest pain [28]. While overall medical costs were similar, the study found that patients assessed with FFR-CT were 22% less likely to undergo ICA. Moreover, when ICA was performed, those in the FFR-CT group had a 52% lower chance of having no obstructive coronary disease identified. These findings suggest that FFR-CT can help avoid unnecessary invasive procedures, while delivering clinical outcomes and quality of life comparable to traditional diagnostic pathways.

The PRECISE trial enrolled 2103 stable patients with suspected CAD across 65 sites, comparing a precision strategy (PS) to the usual testing (UT) [54]. The PS used the PROMISE minimal risk score to defer testing in 20.1% of low-risk patients, while others underwent CCTA with selective FFR-CT. The UT group received standard care, including stress testing or ICA.

At one year, the PS significantly improved clinical efficiency by reducing catheterizations without obstructive CAD from 10.2% in UT to 2.6% (hazard ratio [HR] 0.24; 95% CI, 0.16–0.36). The composite safety outcome of death or nonfatal myocardial infarction was similar between groups (HR 1.52; 95% CI, 0.73–3.15), with death rates of 0.5% vs. 0.7% and nonfatal MI rates of 1.2% vs. 0.5% for PS and UT, respectively. Notably, lipid-lowering (50.0% vs. 41.8%) and antiplatelet (35.7% vs. 27.1%) medication use rates were higher in the PS group (both $p < 0.001$).

These results demonstrate that FFR-CT, combined with risk stratification, effectively acts as a gatekeeper to the catheterization lab, reducing the number of unnecessary invasive procedures without compromising safety. The PRECISE trial supports adopting this approach for stable chest pain evaluation. However, it is important to recognize that most trials to date have enrolled highly selected patient populations, often excluding individuals with arrhythmias, high coronary calcium scores, obesity, renal dysfunction, prior revascularization, or other common comorbidities. These exclusions limit generalizability to real-world settings. Ongoing registry studies and advances in imaging technology are now aiming to address these gaps, and future research will be crucial to determine the effectiveness and scalability of FFR-CT across broader and more complex patient populations.

While FFR-CT demonstrates considerable promise in guiding the evaluation of stable chest pain, it is essential to contextualize its performance against other established and emerging diagnostic modalities. Positron emission tomography (PET), for example, offers superior spatial resolution and quantification of myocardial blood flow and coronary flow reserve, particularly useful in multivessel disease and microvascular dysfunction [55]. Positron emission tomography-derived myocardial flow reserve and invasive coronary flow reserve assess the combined effects of epicardial narrowing, diffuse atherosclerosis, and microvascular dysfunction on coronary blood flow. In contrast, fractional flow reserve primarily reflects the pressure gradient caused by focal and diffuse coronary artery disease. These measures are physiologically related but not interchangeable, with discordance observed in 30–40% of lesions.

Similarly, stress cardiac magnetic resonance imaging (CMR) provides high diagnostic accuracy and prognostic value, especially for identifying ischemia in patients with balanced or diffuse CAD. In a randomized trial of 918 patients with stable angina, CMR-guided care resulted in fewer index revascularizations than FFR-guided care (35.7% vs. 45.0%, $p = 0.005$). The primary outcome, major adverse cardiac events at one year, was similar between groups, meeting noninferiority criteria. These results support CMR as a safe and effective alternative [56].

Invasive pressure-derived indices such as instantaneous wave-free ratio (iFR) have also gained traction as an alternative to FFR, offering lesion-specific physiological assessment without the need for pharmacologic hyperemia. In a randomized trial of 2492 patients with CAD, instantaneous wave-free ratio (iFR)-guided revascularization was compared with FFR-guided revascularization [57]. At one year, major adverse cardiac events occurred in 6.8% of the iFR group and 7.0% of the FFR group, meeting noninferiority criteria. Procedural symptoms were significantly lower with iFR (3.1% vs. 30.8%, $p < 0.001$), and median procedure time was shorter (40.5 vs. 45.0 min, $p = 0.001$). These findings support iFR as a safe, efficient, and adenosine-free alternative to FFR in guiding coronary revascularization.

Hybrid diagnostic strategies combining anatomical and functional data, such as CCTA followed by PET or CMR in equivocal cases, can improve diagnostic accuracy and cost-effectiveness, particularly in complex or intermediate-risk patients. Thus, while FFR-CT offers non-invasive physiological assessment with good negative predictive value, it should be considered as part of a broader diagnostic toolbox rather than a standalone replacement. Tailoring test selection based on patient characteristics, availability, and clinical context remains critical to optimizing care.

14. Conclusions

Coronary computed tomography angiography and computed tomography-derived fractional flow reserve are rapidly redefining the landscape of CAD diagnosis and management, serving as both gatekeepers to the catheterization lab and catalysts for a more precise, noninvasive approach to modern cardiology. When used together, CCTA and FFR-CT deliver comprehensive insights into coronary anatomy, lesion-specific ischemia, high-risk plaque features, vessel wall stress, and volumetric metrics such as the vessel-to-myocardium ratio, none of which can be achieved through traditional noninvasive testing alone.

This integration of detailed anatomical and physiological data enables a more accurate diagnosis and risk stratification, reducing the number of unnecessary invasive coronary angiographies and allowing only truly indicated cases to proceed to the catheterization laboratory. Furthermore, emerging capabilities such as virtual PCI planning and functional SYNTAX scoring elevate these tools from a purely diagnostic function to therapeutic planning platforms. They assist in stent sizing and placement, and in predicting post-intervention flow, all from a noninvasive, pre-procedural standpoint.

Though limitations remain, particularly in patients with prior coronary stents or bypass surgery, the potential for CCTA and FFR-CT to replace invasive coronary angiography as the default diagnostic approach for stable coronary artery disease is becoming increasingly realistic. As image quality improves, costs decline, and computational power increases, the routine application of FFR-CT may become more accessible and widespread.

Author Contributions: Conceptualization: A.P.A. and M.G.-R.; Methodology: A.P.A. and M.G.-R.; Investigation: A.P.A. and M.G.-R.; Writing: A.K., M.A., T.H. and A.P.A.; Writing—review and editing: A.P.A. and M.G.-R.; Visualization: A.P.A. and M.G.-R.; Supervision: A.P.A. and M.G.-R.; Project administration: A.P.A. and M.G.-R. For this review article, research methodology, validation, formal analysis, resource provision, and curation were not separately determined. No software was developed to assist the analysis. All authors have read and agreed to the published version of the manuscript.

Funding: This research received no external funding.

Institutional Review Board Statement: No patients or human subjects were included in this study.

Informed Consent Statement: Not applicable.

Conflicts of Interest: All authors declare that there is no conflict of interest regarding the publication of this article.

References

1. Woodruff, R.C.; Tong, X.; Khan, S.S.; Shah, N.S.; Jackson, S.L.; Loustalot, F.; Vaughan, A.S. Trends in cardiovascular disease mortality rates and excess deaths, 2010–2022. *Am. J. Prev. Med.* **2024**, *66*, 582–589. [CrossRef] [PubMed]
2. Ferencik, M. Complex relationship between plaque characteristics and hemodynamic significance of stenosis: Insights from coronary computed tomography angiography imaging. *Atherosclerosis* **2017**, *260*, 150–152. [CrossRef] [PubMed]
3. Bertolone, D.T.; Gallinoro, E.; Esposito, G.; Paolisso, P.; Bermpeis, K.; De Colle, C.; Fabbricatore, D.; Mileva, N.; Valeriano, C.; Munhoz, D.; et al. Contemporary Management of Stable Coronary Artery Disease. *High. Blood Press. Cardiovasc. Prev.* **2022**, *29*, 207–219. [CrossRef] [PubMed]
4. Meijboom, W.B.; Meijs, M.F.L.; Schuijf, J.D.; Cramer, M.J.; Mollet, N.R.; van Mieghem, C.A.; Nieman, K.; van Werkhoven, J.M.; Pundziute, G.; Weustink, A.C.; et al. Diagnostic accuracy of 64-slice computed tomography coronary angiography. a prospective, multicenter, multivendor study. *J. Am. Coll. Cardiol.* **2008**, *52*, 2135–2144. [CrossRef]
5. Writing Committee Members; Gulati, M.; Levy, P.D.; Mukherjee, D.; Amsterdam, E.; Bhatt, D.L.; Birtcher, K.K.; Blankstein, R.; Boyd, J.; Bullock-Palmer, R.P.; et al. 2021 AHA/ACC/ASE/CHEST/SAEM/SCCT/SCMR Guideline for the Evaluation and Diagnosis of Chest Pain: Executive Summary: A Report of the American College of Cardiology/American Heart Association Joint Committee on Clinical Practice Guide-lines. *J. Am. Coll. Cardiol.* **2021**, *78*, 2218–2261. [CrossRef]
6. Adamson, P.D.; Williams, M.C.; Dweck, M.R.; Mills, N.L.; Boon, N.A.; Daghem, M.; Bing, R.; Moss, A.J.; Mangion, K.; Flather, M.; et al. Guiding therapy by coronary CT angiography improves outcomes in patients with stable chest pain. *J. Am. Coll. Cardiol.* **2019**, *74*, 2058–2070. [CrossRef]
7. DISCHARGE Trial Group; Maurovich-Horvat, P.; Bosserdt, M.; Kofoed, K.F.; Rieckmann, N.; Benedek, T.; Donnelly, P.; Rodriguez-Palomares, J.; Erglis, A.; Štěchovský, C.; et al. CT or invasive coronary angiography in stable chest pain. *N. Engl. J. Med.* **2022**, *386*, 1591–1602.
8. Pijls, N.H.; van Son, J.A.; Kirkeeide, R.L.; De Bruyne, B.; Gould, K.L. Experimental basis of determining maximum coronary, myocardial, and collateral blood flow by pressure measurements for assessing functional stenosis severity before and after percutaneous transluminal coronary angioplasty. *Circulation* **1993**, *87*, 1354–1367. [CrossRef]
9. Pijls, N.H.; De Bruyne, B.; Peels, K.; Van Der Voort, P.H.; Bonnier, H.J.; Bartunek, J.K.J.J.; Koolen, J.J. Measurement of fractional flow reserve to assess the functional severity of coronary-artery stenoses. *N. Engl. J. Med.* **1996**, *334*, 1703–1708. [CrossRef]
10. Pijls, N.H.; Fearon, W.F.; Tonino, P.A.; Siebert, U.; Ikeno, F.; Bornschein, B.; van't Veer, M.; Klauss, V.; Manoharan, G.; Engstrøm, T.; et al. Fractional flow reserve versus angiography for guiding percutaneous coronary intervention in patients with multivessel coronary artery disease: 2-year follow-up of the FAME (Fractional Flow Reserve versus Angiography for Multivessel Evaluation) study. *J. Am. Coll. Cardiol.* **2010**, *56*, 177–184. [CrossRef]
11. Fearon, W.F.; Nishi, T.; De Bruyne, B.; Boothroyd, D.B.; Barbato, E.; Tonino, P.; Jüni, P.; Pijls, N.H.J.; Hlatky, M.A. Clinical outcomes and cost-effectiveness of fractional flow reserve-guided percutaneous coronary intervention in patients with stable coronary artery disease: Three-year follow-up of the FAME 2 trial (fractional flow reserve versus angiography for multivessel evaluation). *Circulation* **2018**, *137*, 480–487.
12. Tröbs, M.; Achenbach, S.; Röther, J.; Redel, T.; Scheuering, M.; Winneberger, D.; Klingenbeck, K.; Itu, L.; Passerini, T.; Kamen, A.; et al. Comparison of fractional flow reserve based on computational fluid dynamics modeling using coronary angiographic vessel morphology versus invasively measured fractional flow reserve. *Am. J. Cardiol.* **2016**, *117*, 29–35. [CrossRef]
13. Narimani-Javid, R.; Moradi, M.; Mahalleh, M.; Najafi-Vosough, R.; Arzhangzadeh, A.; Khalique, O.; Mojibian, H.; Kuno, T.; Mohsen, A.; Alam, M.; et al. Machine learning and computational fluid dynamics derived FFRCT demonstrate comparable diagnostic performance in patients with coronary artery disease; A Systematic Review and Meta-Analysis. *J. Cardiovasc. Comput. Tomogr.* **2025**, *19*, 232–246. [CrossRef]
14. Koo, B.K.; Erglis, A.; Doh, J.H.; Daniels, D.V.; Jegere, S.; Kim, H.S.; Dunning, A.; DeFrance, T.; Lansky, A.; Leipsic, J.; et al. Diagnosis of ischemia-causing coronary stenoses by noninvasive fractional flow reserve computed from coronary computed tomographic angiograms. Results from the prospective multi-center DISCOVER-FLOW (Diagnosis of Ischemia-Causing Stenoses Obtained Via Noninvasive Fractional Flow Reserve) study. *J. Am. Coll. Cardiol.* **2011**, *58*, 1989–1997.
15. Min, J.K.; Leipsic, J.; Pencina, M.J.; Berman, D.S.; Koo, B.K.; van Mieghem, C.; Erglis, A.; Lin, F.Y.; Dunning, A.M.; Apruzzese, P.; et al. Diagnostic accuracy of fractional flow reserve from anatomic CT angiography. *JAMA* **2012**, *308*, 1237–1245. [CrossRef]

16. Nørgaard, B.L.; Leipsic, J.; Gaur, S.; Seneviratne, S.; Ko, B.S.; Ito, H.; Jensen, J.M.; Mauri, L.; De Bruyne, B.; Bezerra, H.; et al. NXT Trial Study Group. Diagnostic performance of noninvasive fractional flow reserve derived from coronary computed tomography angiography in suspected coronary artery disease: The NXT trial (analysis of coronary blood flow using CT angiography: Next steps). *J. Am. Coll. Cardiol.* **2014**, *63*, 1145–1155. [PubMed]
17. Danad, I.; Raijmakers, P.G.; Driessen, R.S.; Driessen, R.S.; Leipsic, J.; Raju, R.; Naoum, C.; Knuuti, J.; Mäki, M.; Underwood, R.S.; et al. Comparison of coronary CT angiography, SPECT, PET, and hybrid imaging for diagnosis of ischemic heart disease determined by fractional flow reserve. *JAMA Cardiol.* **2017**, *2*, 1100–1107. [CrossRef] [PubMed]
18. Douglas, P.S.; Pontone, G.; Hlatky, M.A.; Patel, M.R.; Norgaard, B.L.; Byrne, R.A.; Curzen, N.; Purcell, I.; Gutberlet, M.; Rioufol, G.; et al. Clinical outcomes of fractional flow reserve by computed tomographic angiography-guided diagnostic strategies vs. usual care in patients with suspected coronary artery disease: The prospective longitudinal trial of FFR(CT)—Outcome and resource impacts study. *Eur. Heart J.* **2015**, *36*, 3359–3367. [PubMed]
19. Fairbairn, T.A.; Nieman, K.; Akasaka, T.; Nørgaard, B.L.; Berman, D.S.; Raff, G.; Hurwitz-Koweek, L.M.; Pontone, G.; Kawasaki, T.; Sand, N.P.; et al. Real-world clinical utility and impact on clinical decision-making of coronary computed tomography angiography-derived fractional flow reserve: Lessons from the ADVANCE Registry. *Eur. Heart J.* **2018**, *39*, 3701–3711. [CrossRef]
20. Andreini, D.; Modolo, R.; Katagiri, Y.; Mushtaq, S.; Sonck, J.; Collet, C.; De Martini, S.; Roberto, M.; Tanaka, K.; Miyazaki, Y.; et al. Impact of fractional flow reserve derived from coronary computed tomography angiography on heart team treatment decision-making in patients with multivessel coronary artery disease: Insights from the SYNTAX III REVOLUTION trial. *Circ. Cardiovasc. Interv.* **2019**, *12*, e007607. [CrossRef]
21. Lammens, J.; Motoc, A.; Tanaka, K.; Belsack, D.; Vandeloo, B.; Lochy, S.; Schoors, D.; Van Loo, I.; De Potter, T.; Michiels, V.; et al. Favorable impact of FFR_{CT} on myocardial revascularization outcomes: Results from an observational real-world registry. *Int. J. Cardiol.* **2025**, *15*, 431–133245.
22. Faulder, T.I.; Prematunga, K.; Moloi, S.B.; Faulder, L.E.; Jones, R.; Moxon, J.V. Agreement of fractional flow reserve estimated by computed tomography with invasively measured fractional flow reserve: A systematic review and meta-analysis. *J. Am. Heart Assoc.* **2024**, *13*, e034552. [CrossRef] [PubMed]
23. Takagi, H.; Ishikawa, Y.; Orii, M.; Ota, H.; Niiyama, M.; Tanaka, R.; Morino, Y.; Yoshioka, K. Optimized interpretation of fractional flow reserve derived from computed tomography: Comparison of three interpretation methods. *J. Cardiovasc. Comput. Tomogr.* **2019**, *13*, 134–141. [CrossRef] [PubMed]
24. Cami, E.; Tagami, T.; Raff, G.; Fonte, T.A.; Renard, B.; Gallagher, M.J.; Chinnaiyan, K.; Bilolikar, A.; Fan, A.; Hafeez, A.; et al. Assessment of lesion-specific ischemia using fractional flow reserve (FFR) profiles derived from coronary computed tomography angiography (FFRCT) and invasive pressure measurements (FFRINV): Importance of the site of measurement and implications for patient referral for invasive coronary angiography and percutaneous coronary interventions. *J. Cardiovasc. Comput. Tomogr.* **2018**, *12*, 480–492. [CrossRef]
25. Lu, M.T.; Ferencik, M.; Roberts, R.S.; Lee, K.L.; Ivanov, A.; Adami, E.; Mark, D.B.; Jaffer, F.A.; Leipsic, J.A.; Douglas, P.S.; et al. Noninvasive FFR derived from coronary CT angiography. *JACC Cardiovasc. Imaging* **2017**, *10*, 1350–1358. [CrossRef]
26. Ma, Z.; Tu, C.; Zhang, B.; Zhang, D.; Song, X.; Zhang, H. A meta-analysis comparing the diagnostic performance of computed tomography-derived fractional flow reserve and coronary computed tomography angiography at different levels of coronary artery calcium score. *Eur. Radiol.* **2024**, *34*, 5621–5632. [CrossRef]
27. Hlatky, M.A.; De Bruyne, B.; Pontone, G.; Patel, M.R.; Norgaard, B.L.; Byrne, R.A.; Curzen, N.; Purcell, I.; Gutberlet, M.; Rioufol, G.; et al. Quality-of-life and economic outcomes of assessing fractional flow reserve with computed tomography angiography. *J. Am. Coll. Cardiol.* **2015**, *66*, 2315–2323. [CrossRef]
28. Curzen, N.; Nicholas, Z.; Stuart, B.; Wilding, S.; Hill, K.; Shambrook, J.; Eminton, Z.; Ball, D.; Barrett, C.; Johnson, L.; et al. Fractional flow reserve derived from computed tomography coronary angiography in the assessment and management of stable chest pain: The FORECAST randomized trial. *Eur. Heart J.* **2021**, *42*, 3844–3852. [CrossRef]
29. Ferrag, W.; Scalbert, F.; Adjedj, J.; Dupouy, P.; Ou, P.; Juliard, J.M.; Farnoud, R.; Benadji, A.A.; Du Fretay, X.H.; Wijns, W.; et al. Role of FFR-CT for the evaluation of patients with anomalous aortic origin of coronary artery. *JACC Cardiovasc. Imaging* **2021**, *14*, 1074–1076. [CrossRef]
30. Tang, C.X.; Lu, M.J.; Schoepf, J.U.; Tesche, C.; Bauer, M.; Nance, J.; Griffith, P.; Lu, G.M.; Zhang, L.J. Coronary computed tomography angiography-derived fractional flow reserve in patients with anomalous origin of the right coronary artery from the left coronary sinus. *Korean J. Radiol.* **2020**, *21*, 192–202. [CrossRef]
31. Motoyama, S.; Ito, H.; Sarai, M.; Kondo, T.; Kawai, H.; Nagahara, Y.; Harigaya, H.; Kan, S.; Anno, H.; Takahashi, H.; et al. Plaque characterization by coronary computed tomography angiography and the likelihood of acute coronary events in mid-term follow-up. *J. Am. Coll. Cardiol.* **2015**, *66*, 337–346. [CrossRef] [PubMed]
32. Park, H.B.; Heo, R.; Hartaigh, B.; Cho, I.; Gransar, H.; Nakazato, R.; Leipsic, J.; Mancini, G.B.J.; Koo, B.K.; Otake, H.; et al. Atherosclerotic plaque characteristics by CT angiography identify coronary lesions that cause ischemia. A direct comparison to fractional flow reserve. *J. Am. Coll. Cardiol. Imaging* **2015**, *8*, 1–10. [CrossRef] [PubMed]

33. Tamis-Holland, J.E.; Jneid, H.; Reynolds, H.R.; Agewall, S.; Brilakis, E.S.; Brown, T.M.; Lerman, A.; Cushman, M.; Kumbhani, D.J.; Arslanian-Engoren, C.; et al. Contemporary diagnosis and management of patients with myocardial infarction in the absence of obstructive coronary artery disease. A scientific statement from the American Heart Association. *Circulation* **2019**, *139*, e891–e908. [CrossRef] [PubMed]
34. Canton, L.; Fedele, D.; Bergamaschi, L.; Foà, A.; Di Iuorio, O.; Tattilo, F.P.; Rinaldi, A.; Angeli, F.; Armillotta, M.; Sansonetti, A.; et al. Sex- and age-related differences in outcomes of patients with acute myocardial infarction: MINOCA vs. MIOCA. *Eur. Heart J. Acute Cardiovasc. Care* **2023**, *12*, 604–614. [CrossRef]
35. Kunadian, V.; Chieffo, A.; Camici, P.G.; Berry, C.; Escaned, J.; Maas, A.; Prescott, E.; Karam, N.; Appelman, Y.; Fraccaro, C.; et al. An EAPCI expert consensus document on ischaemia with non-obstructive coronary arteries in collaboration with European society of cardiology working group on coronary pathophysiology & microcirculation endorsed by coronary vasomotor disorders international study group. *Eur. Heart J.* **2020**, *41*, 3504–3520.
36. Taylor, C.A.; Gaur, S.; Leipsic, J.; Achenbach, S.; Berman, D.S.; Jensen, J.M.; Dey, D.; Bøtker, H.E.; Kim, H.J.; Khem, S.; et al. Effect of the ratio of coronary arterial lumen volume to left ventricle myocardial mass derived from coronary CT angiography on fractional flow reserve. *J. Cardiovasc. Comput. Tomogr.* **2017**, *11*, 429–436. [CrossRef]
37. Grover, R.; Leipsic, J.A.; Mooney, J.; Kueh, S.H.; Ohana, M.; Nørgaard, B.L.; Eftekhari, A.; Bax, J.J.; Murphy, D.T.; Hague, C.J.; et al. Coronary lumen volume to myocardial mass ratio in primary microvascular angina. *J. Cardiovasc. Comput. Tomogr.* **2017**, *11*, 423–428. [CrossRef]
38. Kuneman, J.H.; El Mahdiui, M.; van Rosendael, A.R.; van den Hoogen, I.J.; Patel, M.R.; Nørgaard, B.L.; Fairbairn, T.A.; Nieman, K.; Akasaka, T.; Berman, D.S.; et al. Coronary volume to left ventricular mass ratio in patients with diabetes mellitus. *J. Cardiovasc. Comput. Tomogr.* **2022**, *16*, 319–326. [CrossRef]
39. Collet, C.; Sakai, K.; Mizukami, T.; Ohashi, H.; Bouisset, F.; Caglioni, S.; van Hoe, L.; Gallinoro, E.; Bertolone, D.T.; Pardaens, S.; et al. Vascular Remodeling in Coronary Microvascular Dysfunction. *JACC Cardiovasc. Imaging* **2024**, *17*, 1463–1476. [CrossRef]
40. Kim, K.H.; Doh, J.H.; Koo, B.K.; Min, J.K.; Erglis, A.; Yang, H.M.; Park, K.W.; Lee, H.Y.; Kang, H.J.; Kim, Y.J.; et al. A novel noninvasive technology for treatment planning using virtual coronary stenting and computed tomography-derived computed fractional flow reserve. *J. Am. Coll. Cardiol. Interv.* **2014**, *7*, 72–78. [CrossRef]
41. Bom, M.J.; Schumacher, S.P.; Driessen, R.S.; van Diemen, P.A.; Everaars, H.; de Winter, R.W.; van de Ven, P.M.; van Rossum, A.C.; Sprengers, R.W.; Verouden, N.J.W.; et al. Non-invasive procedural planning using computed tomography-derived fractional flow reserve. *Catheter. Cardiovasc. Interv.* **2021**, *97*, 614–622. [CrossRef]
42. Sonck, J.; Nagumo, S.; Norgaard, B.L.; Otake, H.; Ko, B.; Zhang, J.; Mizukami, T.; Maeng, M.; Andreini, D.; Takahashi, Y.; et al. Clinical validation of a virtual planner for coronary interventions based on coronary CT angiography. *J. Am. Coll. Cardiol. Imaging* **2022**, *15*, 1242–1255. [CrossRef]
43. Modi, B.N.; Sankaran, S.; Kim, H.J.; Ellis, H.; Rogers, C.; Taylor, C.A.; Rajani, R.; Perera, D. Predicting the physiological effect of revascularization in serially diseased coronary arteries. *Circ. Cardiovasc. Interv.* **2019**, *12*, e007577. [CrossRef] [PubMed]
44. Collet, C.; Johnson, N.P.; Mizukami, T.; Fearon, W.F.; Berry, C.; Sonck, J.; Collison, D.; Koo, B.K.; Meneveau, N.; Agarwal, S.K.; et al. Impact of Post-PCI FFR Stratified by Coronary Artery. *JACC Cardiovasc. Interv.* **2023**, *16*, 2396–2408. [CrossRef] [PubMed]
45. Fischer, J.J.; Samady, H.; McPherson, J.A.; Sarembock, I.J.; Powers, E.R.; Gimple, L.W.; Ragosta, M. Comparison between visual assessment and quantitative angiography versus fractional flow reserve for native coronary narrowings of moderate severity. *Am. J. Cardiol.* **2002**, *90*, 210–215. [CrossRef] [PubMed]
46. Tonino, P.A.; Fearon, W.F.; De Bruyne, B.; Oldroyd, K.G.; Leesar, M.A.; Ver Lee, P.N.; Maccarthy, P.A.; Van't Veer, M.; Pijls, N.H. Angiographic versus functional severity of coronary artery stenoses in the FAME study fractional flow reserve versus angiography in multivessel evaluation. *J. Am. Coll. Cardiol.* **2010**, *55*, 2816–2821. [CrossRef]
47. Ferguson, T.B.; Chen, C., Jr.; Babb, J.D.; Efird, J.T.; Daggubati, R.; Cahill, J.M. Fractional flow reserve–guided coronary artery bypass grafting: Can intraoperative physiologic imaging guide decision making? *J. Thorac. Cardiovasc. Surg.* **2013**, *146*, 824–835. [CrossRef]
48. Fractional flow reserve to guide to assess coronary artery bypass grafting. *Eur. Heart J.* **2017**, *38*, 1959–1968.
49. Kawashima, H.; Onuma, Y.; Andreini, D.; Mushtaq, S.; Morel, M.A.; Masuda, S.; Taylor, C.A.; Bartorelli, A.L.; Serruys, P.W.; Pompilio, G. Successful coronary artery bypass grafting based solely on non-invasive coronary computed tomography angiography. *Cardiovasc. Revasc. Med.* **2022**, *40*, 187–189. [CrossRef]
50. Sonck, J.; Miyazaki, Y.; Collet, C.; Onuma, Y.; Asano, T.; Takahashi, K.; Kogame, N.; Katagiri, Y.; Modolo, R.; Serruys, P.W.; et al. Feasibility of planning coronary artery bypass grafting based only on coronary computed tomography angiography and CT-derived fractional flow reserve: A pilot survey of the surgeons involved in the randomized SYNTAX III Revolution trial. *Interact. Cardiovasc. Thorac. Surg.* **2019**, *29*, 209–216. [CrossRef]
51. Knuuti, J.; Wijns, W.; Saraste, A.; Capodanno, D.; Barbato, E.; Funck-Brentano, C.; Prescott, E.; Storey, R.F.; Deaton, C.; Cuisset, T.; et al. 2019 ESC Guidelines for the diagnosis and management of chronic coronary syndromes. *Eur. Heart J.* **2020**, *41*, 407–477. [CrossRef]

52. Moss, A.J.; Williams, M.C.; Newby, D.E.; Nicol, E.D. The updated NICE guidelines: Cardiac CT as the first-line test for coronary artery disease. *Curr. Cardiovasc. Imaging Rep.* **2017**, *10*, 15. [CrossRef]
53. Kawashima, H.; Pompilio, G.; Andreini, D.; Bartorelli, A.L.; Mushtaq, S.; Ferrari, E.; Maisano, F.; Buechel, R.R.; Tanaka, K.; La Meir, M.; et al. Safety and feasibility evaluation of planning and execution of surgical revascularisation solely based on coronary CTA and FFRCT in patients with complex coronary artery disease: Study protocol of the FASTTRACK CABG study. *BMJ Open* **2020**, *10*, e038152. [CrossRef]
54. Douglas, P.S.; Nanna, M.G.; Kelsey, M.D.; Yow, E.; Mark, D.B.; Patel, M.R.; Rogers, C.; Udelson, J.E.; Fordyce, C.B.; Curzen, N.; et al. Comparison of an initial risk-based testing strategy vs usual testing in stable symptomatic patients with suspected coronary artery disease. *JAMA Cardiol.* **2023**, *8*, 904–914. [CrossRef]
55. Murthy, V.L.; Bateman, T.M.; Beanlands, R.S.; Berman, D.S.; Borges-Neto, S.; Chareonthaitawee, P.; Cerqueira, M.D.; deKemp, R.A.; DePuey, E.G.; Dilsizian, V.; et al. Clinical Quantification of Myocardial Blood Flow Using PET: Joint Position Paper of the SNMMI Cardiovascular Council and the ASNC. *J. Nucl. Med.* **2018**, *59*, 273–293. [CrossRef] [PubMed]
56. Nagel, E.; Greenwood, J.P.; McCann, G.P.; Bettencourt., N.; Shah, A.M.; Hussain, S.T.; Perera, D.; Plein, S.; Bucciarelli-Ducci, C.; Paul, M.; et al. Magnetic Resonance Perfusion or Fractional Flow Reserve in Coronary Disease. *N. Engl. J. Med.* **2019**, *380*, 2418–2428. [CrossRef] [PubMed]
57. Davies, J.E.; Sen, S.; Dehbi, H.M.; Al-Lamee, R.; Petraco, R.; Nijjer, S.S.; Bhindi, R.; Lehman, S.J.; Walters, D.; Sapontis, J.; et al. Use of the Instantaneous Wave-free Ratio or Fractional Flow Reserve in PCI. *N. Engl. J. Med.* **2017**, *376*, 1824–1834. [CrossRef] [PubMed]

Journal of
Cardiovascular Development and Disease

MDPI

Review

Advancements in Acute Pulmonary Embolism Diagnosis and Treatment: A Narrative Review of Emerging Imaging Techniques and Intravascular Interventions

Michaela Cellina [1,*], Matilde Pavan [2], Niccolò Finardi [2], Francesco Cicchetti [2], Maurizio Cè [3], Pierpaolo Biondetti [3], Carolina Lanza [3], Serena Carriero [3] and Gianpaolo Carrafiello [2,3]

1 Radiology Department, ASST Fatebenefratelli Sacco, Ospedale Fatebenefratelli, Piazza Principessa Clotilde 3, 20121 Milan, Italy
2 Postgraduate School in Radiodiagnostics, Università degli Studi di Milano, Via Festa del Perdono 7, 20122 Milan, Italy; matilde.pavan@unimi.it (M.P.); niccolo.finardi@unimi.it (N.F.); francesco.cicchetti@unimi.it (F.C.)
3 Radiology Department, Fondazione IRCCS Ca' Granda Ospedale Maggiore Policlinico, Via Francesco Sforza 35, 20122 Milano, Italy; maurizioce.md1@gmail.com (M.C.); carolina.lanza@policlinico.mi.it (C.L.); serena.carriero@policlinico.mi.it (S.C.)
* Correspondence: michaela.cellina@asst-fbf-sacco.it; Tel.: +39-0263632424

Abstract: Acute pulmonary embolism (APE) represents a significant cause of morbidity and mortality worldwide, requiring rapid and precise diagnosis and effective therapy strategies. Computed Tomography Pulmonary Angiography (CTPA) is currently the gold standard technique for diagnosing PE; however, it presents some disadvantages, including limited sensitivity in detecting sub-segmental emboli and contrast-related risks. Recent advancements in imaging technologies, including Dual-Energy Computed Tomography (DECT) and Photon Counting (PC), offer improved sensitivity and specificity for APE and perfusion abnormalities detection. Digital Dynamic Radiography (DDR) perfusion imaging represents a novel imaging that allows pulmonary perfusion assessment without contrast medium administration, able to detect anomalies at the patient's bedside, representing a promising advancement, particularly for critically ill or contrast-allergic patients. In parallel, interventional radiology has become integral to APE management, particularly for high-risk and intermediate–high-risk patients, with evolving intravascular treatment techniques such as catheter-directed thrombolysis, mechanical thrombectomy, and thrombus aspiration. This narrative review provides an overview of the latest developments in APE diagnostic imaging and interventional radiology, contextualizing them within current guideline recommendations for endovascular treatment.

Keywords: pulmonary embolism; photon counting CT; DECT; mechanical thrombectomy; catheter-directed thrombolysis

1. Introduction

Acute pulmonary embolism (APE) is a serious condition characterized by the obstruction of blood circulation in the pulmonary arteries or their branches, mainly caused by a blood clot, which typically originates in the deep venous system of the legs [1]. This condition places a significant strain on healthcare systems, with an estimated occurrence of 39 to 115 cases per 100,000 individuals annually in the United States, and a steady rise over the last ten years [2]. Additionally, the literature reports that around one-third of patients with APE will experience a recurrence within a decade [2].

Although APE is the third leading cause of cardiovascular-related deaths, after coronary artery disease and stroke [3], estimating the precise case/fatality rates for PE can be challenging, with a mortality rate that varies between 60% to less than 1% [4]. This variability highlights the need for effective and timely diagnostic and therapeutic strategies, with early detection being crucial. Early and accurate diagnosis is essential for prompt, life-saving therapy while avoiding unnecessary anticoagulation treatments in patients without APE. The clinical presentation of APE is highly variable and often nonspecific, overlapping with other cardiopulmonary conditions such as pneumonia, acute coronary syndrome, and heart failure [5], making diagnosis highly dependent on imaging techniques [6]. However, despite the often non-specific clinical signs, the introduction of clinical prediction tools, such as the Wells Score, the Geneva Score and the YEARS algorithm, has significantly aided clinicians in identifying patients who are more likely to have APE and should therefore undergo further diagnostic imaging [7].

Incidental APE detection on CT scans across different populations is approximately 2.6%, with elevated rates in cancer patients (up to 5%) and hospitalized individuals [5], with most incidental APEs clinically relevant [5].

Throughout the years, computed tomography pulmonary angiography (CTPA) has emerged as the reference standard imaging method for diagnosing APE [2]. CTPA is a non-invasive procedure characterized by high sensitivity (96–100%) and specificity (89–98%) [8], but despite its accuracy, CTPA has drawbacks, as it heavily depends on optimal contrast opacification of the pulmonary arterial tree, which can be affected in patients with poor cardiac output, improper timing of contrast bolus and other technical issues, leading to non-diagnostic results. Additionally, the use of ionizing radiation and iodinated contrast media presents cumulative risks, especially in younger patients, pregnant women, and those with existing renal issues or contrast allergies [9]. These constraints underscore the necessity for ongoing enhancement of diagnostic approaches and the investigation of new imaging techniques.

Recent imaging methods have proven valuable for diagnosing APE. Dual-Energy CT (DECT) enables the generation of pulmonary perfusion maps, offering functional data alongside anatomical details, enhancing diagnostic precision, while minimizing the volume of contrast agent [10,11]. Likewise, photon-counting detector CT (PC) demonstrates distinct advantages, such as decreased radiation exposure and minimized contrast agent needs, while maintaining superior image quality [12]. Additionally, Dynamic Digital Radiography (DDR) is emerging as a valuable non-invasive method for evaluating pulmonary function and blood flow, demonstrating a strong ability to identify chronic thromboembolic pulmonary hypertension, akin to ventilation/perfusion scans [13].

Along with these imaging innovations, the management of APE is also evolving, with the emergence of risk-stratification tools and interventional radiology-based treatments [14]. These techniques, including catheter-directed thrombolysis and mechanical thrombectomy, have emerged as effective alternatives, especially for patients with contraindications to systemic thrombolysis or those who have not responded to it [15]. Recent studies have not only demonstrated the safety and efficacy of these interventional approaches but also aim to further evaluate the role of interventional radiology for intermediate–high-risk APE patients, expanding the therapeutic indications of these techniques [16].

This review explores emerging imaging and interventional techniques that are playing an increasingly important role in both the diagnosis and treatment of APE, with a focus on their recent developments and potential clinical applications.

2. Search Strategy and Methodology

We conducted a review of the literature by searching the PubMed database up to May 2025 using the following key terms, individually and in combination: 'pulmonary embolism', 'computed tomography pulmonary angiography', 'dual-energy CT', 'photon-counting CT', 'dynamic digital radiography', 'catheter-directed thrombolysis', 'mechanical thrombectomy', 'low-dose systemic thrombolysis' and 'artificial intelligence'. Additional relevant articles were identified through manual reference checks of selected papers and recent guidelines.

3. Diagnostic Imaging

Recent advances in imaging technology have emerged to address some of the inherent limitations of CTPA, which, despite these developments, remains the current gold standard for the diagnosis of APE.

3.1. High-Pitch CT

High-pitch helical CT scanning enables rapid acquisition of thoracic images, which is particularly useful in the emergency setting for patients who are dyspneic or unable to cooperate. A recent study analyzed 81 normal-weight patients referred for CTPA for suspected APE: forty-one patients underwent the high-pitch CTPA protocol, while 40 underwent the standard CTPA protocol, both on a second-generation dual-source CT scanner [17]. The key differences between the protocols included the scan pitch (3.2 for high-pitch vs. 1.2 as a standard), scan time (<1 s for high-pitch vs. ~2 s as standard), breathing instructions (free-breathing for high-pitch vs. breath-hold as a standard), and contrast medium volume (20 mL for high-pitch vs. 50 mL). The detection rate of APE was also similar in both groups, and subjective image quality was rated as good to excellent (rating score 1) in over 90% of all exams for both protocols. Contrast opacification was systematically above 250 HU in the high-pitch group, which is considered sufficient for differentiating clots from surrounding tissues. High-pitch CTPA with ultra-low contrast volume resulted in significantly lower mean contrast opacification and noise values in all segmental pulmonary arteries compared to standard CTPA. The median effective dose was significantly lower for high-pitch CTPA (1.04 mSv) than for standard CTPA (1.49 mSv) ($p < 0.0001$), with a dose saving of approximately 30% [17]. The high-pitch mode's short acquisition time can also mitigate or avoid motion artifacts.

3.2. Dual Energy CT

3.2.1. Principles of DECT

DECT relies on the differences in the photoelectric effect and Compton scattering at different energetic levels to generate material-specific maps for the characterization of different tissues and components. Several dual-energy acquisition techniques are currently in clinical use, including dual-source systems, rapid kVp-switching single-source scanners, and layered detector configurations.

Post-processing techniques enable the generation of virtual monoenergetic images (VMIs), virtual non-contrast images (VNC), and iodine distribution maps, all of which contribute to enhanced diagnostic confidence and potentially reduce the need for additional imaging [18]. Iodine maps derived from DECT datasets allow for the visualization of regional pulmonary perfusion by quantifying iodine distribution within the lung parenchyma [19]. these color-coded blood volume maps can reveal perfusion defects corresponding to embolized pulmonary arterial territories, supporting or clarifying vascular findings [20]. DECT integrates both anatomic and functional assessments: the CT angiogram visualizes the clot anatomically, while the iodine map reveals the resulting perfusion deficit, similar to what is seen in a nuclear perfusion scan. This allows for an improved reader detection of segmental and sub-segmental emboli and enables functional assessment of perfusion [21].

3.2.2. Accuracy of DECT

Thieme et al. [22] examined the diagnostic accuracy of DECT perfusion imaging in relation to perfusion scintigraphy. They found a sensitivity and specificity of 75% and 80% per patient, respectively, and a good agreement with scintigraphic findings. In a later investigation [23], the authors explored the diagnostic performance DECT iodine maps (which analyze perfusion defects) against SPECT/CT, finding a sensitivity of 76.7% and a specificity of 98.2%. When evaluating a consensus interpretation of all imaging techniques as the reference standard, DECT-CTPA exhibited 100% sensitivity and specificity in identifying APE, surpassing the combination of SPECT/CT and ventilation scintigraphy (85.7% sensitivity, 87.5% specificity). Grob et al. [24] conducted a prospective study comparing subtraction CT and DECT iodine maps to conventional CTPA. DECT achieved a specificity of 95% and a sensitivity of 85%, which was not significantly different from that of CTPA alone (80% sensitivity).

A meta-analysis by Monti et al. [25] assessed the diagnostic performance of DECT for APE detection, focusing exclusively on lobar and segmental emboli. The analysis stratified results based on different DECT post-processing techniques: linear blending (LB) alone showed a pooled sensitivity of 0.87 (95% CI: 0.76–0.95) and specificity of 0.93 (95% CI: 0.87–0.97) across six study components involving 348 patients; LB combined with iodine maps showed a slightly improved sensitivity of 0.89 (95% CI: 0.82–0.94) and specificity of 0.90 (95% CI: 0.86–0.94), based on 14 study components and 1007 patients; the combination of LB, iodine maps, and VMIs achieved a sensitivity of 0.90 (95% CI: 0.70–0.98) and specificity of 0.90 (95% CI: 0.77–0.97), although data were limited to two studies totaling 144 patients. Despite these encouraging results, the meta-analysis concluded that DECT, regardless of the reconstruction approach used, did not demonstrate a substantial diagnostic advantage over conventional single-energy CT (SECT) [26].

Finally, Foti et al. [27] prospectively evaluated the diagnostic performance of venous-phase DECT in oncology patients, using standard CTPA as the reference standard. Among 61 patients (30 with confirmed APE), venous phase DECT demonstrated a per-patient sensitivity of 90.0% and specificity of 100% for both readers; lung perfusion imaging showed lower performance, with a per-patient sensitivity of 73.3% and specificity of 67.7%.

In addition to detection, DECT offers further characterization and prognostic information; perfusion defect scoring has been suggested to measure APE severity, and research has indicated a link to right ventricular dysfunction and negative outcomes [28,29]. It provides considerable benefits concerning the creation of VNC and virtual VMIs from one contrast-enhanced acquisition. VNC images are produced by subtracting the iodine-attenuation component from the contrast-enhanced dataset using material decomposition algorithms, thereby simulating a non-contrast examination [30], and eliminating the need for an additional scan, significantly reducing radiation exposure, particularly important for young patients and those undergoing repeated imaging. Additionally, VNC images enhance the assessment of incidental pulmonary nodules, vascular calcifications, or hemorrhage by allowing a thorough examination of lung parenchyma, calcifications, and mediastinal structures revealed by intravenous contrast.

VMIs are images synthesized at different energy levels, usually ranging from 40 to 190 keV (Figures 1 and 2). VMIs at low-keV levels (e.g., 40–60 keV) increase the attenuation of iodine within the pulmonary arteries, improving the contrast-to-noise ratio and the conspicuity of emboli in pulmonary arteries, also compensating for suboptimal contrast opacification due to low cardiac output, poor injection technique, or delayed bolus timing. VMIs also allow for the reduction in the administered contrast medium amount without compromising vascular visualization, particularly useful in patients with impaired renal function.

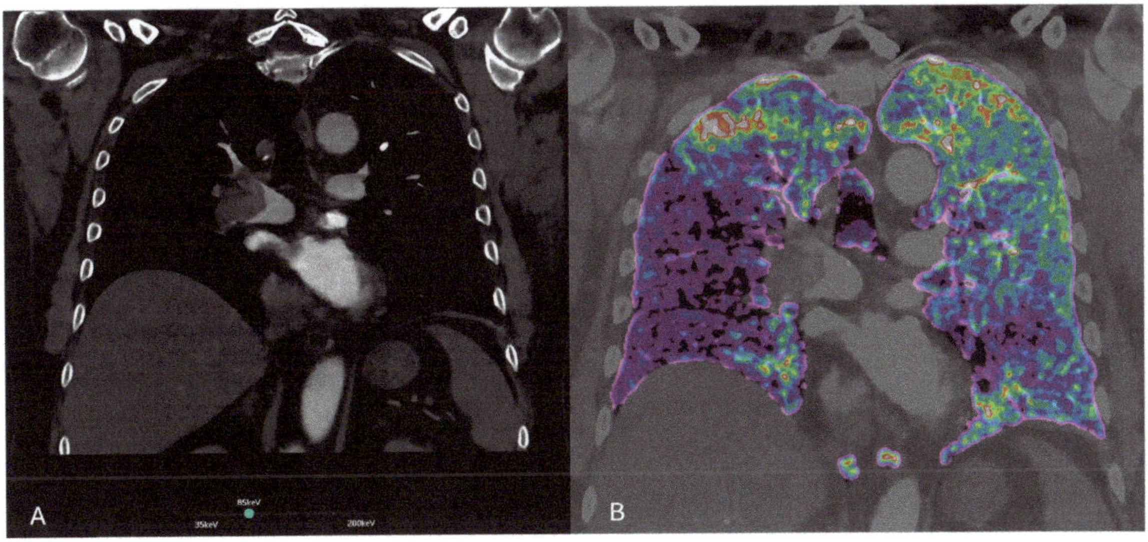

Figure 1. (**A**) Dual-energy CT. Virtual monochromatic at 85 keV image enhances vascular contrast while minimizing noise and beam-hardening artifacts. This reconstruction optimizes visualization of pulmonary embolism within the pulmonary arteries. (**B**) Iodine perfusion map demonstrates the regional lung perfusion. Areas of reduced iodine uptake (shown in purple) correspond to perfusion defects due to embolic obstruction of the pulmonary arteries.

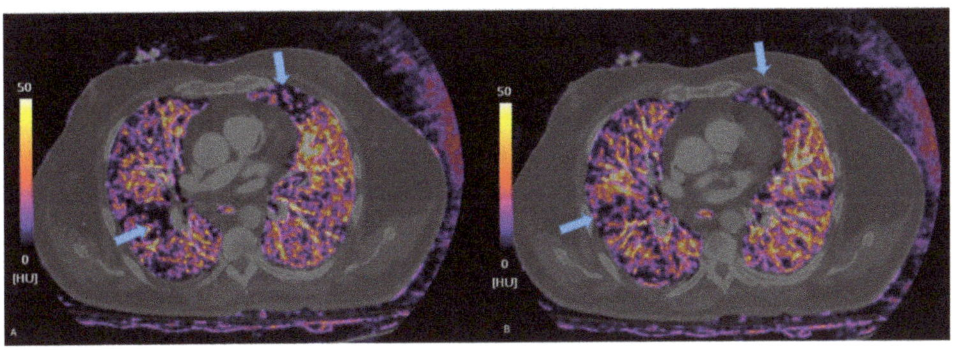

Figure 2. Iodine maps help detect segmental perfusion deficits, hard to detect on traditional CTPA, visible as defects in iodine contents (blue arrows, (**A**,**B**)), whiting the lung parenchyma.

Finally, the use of high-energy VMIs (e.g., 100–140 keV) can mitigate beam-hardening artifacts from dense contrast or metallic implants, improving overall image quality.

3.3. *Photon-Counting CT*

3.3.1. Principles of Photon Counting

PC is a new imaging technique that greatly improves traditional CT and depends on energy-integrating detectors (EIDs). PC provides enhanced spatial and contrast resolution, lower electronic noise, and the possibility for a decrease in radiation dose [19,31].

The key distinction lies in the use of PC Detectors (PCDs), which work in a completely different way compared to EIDs: while EIDs convert X-rays into light, and then converts this light into electrical signals using a photodiode [32], PCDs, made of special materials like cadmium telluride or silicon, directly convert X-rays into electrons and receive them as electrical signals. PCDs count each photon and measure its energy by sorting it into multiple energy bins (typically three to eight) based on the height of the generated electrical pulse, thereby filtering out electronic noise below a certain threshold. This energy-resolving capability enables accurate multi-energy imaging, overcoming the dual-energy limitations of current spectral CT systems [10]. It allows the decomposition of materials using the energy-dependent attenuation characteristics of each voxel, producing basis image maps that measure substances such as iodine or calcium. These maps are applicable for generating VMIs, VNC images, or images specific to materials [31]. PC additionally facilitates quantitative imaging by delivering physical characteristics at the voxel level, enabling more precise measurement of contrast agents compared to DECT.

PCDs enable a significant reduction in contrast medium administration and radiation dose for diagnosing APE compared to conventional EID-CT while maintaining good to excellent image quality [32].

3.3.2. Diagnostic Accuracy of of Photon Counting-CTPA

Pennenbecker et al. [12] found that PC-CTPA offered better subjective and objective image quality compared to SECT, even with an ultra-low contrast and radiation dose protocol, enabling a 50% reduction in contrast medium and a markedly lower effective dose (1.4 mSv versus 3.3 mSv). In a different study, the authors [33] showed that PC scans provided better subjective and objective image quality than EID images and a 28% decrease in radiation dose when compared to corresponding EID-CTPA, with enhanced CT attenuation in all examined pulmonary vessels.

Morevoer, when working with PC, VMIs help APE diagnosis by optimizing contrast resolution and reducing artifacts [34]. Lower keV VMI reconstructions (40–50 keV) improve vascular attenuation in pulmonary arteries, increasing iodine signal intensity and enhancing thrombus detection sensitivity [35]. This is particularly useful for subsegmental APE identification, where traditional CT may struggle due to limited contrast resolution (Figure 3). VMI generation allows a significant reduction in radiation dose by 46–47% compared to SECT.

Although 40 keV VMIs achieve peak signal-to-noise ratios, 50 keV balances noise reduction and artifact mitigation, with studies demonstrating superior APE visibility at this energy level due to fewer beam-hardening artifacts [35]. Additionally, VMIs enable diagnostic salvage of suboptimal enhanced studies through contrast boost effects, maintaining diagnostic confidence even in technically challenging cases [35].

PC CTPA is now being used routinely in clinical settings, with continuing research aiming to evaluate its diagnostic performance compared with traditional CTPA. Recent prospective investigations have shown that PC produces 95–100% of tests classified as diagnostic for PE, with some series reporting no non-diagnostic scans. In most situations, subjective image quality was rated excellent or good, exceeding EID-CT and DECT [12,33]. Furthermore, PC improves contrast-to-noise and signal-to-noise ratios, reduces motion aberrations, and increases CT attenuation in pulmonary arteries, all of which are crucial for effective PE identification. However, most published studies use diagnostic yield and picture quality as surrogates for accuracy, with few reporting sensitivity and specificity against a reference standard [12,33].

In a recent prospective study, Remy-Jardin et al. [36] found a high diagnosis rate (95.3%) for PC scans, since most non-diagnostic instances, mostly due to inadequate vascular opacification, could be efficiently rectified using low-energy VMI reconstructions. Fletcher et al. [37] found that PC's greater spatial resolution and contrast-to-noise ratio could provide similar or even better diagnostic accuracy for APE than DECT.

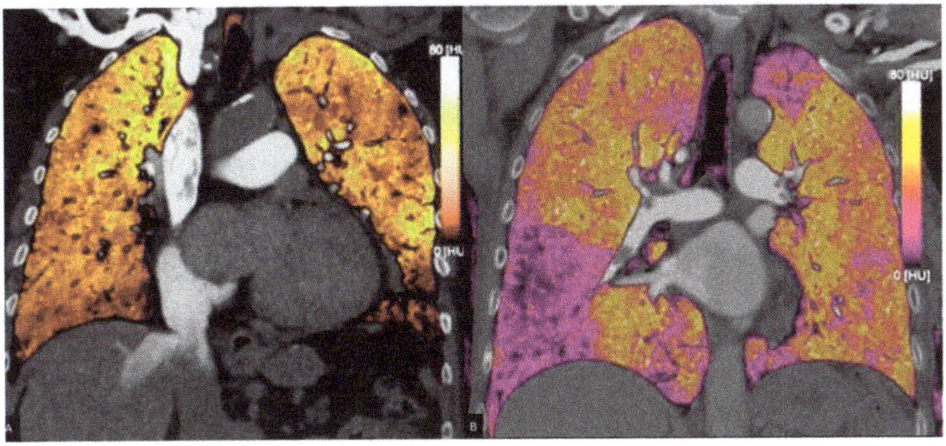

Figure 3. Pulmonary blood volume map derived from PC acquisition, showing iodine distribution. The perfusion is almost homogeneous in (**A**), whereas in (**B**), perfusion deficits are bilaterally present. Areas of reduced perfusion appear in darker shades (**B**), assisting in the identification of embolic territories and functional assessment of the pulmonary circulation.

3.4. Dynamic Digital Radiography

3.4.1. Principles of Dynamic Digital Radiography

DDR is an emerging low-radiation method for assessing pulmonary perfusion that applies a flat-panel detector and a conventional radiography system with a pulsed X-ray generator, allowing for the capture of sequential high-resolution images over time., creating a dynamic sequence that represents motion and functional changes, such as airflow and blood flow in the lungs.

Patients are imaged in a standing or supine position over a breath-hold of 6 s, and the obtained images are processed to highlight temporal changes in pixel intensity corresponding to pulmonary blood flow from the baseline timing (end-diastolic phase) [38] (Figures 4 and 5). The resulting images reveal blood flow dynamics within the lungs and a color-coded map that represents the lung perfusion [39].

APE is visible on DDR examinations as well-defined triangular or wedge-shaped perfusion defects, similar to those observed in traditional imaging modalities such as lung perfusion scintigraphy [40].

DDR obtains lung perfusion without utilizing intravenous contrast media, providing a secure option for patients with contraindications to contrast agents and presenting benefits regarding radiation exposure and patient comfort. The low radiation doses (0.2 mSv) compared to traditional imaging techniques make DDR a promising option for functional analysis of pulmonary circulation, especially in patients who require repeated imaging or have limited tolerance for more invasive procedures.

The availability of DDR portable equipment allows the acquisition also at the patients' bed, speeding up the workflow in the emergency setting.

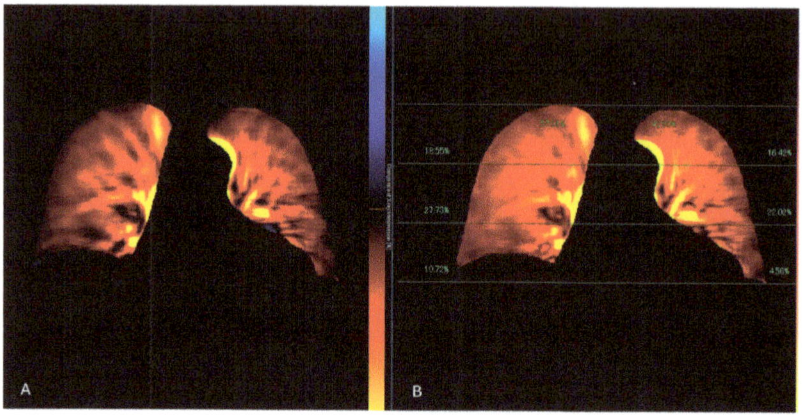

Figure 4. The perfusion algorithm uses the reference frame subtraction method to analyze the degree of pixel value change from the baseline timing (end-diastolic phase) (**A**). After removing the respiratory-related temporal changes in pixel values using a band-pass filter, a color-coded map representing the pixel value change rate and a map showing the contribution of the different lung areas to the global perfusion are obtained (**B**).

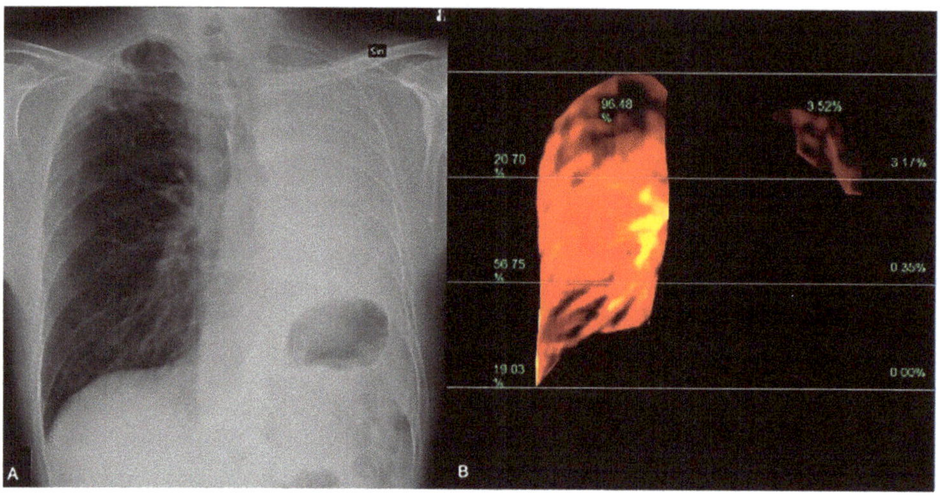

Figure 5. DDR perfusion assessment of a lung cancer patient, presenting dyspnea and raised D-dimer values. The traditional X-Ray (**A**) shows a pleural effusion extending to the apex. The perfusion study (**B**) demonstrated a regular perfusion of the right lung parenchyma and left apex.

3.4.2. Accuracy of Dynamic Digital Radiography

Studies have demonstrated the efficacy of DDR in detecting chronic thromboembolic pulmonary hypertension (CTEPH), a pathological condition related to unresolved pulmonary embolism. Research indicates that DDR has comparable sensitivity and specificity to ventilation/perfusion (V/Q) scanning in identifying CTEPH, suggesting its potential as a reliable diagnostic tool in clinical practice [13].

The main advantages of the different imaging techniques are listed in Table 1.

Table 1. Advantages and disadvantages of the different imaging techniques in APE diagnosis. CTPA: Computed Tomography Pulmonary Angiography; VMI: Virtual Monochromatic Image; VNC: Virtual Non-Contrast; RV: Right Ventricle; APE: Acute Pulmonary Embolism.

Technique	Pros	Cons
High-Pitch CT	- Very fast scan time (<1 s) - Low radiation dose (~30% lower than standard CTPA) - Lower contrast volume (20 mL) - Reduced motion artifacts - Good for dyspnoic or uncooperative patients - Excellent image quality in >90% cases	- Slightly lower contrast opacification and increased noise in segmental arteries
Dual-Energy CT (DECT)	- Combines anatomical and perfusion imaging - Enables iodine perfusion maps, VMIs, VNC - Detects subsegmental emboli better - Can reduce need for additional imaging - High sensitivity/specificity when combined with advanced post-processing - Allows contrast and dose reduction - Helps assess severity (e.g., RV dysfunction correlation)	- Variable diagnostic performance depending on protocol and post-processing - No substantial advantage over SECT in meta-analysis - Complexity and cost of post-processing - Limited widespread availability and standardization
Photon-Counting CT (PC)	- Superior spatial and contrast resolution - Significantly lower contrast and radiation doses (up to 50% reduction) - Improved image quality and emboli conspicuity - Effective for subsegmental APE detection - Less electronic noise - Compatible with high-pitch and spectral modes - Approaching clinical use in 2025	- Expensive and limited current availability - Few studies report sensitivity/specificity against gold standard - Clinical validation still ongoing despite promising results
Dynamic Digital Radiography (DDR)	- No contrast medium required - Very low radiation dose (~0.2 mSv) - Simple, quick, and non-invasive - Useful in patients with contrast allergies or renal impairment - Effective for functional assessment - Portable and usable bedside	- Limited spatial resolution - Not yet standard for APE diagnosis - Mainly validated for chronic thromboembolic disease - Primarily functional, not anatomical imaging

4. Artificial Intelligence

4.1. Automated Detection

Artificial intelligence (AI) is transforming medical imaging and diagnostics, significantly enhancing precision and efficiency. Recent advancements have focused on developing AI algorithms that efficiently and accurately evaluate medical images [41]. Specifically for APE, AI improves the interpretation of imaging studies such as CTPA, aiding radiologists in detecting subtle PE signs that could otherwise be missed or misinterpreted [42]. By analyzing vast amounts of imaging data, these systems significantly advance CTPA-based APE detection, leading to better diagnostic performance [43]. While diagnosing APE remains challenging due to other conditions that can mimic its appearance and variability in imaging interpretation, AI, particularly deep learning (DL), has emerged as a promising addition to traditional diagnostic pathways [44].

Previous studies utilized machine learning (ML) to create Computer-Assisted Detection (CAD) programs that supported radiologists in identifying APE. Although CAD software exhibited low sensitivity and specificity and necessitated manual verification by radiologists, its incorporation into radiologist workflows greatly enhanced detection rates [45]. Recent deep learning algorithms, particularly Convolutional Neural Networks (CNNs), have demonstrated high accuracy in identifying and localizing pulmonary emboli on CTPA images. These networks analyze different image features, such as shapes, edges, and textures, and gradually learn to identify more complex patterns, like clots inside pulmonary arteries [46,47].

Different AI models have been explored for the APE detection on CTPA [41]. Among the most common AI architectures are U-Net variants, which are convolutional neural networks originally developed for biomedical image analysis [44]. In APE detection, U-Net-based models are used to highlight areas likely to contain emboli by learning spatial patterns across CT slices. These networks can be implemented in different formats: 2D models analyze each slice independently; 2.5D models examine a few adjacent slices simultaneously to capture limited depth information; and 3D models process the entire volumetric scan, providing a more comprehensive spatial understanding of the pulmonary vasculature.

To enhance the performance of these base models, researchers often integrate DenseNet or ResNet components [48], which are DL architectures known for their ability to extract many additional features from medical images. These hybrid models frequently use transfer learning approaches, meaning they are partially pre-trained on large general image datasets and then fine-tuned on APE-specific scans. In some cases, attention mechanisms are added to guide the network's focus toward areas most likely to contain emboli, improving both accuracy and interpretability [49].

Another important class of models focuses on object detection, which aims to locate and mark the position of emboli within the pulmonary arteries. Examples include Faster R-CNN and Mask R-CNN [49], which generate bounding boxes around suspected emboli by scanning the image for candidate regions.

Numerous studies have evaluated the performance of AI algorithms for APE detection using metrics such as sensitivity, specificity, Area Under the Curve (AUC), and accuracy [41,42,46,50–54]. A systematic review and meta-analysis of DL-based AI algorithms for APE detection on CTPA showed a pooled sensitivity of 88% and a specificity of 86% per scan [55]. A recent meta-analysis [56] examined the effectiveness of DL algorithms for identifying APE on CTPA scans. Analyzing data from twenty-four studies encompassing almost 23,000 patients, the research finds that DL models exhibit high diagnostic accuracy. Specifically, U-Net architecture shows higher sensitivity for detecting true positives, while CNN models demonstrate better specificity with fewer false positives.

Specific AI tools have been evaluated and received regulatory approval. In particular, CINA-PE (Avicenna.AI), an FDA-cleared and CE-marked DL-based algorithm, demonstrated high performance in different studies, with a per-case sensitivity and specificity that range between 93.9–91.4% and 94.8–91.5%, respectively, and an AUC-ROC of 0.92 [57,58]. Notably, the algorithm detected 22 out of 29 (76%) APE cases that were not mentioned in the initial clinical report, leading to a reduction in the overall missing rate from 15.6% to 3.8%. Another study showed CINA-PE reduced the incidental APE missing rate from 50% to 7.1% compared to no AI assistance [59].

Another FDA-approved AI model is Aidoc, which has been tested in real hospitals showing high levels of accuracy, with sensitivity reaching 96.8% and specificity up to 99.9% [60].

Zsarnoczay et al. [50] analyzed the performance of another Deep Neural Network (DNN)-based prototype algorithm that showed a sensitivity of 84.6% and a specificity of 95.1% for PE detection, with an overall accuracy of 93.8%. This DNN algorithm demonstrated excellent sensitivity for detecting central (100%) and lobar (96.7%) APE and achieved a sensitivity of 72.9% for peripheral APE.

When using AI, common sources of false positives included lung masses, pneumonia, and contrast flow artifacts, while false negatives often involved chronic and subsegmental APE. Detecting peripheral and small emboli poses a significant challenge, and current AI initiatives aim to enhance precision in these regions, while earlier research typically concentrated only on major arteries [61]. A SPE-YOLO model, designed specifically for recognizing small APE, reached a sensitivity of 90.70% and an accuracy of 86.45% on an external validation dataset [62].

Beyond contrast-enhanced CTPA, the possible role of automated APE detection on unenhanced chest CT has also been explored [63]. A prototype AI algorithm utilizing nnDetection, based on the Retina U-Net architecture, demonstrated the potential to detect APE on non-contrast CT scans. This algorithm showed varying sensitivity based on location: 54.5% for central, 81.9% for segmental, and 80.0% for subsegmental APE. While sensitivity on unenhanced scans may be lower than on CTPA, such AI tools could potentially guide the decision on whether a follow-up contrast-enhanced scan is necessary. However, external validation with larger sample sizes is needed to confirm these findings and assess reliability in real-world settings. These AI tools can support the radiologist's workflow by automatically flagging suspicious cases, generating annotated images with bounding boxes highlighting potential emboli, and therefore prioritizing review cases [57]. In some models, these bounding boxes are intentionally expanded to include surrounding vascular structures, offering the algorithm additional anatomical context to refine its predictions. This approach can improve detection accuracy by helping the AI differentiate emboli from normal variants or artifacts [41].

A summary of the performance of the main DL algorithms is presented in Table 2.

Table 2. This table provides a summary based on the specific performance metrics (Sensitivity, Specificity, Area Under the Curve—AUC) available for each mentioned AI tool.

Name of the Tool	Specificity	Sensitivity	AUC
CINA-PE (Avicenna.AI) [57,58]	94.8%	93.9%	AUC: 0.92
Aidoc [60]	95.8%	92.6%	AUC: 0.87
Retina U-Net/nnDetection (unenhanced CT) [56]	N/A	Varies by location: Central 54.5%, Segmental 81.9%, Subsegmental 80.0%	N/A
Deep Learning Algorithm (Liu et al.) [52]	76.5%	94.6%	AUC: 0.92
Deep Learning Model (Huhtanen et al.) [51]	86.6%	93.5%	AUC: 0.91
End-to-end DL Model (Huang et al.) [48]	N/A	N/A	AUC: 0.84–0.85
Deep Learning Algorithm (Li et al.) [59]	95.5%	92.7%	AUC: 0.95
nnU-Net-based Algorithm (Kahraman et al.) [53]	94.6%	96.1%	N/A

4.2. *Segmentation and Quantification*

Beyond detection, AI also plays an important role in segmenting anatomical structures and embolic material. CNNs are often used for segmenting lung lobes, the heart, and pulmonary arteries, regions critical for accurately localizing and quantifying APE. Common architectures include 2D, 2.5D, and 3D U-Nets, alongside advanced models like Retina U-Net, nnU-Net, and MP-Net, all engineered to delineate features at a pixel level [44]. Segmentation facilitates not only the identification and volumetric analysis of pulmonary arterial thrombi but also of cardiac structures, particularly the right and left ventricles. This capability assists in determining the RV/LV diameter ratio, a widely used prognostic marker in APE reflecting right heart strain [64]. Several AI models have demonstrated the capacity to automate both clot and cardiac segmentation without requiring manual annotation [51]. Nevertheless, clot segmentation can occasionally be incomplete or inaccurate, especially in subsegmental branches. Moreover, certain training datasets may lack the high-quality, voxel-level annotations essential for intricate calculations such as the Qanadli score, a severity metric. An ongoing focus of current research involves addressing these limitations by incorporating larger and more diverse annotated datasets [43].

4.3. Prediction

Segmentation is useful to establish the APE severity, including estimating the Qanadli score [44], an index that quantifies the arterial obstruction based on the number and location of occluded segmental branches, and the right ventricle-to-left ventricle diameter ratio (RV/LV ratio) [65]. These are crucial metrics for assessing APE severity and predicting mortality. An AI-based approach has demonstrated the feasibility of estimating the Qanadli score with a coefficient of determination (R2) of 0.717 and the RV/LV ratio with an R2 of 0.723 on the test set. This suggests the potential of AI in providing reliable and useful predictions for these important clinical metrics and potentially promoting the use of the Qanadli score as an APE marker in clinical practice [44].

AI is also a promising tool for outcome prediction and risk stratification [66]. ML models surpass traditional risk scoring systems in risk stratification performance. The integration of different data inputs, such as laboratory results, medical history, and vital signs, makes AI capable of predicting APE probability.

Finally, Natural Language Processing (NLP), a branch of AI that focuses on processing written or spoken language by extracting relevant information from radiology reports, medical history and admission notes, can be used to identify patients with a potential diagnosis [67].

5. Therapeutic Strategies

5.1. Risk Stratification and Interventional Procedure for Pulmonary Embolism

Risk stratification is a cornerstone of managing APE as it determines the appropriate diagnostic and therapeutic strategies [68] and identifies patients who may benefit from advanced therapies such as catheter-directed treatment (CDT) or mechanical thrombectomy. Risk assessment stratifies patients into high-, intermediate-, and low-risk categories, based on hemodynamic status, RV function, and biomarker evidence of myocardial injury [69]. Among these, high-risk and selected intermediate-risk patients are the most relevant populations for interventional approaches [68,69].

High-risk APE is characterized by hemodynamic instability, including cardiac arrest, obstructive shock (systolic blood pressure <90 mmHg or vasopressor use with signs of end-organ hypoperfusion), or persistent hypotension unresponsive to volume resuscitation [69–71]. This population has the highest early mortality and requires urgent reperfusion [68]. Current guidelines from the ACCP (2021) recommend systemic thrombolysis via a peripheral vein over catheter-directed thrombolysis for high-risk PE [72]. However, while systemic thrombolysis remains the recommended first-line treatment, CDT and surgical embolectomy remain critical valid options for patients with contraindications to thrombolysis, failed thrombolysis, or shock likely to be fatal before systemic therapy can act [72].

The ESC 2019 guidelines similarly recommend systemic thrombolysis as first-line therapy, with catheter-based options reserved for selected high-risk patients with contraindications or failure of thrombolysis [71]. In such cases, interventional radiology plays a pivotal role by providing minimally invasive alternatives that rapidly restore pulmonary perfusion and improve right heart function, often with a lower risk of bleeding [69].

Although hemodynamically stable patients may not fulfill the criteria for massive APE, they can exhibit severity markers such as increased troponin or brain natriuretic peptide levels, along with RV dysfunction detected through echocardiography or CTPA [71]. Within this group, intermediate–high-risk APE, defined by combined RV dysfunction and elevated cardiac biomarkers, represents the subgroup most likely to benefit from advanced therapies [16,73].

Systemic thrombolysis is not routinely recommended; however, interventional radiology-guided CDT or mechanical thrombectomy may be considered for patients whose clinical condition deteriorates despite anticoagulation, or for those with persistent signs of RV overload and hypoxia [72]. In such cases, "rescue reperfusion" has garnered clinical support, especially since CDT techniques provide effective reperfusion while minimizing systemic thrombolytic exposure [71]. Recent guidelines from the PERT Consortium (2023) [71] also highlight the potential role of reduced-dose systemic thrombolysis in intermediate-risk PE, especially for patients at elevated bleeding risk, reinforcing the need for individualized decision-making.

Interventional radiology plays a limited role in low-risk APE, which includes hemodynamically stable patients, lack of RV dysfunction, and a PESI class I–II or a simplified PESI score of 0 [71]. These patients are typically treated successfully with anticoagulation alone, and many may be managed in outpatient settings [69].

5.2. EkoSonic Endovascular System (EKOS)

The EkoSonic Endovascular System (EKOS) is a directed thrombolysis platform that combines ultrasound energy with low-dose fibrinolytic infusion to accelerate thrombus dissolution. Its efficacy was evaluated through different trials, such as the ULTIMA trial, a randomized controlled trial enrolling 59 patients with intermediate-risk APE, which showed that ultrasound-assisted CDT using EKOS was significantly more effective than anticoagulation alone in reducing RV/LV ratio at 24 h, with no major bleeding events reported [73]. Another study on EKOS was the SEATTLE II study, a prospective multicenter trial involving 150 patients with massive or submassive APE. This study demonstrated a significant reduction in the RV/LV diameter ratio (mean change from 1.55 to 1.13) and a decrease in mean pulmonary artery pressure (from 51.4 mmHg to 36.9 mmHg) following EKOS treatment [74]. However, the significant bleeding rate was 10%. Importantly, this trial lacked a control group, limiting the strength of conclusions regarding efficacy relative to standard care.

The OPTALYSE-PE trial aimed to determine the optimal duration and dose of thrombolytic delivery using EKOS in intermediate-risk patients [75]. This randomized, multicenter trial enrolled 101 patients into four groups receiving different combinations of recombinant tissue plasminogen activator (rtPA) doses (4–12 mg) and durations (2–6 h). All regimens demonstrated rapid improvement in the RV/LV ratio and thrombus burden, with a significant bleeding rate of 4%, which included two intracranial hemorrhages, with one attributed to rtPA. These findings support the feasibility of shorter, lower-dose thrombolytic protocols that may improve safety while preserving efficacy. The SUNSET sPE trial highlighted a different outcome; another randomized study of 81 patients compared EKOS with standard CDT devices and found no significant difference in thrombus score reduction, suggesting that the benefits of ultrasound facilitation may be less pronounced than initially thought. However, the trial was limited by a small sample size [76].

A highly anticipated trial is the HI-PEITHO study, a large, prospective, multicenter, randomized controlled trial designed to compare EKOS-based CDT plus anticoagulation versus anticoagulation alone in 406 patients with intermediate–high-risk APE. The trial's primary outcomes include PE-related death, recurrence, and cardiorespiratory decompensation at 7 days. The results will significantly influence future guideline recommendations regarding CDT use in intermediate-risk patients [16].

Recent case reports also highlight the clinical applicability of catheter-directed therapies such as EKOS in complex APE scenarios, where systemic thrombolysis poses significant risks. For example, a 50-year-old female patient with May–Thurner Syndrome and extensive thrombotic burden was successfully treated using bilateral EkoSonic Endovascular System (EKOS) catheters without the use of systemic thrombolysis [77]. The patient presented a bilateral submassive pulmonary embolism and a large right atrial thrombus, conditions that, combined with her comorbidities, would traditionally complicate treatment decisions, even if she was hemodynamically stable. EKOS therapy resulted in complete resolution of the atrial thrombus within 30 h, and the patient was discharged home on anticoagulation by day five. This case illustrates how ultrasound-assisted catheter-directed thrombolysis may offer a safer and effective alternative in patients at higher risk of bleeding or those with anatomically complex thrombi. Such real-world outcomes further support the consideration of CDT in intermediate–high-risk PE patients where systemic fibrinolysis is contraindicated or not recommended.

5.3. *FlowTriever System (Inari Medical)*

The FlowTriever System (Inari Medical, Irvine, CA, USA) is a mechanical thrombectomy device using a large-bore catheter, available in 16F, 20F, and 24F sizes, and a 60 mL syringe with a locking mechanism to create a vacuum, designed to remove thrombus from the pulmonary arteries without thrombolytics. It uses aspiration through the Triever catheter (Inari Medical, Irvine, CA, USA) and mechanical engagement tools with self-expanding nitinol disks, offering immediate hemodynamic benefits compared to the gradual improvements seen with CDT. Although technically more demanding, effective outcomes have been favorable, regardless of operator experience.

Significant evidence from various studies highlights the efficacy and safety of FlowTriever across different patient settings. The FLARE study, a prospective, single-arm trial of 106 intermediate-risk PE patients, demonstrated a significant average reduction (25%) in the RV/LV ratio at 48 h post-procedure, along with a low rate (3.8%) of composite adverse safety outcomes and minimal bleeding complications [74]. The FLASH registry, encompassing a larger, real-world cohort of over 800 patients (primarily intermediate- and high-risk APE), reported immediate improvements including a 23% decrease in mean pulmonary artery pressure, enhanced oxygenation, and heart rate stabilization [78,79]. FLASH further confirmed excellent safety, with a 30-day mortality of only 0.9% and major bleeding rates under 1%, supporting FlowTriever as particularly valuable in patients contraindicated to thrombolysis.

In the high-risk APE setting, the FLAME study compared 53 patients treated with FlowTriever (Figure 6) to historical controls, revealing notably lower in-hospital adverse clinical events, primarily driven by an impressively low mortality rate (1.9%) [80].

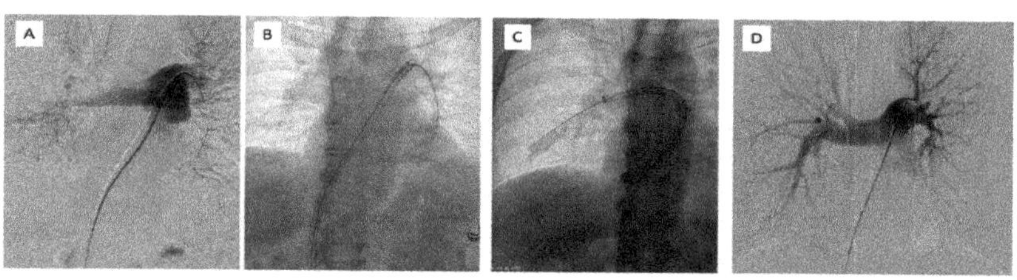

Figure 6. 65-year-old male affected by bilateral pulmonary embolism treated with FlowTriever system. (**A**) Left pulmonary artery catheterism and phlebography demonstrated the presence of right main pulmonary artery thrombus and lack of opacification of lower left lobar pulmonary branches. (**B**) Placement of 24F inari device in the left pulmonary artery and (**C**) in the right pulmonary artery with the aspiration of clots. (**D**) Final phlebography demonstrated the patency of the pulmonary artery on both systems with good peripheral vascularization.

The PEERLESS study further strengthens FlowTriever's evidence base as the first randomized controlled trial (RCT) to directly compare two advanced catheter-based therapies,

FlowTriever versus CDT, in intermediate-risk APE patients. Enrolling 550 patients, PEERLESS demonstrated a significantly favorable primary endpoint for FlowTriever, primarily driven by fewer cases of clinical deterioration, lower need for bailout therapies, and reduced ICU admissions and lengths of stay [81]. Notably, there was no significant difference between groups in mortality, major bleeding, or intracranial hemorrhage. FlowTriever was also associated with fewer all-cause readmissions within 30 days compared to CDT.

These studies underscore FlowTriever's capacity for rapid thrombus removal, significant acute improvement in right ventricular function, and an impressive safety profile, making it a compelling therapeutic choice for a broad spectrum of APE patients.

5.4. Indigo Aspiration System (Penumbra Inc.)

The Indigo Aspiration System (Penumbra Inc., Alameda, CA, USA) is a mechanical thrombectomy device designed to rapidly remove thrombus in APE using continuous aspiration and mechanical fragmentation. The system features a computer-assisted vacuum thrombectomy (CAVT), regulated by a microprocessor, facilitating precise thrombus extraction while minimizing blood loss. The device comprises aspiration catheters of various sizes (8–12 Fr), a suction pump, and an optional separator wire for enhanced thrombus disruption.

Clinical evaluation through the EXTRACT-PE study—a prospective, multicenter, single-arm trial with 119 intermediate-risk PE patients—demonstrated significant efficacy, showing a mean reduction of 0.43 (27.3%) in the RV/LV ratio at 48 h. Safety outcomes were favorable, with a major adverse event rate of only 1.7%, major bleeding occurring in 1.7%, and no cases of intracranial hemorrhage reported. Notably, 98.3% of patients underwent the procedure without adjunctive thrombolytic therapy. The median procedural duration of 37 min and minimal blood loss further underscored the efficiency and safety of this system [82].

Additional support comes from interim results of the STRIKE-PE trial, a larger prospective, international study evaluating Indigo Aspiration in intermediate- and high-risk APE patients. Interim findings from 150 patients confirmed significant acute hemodynamic improvements, including a 25.7% reduction in the RV/LV ratio and reduced pulmonary artery pressures at 48 h, alongside low complication rates (2.7% composite major adverse events) and notable functional and quality-of-life benefits at 90 days [83]. The ongoing STRIKE-PE trial plans to enroll 600 patients, offering extended follow-up data for up to one year.

Together, these studies position the Indigo Aspiration System as an effective, safe, and versatile mechanical thrombectomy option for managing APE, particularly in populations where thrombolysis is contraindicated or undesirable.

Clinical case reports further emphasize the role of the Indigo Aspiration System in high-risk pulmonary embolism scenarios, particularly where thrombolysis is contraindicated. Angelini et al. [84] described the case of a 75-year-old male presenting with extensive bilateral pulmonary emboli and right ventricular dysfunction, but without hemodynamic instability. Given the patient's older age and risk of bleeding, catheter-directed aspiration with the Penumbra Indigo system was chosen. A successful removal of 40% of the thrombus burden occurred without any procedural complications, and the patient showed quick clinical improvement, leading to discharge just two days after the intervention. This case exemplifies how aspiration thrombectomy may provide a safe and effective alternative to systemic thrombolysis in intermediate- to high-risk APE patients, especially those with comorbidities that increase bleeding risk. These findings support trial data and highlight the growing role of mechanical thrombectomy in modern APE management algorithms.

5.5. Other Devices

Other devices include the AngioJet rheolytic thrombectomy system (Boston Scientific, Marlborough, MA, USA), which utilizes high-pressure saline jets to fragment and aspirate thrombi and allows local thrombolytic injections. The AngioJet system has primarily been assessed in small, retrospective studies involving intermediate- and high-risk APE patients. One retrospective study of 44 patients (21 high-risk and 23 intermediate–high-risk) showed significant short-term clinical and hemodynamic improvements. However, mortality was relatively high (six in-hospital deaths), and complications such as significant bleeding occurred in 4.5% of patients [85]. Another single-center experience with 56 patients noted a significant bleeding rate of 7.1% and mortality of 8.9% [86]. Due to complications like bradyarrhythmia, hemolysis-related acute kidney injury, and hemoptysis, the FDA issued a black box warning for its use in pulmonary arteries, emphasizing the need for careful patient selection and procedure management.

The AngioVac (AngioDynamics, Oakville, ON, USA) is a large-bore (24 Fr) catheter system designed for venous thrombus removal via extracorporeal venovenous bypass. It allows filtration of aspirated thrombus before reinfusion into the systemic circulation. However, the available literature does not provide detailed evidence from specific randomized trials or robust clinical studies conclusively demonstrating its efficacy in treating PE, relying instead on limited single-center experiences and case reports.

The BASHIR endovascular catheter (Thrombolex, New Britain, PA, USA) introduces a unique concept of mechanical expansion and local thrombolysis via an expandable infusion basket with multiple orifices. Preliminary data have shown significant improvements in RV function and thrombus burden with a favorable safety profile [87]. While not yet supported by large-scale randomized trials, its use is increasing in specialized centers.

6. Systemic Thrombolysis

The mortality rate from an APE primarily depends on how well the right ventricle (RV) can cope with the sudden strain placed upon it, and quick intervention is vital for APE patients showing signs of RV failure. Anticoagulation treatment is effective in preventing clot progression; however, it does not significantly improve RV function or pulmonary perfusion in the early stages of treatment [88]. Several studies have shown that anticoagulant therapy alone does not lead to marked improvements in RV function or lung perfusion in the initial phase of management [89,90].

Thrombolytic therapy has instead demonstrated more immediate benefits, including significant improvements in both RV function and pulmonary perfusion.

The impact of low-dose systemic tissue plasminogen activator (tPA) thrombolysis on patient outcomes remains a subject of debate, as thrombolytic therapy carries an increased risk of bleeding complications [91].

To minimize this risk while retaining therapeutic benefits, low-dose, prolonged thrombolysis using alteplase or tPA has been proposed as an alternative for patients with intermediate- or high-risk APE [92]. This strategy involves administering reduced doses of tPA over an extended duration, as opposed to conventional full-dose regimens.

Low-dose systemic tPA has emerged as a promising treatment option for APE, particularly in intermediate-risk patients. Compared to anticoagulation alone, this approach seeks to achieve more rapid clot resolution and improved RV function, with a lower bleeding risk than traditional high-dose thrombolytic therapy [93].

Common regimens include a 6 h infusion of low-dose tPA (e.g., 50 mg total, sometimes given as a 10 mg bolus followed by infusion) to balance thrombolytic efficacy with bleeding risk reduction [94]. This administration has proven to be effective in reducing hospital length of stay and decreasing hemodynamic decompensation in intermediate-risk APE patients [95].

7. Pulmonary Embolism Response Teams (PERTs)

Many institutions have established Pulmonary Embolism Response Teams (PERTs) to support decision-making in this increasingly complex therapeutic landscape. These multidisciplinary teams typically include pulmonologists, cardiologists, emergency medicine physicians, hematologists, interventional radiologists, cardiothoracic surgeons, and pharmacists. PERTs provide rapid consultation, often via virtual or in-person meetings, and facilitate real-time clinical, imaging, and laboratory data analysis to guide optimal treatment strategies [96].

Their role is particularly vital in intermediate- and high-risk APE cases, or in low-risk patients with complicating factors such as significant comorbidities or contraindications to standard therapies.

Studies assessing the impact of PERT implementation have demonstrated notable benefits. Direct PERT consultation has been associated with reductions in 30-day mortality, hospital length of stay, time to therapeutic anticoagulation, and bleeding complications, even though patients receiving PERT consultation were more likely to undergo advanced interventions such as thrombolysis or thrombectomy [96,97]. The advantages stem from the process of coordinated multidisciplinary decision-making rather than the mere presence of a PERT at the institution. In addition to improving clinical outcomes, PERTs promote the judicious use of resources, such as avoiding unnecessary placement of inferior vena cava (IVC) filters and facilitating patient enrollment into clinical trials [98]. Through registries like KNOCOUT PE [99] and trials such as PE-TRACT [100], PERTs generate high-quality data that may shape future guidelines and standards of care.

8. Discussion

The management of APE has evolved remarkably over the past decade, driven by innovations in diagnostic imaging, interventional radiology, AI, and structured clinical management frameworks such as PERTs. While CTPA remains the reference standard for diagnosis [8,9], its limitations, particularly in detecting subsegmental emboli and in patients contraindicated for iodinated contrast, have spurred the development of advanced imaging modalities. Technologies such as DECT, PC, and Dynamic Digital Radiography (DDR) [10,12,13] offer functional insights into pulmonary perfusion and enhanced image quality at lower contrast and radiation doses. However, while promising, most of these technologies require further validation in large, prospective multicenter studies to establish their impact on clinical outcomes, management decisions, and health economics.

Simultaneously, AI has begun to integrate into APE diagnostics, with deep learning algorithms showing high diagnostic accuracy and support in CTPA interpretation. FDA-cleared tools like CINA-PE and Aidoc have demonstrated improved detection rates of APE and potential reductions in missed diagnoses, particularly for incidental and peripheral emboli [55]. AI applications in image segmentation, Qanadli score estimation, and outcome prediction are also expanding, offering future opportunities for comprehensive, automated PE severity assessment.

From a therapeutic perspective, the field of interventional radiology has made substantial progress in addressing high- and intermediate–high-risk APE, especially in patients contraindicated for systemic thrombolysis. Catheter-directed therapies (CDTs) such as the EkoSonic Endovascular System (EKOS), FlowTriever System, Indigo Aspiration System, and emerging devices like the BASHIR catheter have demonstrated safety and efficacy in clinical trials. Notably, randomized evidence from trials like PEERLESS [81] and upcoming data from HI-PEITHO [16] will help clarify the optimal role of these interventions in guideline-based practice.

APE treatment is complex and should be formulated by an experienced interdisciplinary clinician team and based on careful risk stratification, including different factors, such as patient characteristics, cardio-pulmonary reserve, bleeding risk, and available interventional resources.

Recent guidelines (ESC 2019, ACCP 2021, and the PERT Consortium recommendations) [72,77] continue to support systemic thrombolysis as the first-line reperfusion therapy for high-risk PE, reserving CDT for specific clinical scenarios. Low-dose systemic tPA has emerged as a promising treatment option for acute pulmonary embolism (PE), particularly in intermediate-risk patients. Risk stratification remains the cornerstone of APE management, but as reviewers appropriately noted, definitions for acute right ventricular dysfunction lack standardization, and the prognostic distinction between intermediate–low- and intermediate–high-risk groups remains debated.

9. Limitations

As a narrative review inherently carries selection bias, studies were chosen based on relevance and author expertise rather than a systematic or meta-analytic methodology. Although we endeavored to present balanced and current evidence, some emerging technologies and trials may have been inadvertently overlooked.

Moreover, much of the supporting evidence for newer imaging modalities like PC, DDR, and AI-based tools derives from single-center studies or early-phase trials with limited patient cohorts. Consequently, the generalizability of these findings to broader clinical practice remains uncertain.

Finally, interventional radiology techniques, while increasingly utilized, lack extensive randomized controlled trial data in intermediate-risk PE populations, with most published studies being observational or single-arm registries. The forthcoming results from pivotal trials such as HI-PEITHO will be crucial in refining recommendations and clinical indications.

10. Conclusions

APE is a complex and potentially life-threatening condition that demands a multidisciplinary and personalized approach. Recent advances in imaging technologies have improved diagnostic accuracy while minimizing patient risk. Minimally invasive endovascular therapies are becoming increasingly central for managing high- and intermediate-risk cases, offering effective alternatives to systemic thrombolysis. Pulmonary Embolism Response Teams facilitate tailored decision-making and improve outcomes through structured collaboration. Continued integration of artificial intelligence, risk stratification models, and clinical expertise will be critical to advancing APE care and improving long-term patient outcomes.

Author Contributions: Conceptualization, M.C. (Michaela Cellina) and M.P.; methodology, M.C. (Michaela Cellina), M.P. and M.C. (Maurizio Cè); investigation, S.C., C.L. and P.B.; writing—original draft preparation, M.C. (Michaela Cellina), M.P., N.F., F.C., M.C. (Maurizio Cè) and P.B.; writing—review and editing, M.C. (Michaela Cellina), M.C. (Maurizio Cè), M.P., N.F., F.C. and P.B.; visualization, S.C. and G.C.; supervision, G.C.; project administration, S.C. and G.C. All authors have read and agreed to the published version of the manuscript.

Funding: This research received no external funding.

Institutional Review Board Statement: Not applicable.

Informed Consent Statement: Not applicable.

Data Availability Statement: No new data were created or analyzed in this study. Data sharing is not applicable to this article.

Conflicts of Interest: The authors declare no conflicts of interest.

Abbreviations

The following abbreviations are used in this manuscript:

APE	Acute Pulmonary Embolism
CTPA	Computed Tomography Pulmonary Angiography
DECT	Dual-Energy Computed Tomography
PC	Photon Counting
DDR	Dynamic Digital Radiography
RV	Right Ventricle
VNC	Virtual Non-Contrast
VMIs	Virtual Monoenergetic Images
EID-CT	Energy-Integrating Detector CT
PCDs	Photon-Counting Detectors
DL	Deep Learning
CNNs	Convolutional Neural Networks
CAD	Computer-Assisted Detection
ML	Machine Learning
AUC	Area Under the Curve
DNN	Deep Neural Network
NLP	Natural Language Processing
CT	Computed Tomography
PE	Pulmonary Embolism
V/Q	Ventilation/Perfusion (referring to V/Q scanning)
CTEPH	Chronic Thromboembolic Pulmonary Hypertension
SECT	Single-Energy CT
LB	Linear Blending
RV/LV	Right Ventricle-to-Left Ventricle diameter ratio

References

1. Peracaula, M.; Sebastian, L.; Francisco, I.; Vilaplana, M.B.; Rodríguez-Chiaradía, D.A.; Tura-Ceide, O. Decoding Pulmonary Embolism: Pathophysiology, Diagnosis, and Treatment. *Biomedicines* **2024**, *12*, 1936. [CrossRef]
2. Teissandier, D.; Roussel, M.; Bannelier, H.; Freund, Y.; Catoire, P. Contemporary approaches to pulmonary embolism diagnosis: A clinical review. *Korean Soc. Emerg. Med.* **2024**, *11*, 127–135. [CrossRef]
3. Raskob, G.E.; Angchaisuksiri, P.; Blanco, A.N.; Buller, H.; Gallus, A.; Hunt, B.J.; Hylek, E.M.; Kakkar, A.; Konstantinides, S.V.; McCumber, M.; et al. Thrombosis: A major contributor to global disease burden. *Arter. Thromb. Vasc. Biol.* **2014**, *34*, 2363–2371. [CrossRef]
4. Faluk, M.; Hasan, S.M.; Chacko, J.J.; Abdelmaseih, R.; Patel, J. Evolution of Acute Pulmonary Embolism Management: Review Article. *Curr. Probl. Cardiol.* **2021**, *46*, 100551. [CrossRef]
5. Pollack, C.V.; Schreiber, D.; Goldhaber, S.Z.; Slattery, D.; Fanikos, J.; O'Neil, B.J.; Thompson, J.R.; Hiestand, B.; Briese, B.A.; Pendleton, R.C.; et al. Clinical characteristics, management, and outcomes of patients diagnosed with acute pulmonary embolism in the emergency department: Initial report of EMPEROR (Multicenter Emergency Medicine Pulmonary Embolism in the Real World Registry). *J. Am. Coll. Cardiol.* **2011**, *57*, 700–706. [CrossRef]
6. Noschang, J.; Guimarães, M.D.; Teixeira, D.F.D.; Braga, J.C.D.; Hochhegger, B.; Santana, P.R.P.; Marchiori, E. Pulmonary thromboembolism: New diagnostic imaging techniques. *Radiol. Bras.* **2018**, *51*, 178–186. [CrossRef] [PubMed]
7. Thomas, S.E.; Weinberg, I.; Schainfeld, R.M.; Rosenfield, K.; Parmar, G.M. Diagnosis of Pulmonary Embolism: A Review of Evidence-Based Approaches. *Biomedicines* **2024**, *13*, 3722. [CrossRef]
8. Zantonelli, G.; Cozzi, D.; Bindi, A.; Cavigli, E.; Moroni, C.; Luvarà, S.; Grazzini, G.; Danti, G.; Granata, V.; Miele, V. Acute Pulmonary Embolism: Prognostic Role of Computed Tomography Pulmonary Angiography (CTPA). *Tomography* **2022**, *8*, 529–539. [CrossRef]

9. Patel, P.; Bhatt, M.; Braun, C.; Begum, H.; Wiercioch, W.; Varghese, J.; Wooldridge, D.; Alturkmani, H.; Thomas, M.; Baig, M.; et al. Systematic review and meta-analysis of test accuracy for the diagnosis of suspected pulmonary embolism. *Blood Adv.* **2020**, *4*, 4296–4311. [CrossRef]
10. Vlahos, I.; Jacobsen, M.C.; Godoy, M.C.; Stefanidis, K.; Layman, R.R. Dual-energy CT in pulmonary vascular disease. *Br. J. Radiol.* **2021**, *95*, 20210699. [CrossRef]
11. Guerrini, S.; Zanoni, M.; Sica, C.; Bagnacci, G.; Mancianti, N.; Galzerano, G.; Garosi, G.; Cacioppa, L.M.; Cellina, M.; Zamboni, G.A.; et al. Dual-Energy CT as a Well-Established CT Modality to Reduce Contrast Media Amount: A Systematic Review from the Computed Tomography Subspecialty Section of the Italian Society of Radiology. *J. Clin. Med.* **2024**, *13*, 6345. [CrossRef]
12. Pannenbecker, P.; Huflage, H.; Grunz, J.P.; Gruschwitz, P.; Patzer, T.S.; Weng, A.M.; Heidenreich, J.F.; Bley, T.A.; Petritsch, B. Photon-counting CT for diagnosis of acute pulmonary embolism: Potential for contrast medium and radiation dose reduction. *Eur. Radiol.* **2023**, *33*, 7830–7839. [CrossRef]
13. Yamasaki, Y.; Abe, K.; Kamitani, T.; Hosokawa, K.; Hida, T.; Sagiyama, K.; Matsuura, Y.; Baba, S.; Isoda, T.; Maruoka, Y.; et al. Efficacy of Dynamic Chest Radiography for Chronic Thromboembolic Pulmonary Hypertension. *Radiology* **2023**, *306*, e220908. [CrossRef] [PubMed]
14. Marti, C.; John, G.; Konstantinides, S.; Combescure, C.; Sanchez, O.; Lankeit, M.; Meyer, G.; Perrier, A. Systemic thrombolytic therapy for acute pulmonary embolism: A systematic review and meta-analysis. *Eur. Heart J.* **2015**, *36*, 605–614. [CrossRef] [PubMed]
15. Harvey, J.J.; Huang, S.; Uberoi, R. *Catheter-Directed Therapies for the Treatment of High Risk (Massive) and Intermediate Risk (Submassive) Acute Pulmonary Embolism*; John Wiley and Sons Ltd.: Hoboken, NJ, USA, 2022.
16. Klok, F.A.; Piazza, G.; Sharp, A.S.P.; Ní Ainle, F.; Jaff, M.R.; Chauhan, N.; Patel, B.; Barco, S.; Goldhaber, S.Z.; Kucher, N.; et al. Ultrasound-facilitated, catheter-directed thrombolysis vs anticoagulation alone for acute intermediate-high-risk pulmonary embolism: Rationale and design of the HI-PEITHO study. *Am. Heart J.* **2022**, *251*, 43–53. [CrossRef]
17. Schönfeld, T.; Seitz, P.; Krieghoff, C.; Ponorac, S.; Wötzel, A.; Olthoff, S.; Schaudt, S.; Steglich, J.; Gutberlet, M.; Gohmann, R.F. High-pitch CT pulmonary angiography (CTPA) with ultra-low contrast medium volume for the detection of pulmonary embolism: A comparison with standard CTPA. *Eur. Radiol.* **2024**, *34*, 1921–1931. [CrossRef]
18. D'Angelo, T.; Bucolo, G.M.; Yel, I.; Koch, V.; Gruenewald, L.D.; Martin, S.S.; Alizadeh, L.S.; Vogl, T.J.; Ascenti, G.; Lanzafame, L.R.M.; et al. Dual-energy CT late arterial phase iodine maps for the diagnosis of acute non-occlusive mesenteric ischemia. *Radiol. Med.* **2024**, *129*, 1611–1621. [CrossRef]
19. Rajiah, P.; Parakh, A.; Kay, F.; Baruah, D.; Kambadakone, A.R.; Leng, S. Update on multienergy CT: Physics, principles, and applications. *Radiographics* **2020**, *40*, 1284–1308. [CrossRef]
20. Borgheresi, A.; Cesari, E.; Agostini, A.; Badaloni, M.; Balducci, S.; Tola, E.; Consoli, V.; Palucci, A.; Burroni, L.; Carotti, M.; et al. Pulmonary emphysema: The assessment of lung perfusion with Dual-Energy CT and pulmonary scintigraphy. *Radiol. Med.* **2024**, *129*, 1622–1632. [CrossRef] [PubMed]
21. Grob, D.; Smit, E.; Prince, J.; Kist, J.; Stöger, L.; Geurts, B.; Snoeren, M.M.; van Dijk, R.; Oostveen, L.J.; Prokop, M.; et al. Iodine Maps from Subtraction CT or Dual-Energy CT to Detect Pulmonary Emboli with CT Angiography: A Multiple-Observer Study. *Radiology* **2019**, *292*, 197–205. [CrossRef] [PubMed]
22. Thieme, S.F.; Becker, C.R.; Hacker, M.; Nikolaou, K.; Reiser, M.F.; Johnson, T.R.C. Dual energy CT for the assessment of lung perfusion-Correlation to scintigraphy. *Eur. J. Radiol.* **2008**, *68*, 369–374. [CrossRef]
23. Thieme, S.F.; Graute, V.; Nikolaou, K.; Maxien, D.; Reiser, M.F.; Hacker, M.; Johnson, T.R. Dual Energy CT lung perfusion imaging—Correlation with SPECT/CT. *Eur. J. Radiol.* **2012**, *81*, 360–365. [CrossRef]
24. Grob, D.; Smit, E.; Oostveen, L.J.; Snoeren, M.M.; Prokop, M.; Schaefer-Prokop, C.M.; Sechopoulos, I.; Brink, M. Image Quality of Iodine Maps for Pulmonary Embolism: A Comparison of Subtraction CT and Dual-Energy CT. *AJR Am. J. Roentgenol.* **2019**, *212*, 1253–1259. [CrossRef]
25. Monti, C.B.; Zanardo, M.; Cozzi, A.; Schiaffino, S.; Spagnolo, P.; Secchi, F.; De Cecco, C.N.; Sardanelli, F. Dual-energy CT performance in acute pulmonary embolism: A meta-analysis. *Eur. Radiol.* **2021**, *31*, 6248–6258. [CrossRef] [PubMed]
26. Stein, P.D.; Fowler, S.E.; Goodman, L.R.; Gottschalk, A.; Hales, C.A.; Hull, R.D.; Leeper, K.V., Jr.; Popovich, J., Jr.; Quinn, D.A.; Sos, T.A.; et al. PIOPED II Investigators. Multidetector computed tomography for acute pulmonary embolism. *N. Engl. J. Med.* **2006**, *354*, 2317–2327. [CrossRef]
27. Foti, G.; Silva, R.; Faccioli, N.; Fighera, A.; Menghini, R.; Campagnola, A.; Carbognin, G. Identification of pulmonary embolism: Diagnostic accuracy of venous-phase dual-energy CT in comparison to pulmonary arteries CT angiography. *Eur. Radiol.* **2021**, *31*, 1923–1931. [CrossRef] [PubMed]
28. Im, D.J.; Hur, J.; Han, K.H.; Lee, H.J.; Kim, Y.J.; Kwon, W.; Choi, B.W. Acute Pulmonary Embolism: Retrospective Cohort Study of the Predictive Value of Perfusion Defect Volume Measured with Dual-Energy CT. *AJR Am. J. Roentgenol.* **2017**, *209*, 1015–1022. [CrossRef] [PubMed]

29. Chae, E.J.; Seo, J.B.; Jang, Y.M.; Krauss, B.; Lee, C.W.; Lee, H.J.; Song, K.S. Dual-energy CT for assessment of the severity of acute pulmonary embolism: Pulmonary perfusion defect score compared with CT angiographic obstruction score and right ventricular/left ventricular diameter ratio. *AJR Am. J. Roentgenol.* **2010**, *194*, 604–610. [CrossRef] [PubMed]
30. Cellina, M.; Cè, M.; Grimaldi, E.; Mastellone, G.; Fortunati, A.; Oliva, G.; Martinenghi, C.; Carrafiello, G. The role of dual-energy computed tomography (DECT) in emergency radiology: A visual guide to advanced diagnostics. *Clin. Radiol.* **2025**, *83*, 106836. [CrossRef]
31. Schwartz, F.R.; Bache, S.; Lee, R.; Maxfield, C.M.; Fadell, M.F., 2nd; Gaca, A.M.; Samei, E.; Frush, D.P.; Cao, J.Y. Photon-counting CT yields superior abdominopelvic image quality at lower radiation and iodinated contrast doses. *Pediatr. Radiol.* **2025**, *55*, 1202–1211. [CrossRef] [PubMed]
32. Willemink, M.J.; Persson, M.; Pourmorteza, A.; Pelc, N.J.; Fleischmann, D. Photon-counting CT: Technical principles and clinical prospects. *Radiol. Soc. N. Am. Inc.* **2018**, *289*, 293–312. [CrossRef]
33. Pannenbecker, P.; Heidenreich, J.F.; Huflage, H.; Gruschwitz, P.; Patzer, T.S.; Weng, A.M.; Grunz, J.P.; Kunz, A.S.; Bley, T.A.; Petritsch, B. The Best of Both Worlds: Ultra-high-pitch Pulmonary Angiography with Free-Breathing Technique by Means of Photon-Counting Detector CT for Diagnosis of Acute Pulmonary Embolism. *Acad. Radiol.* **2024**, *31*, 5280–5288. [CrossRef] [PubMed]
34. Pallasch, F.B.; Rau, A.; Reisert, M.; Rau, S.; Diallo, T.; Stein, T.; Faby, S.; Bamberg, F.; Weiss, J. Photon-counting detector computed tomography for metal artifact reduction: A comparative study of different artifact reduction techniques in patients with orthopedic implants. *Radiol. Med.* **2024**, *129*, 890–900. [CrossRef]
35. Yalynska, T.; Polacin, M.; Frauenfelder, T.; Martini, K. Impact of Photon Counting Detector CT Derived Virtual Monoenergetic Images on the Diagnosis of Pulmonary Embolism. *Diagnostics* **2022**, *12*, 2715. [CrossRef]
36. Remy-Jardin, M.; Oufriche, I.; Guiffault, L.; Duhamel, A.; Flohr, T.; Schmidt, B.; Remy, J. Diagnosis of acute pulmonary embolism: When photon-counting-detector CT replaces energy-integrating-detector CT in daily routine. *Eur. Radiol.* **2024**, *34*, 6544–6555. [CrossRef]
37. Nehra, A.K.; Rajendran, K.; Baffour, F.I.; Mileto, A.; Rajiah, P.S.; Horst, K.K.; Inoue, A.; Johnson, T.F.; Diehn, F.E.; Glazebrook, K.N.; et al. Seeing More with Less: Clinical Benefits of Photon-counting Detector CT. *Radiographics* **2023**, *43*, e220158. [CrossRef] [PubMed]
38. Cè, M.; Oliva, G.; Rabaiotti, F.L.; Macrì, L.; Zollo, S.; Aquila, A.; Cellina, M. Portable Dynamic Chest Radiography: Literature Review and Potential Bedside Applications. *Med. Sci.* **2024**, *12*, 10. [CrossRef] [PubMed]
39. Yamasaki, Y.; Abe, K.; Hosokawa, K.; Kamitani, T. A novel pulmonary circulation imaging using dynamic digital radiography for chronic thromboembolic pulmonary hypertension. *Eur. Heart J.* **2020**, *41*, 2506. [CrossRef]
40. Yamasaki, Y.; Kamitani, T.; Sagiyama, K.; Hino, T.; Kisanuki, M.; Tabata, K.; Isoda, T.; Kitamura, Y.; Abe, K.; Hosokawa, K.; et al. Dynamic chest radiography for pulmonary vascular diseases: Clinical applications and correlation with other imaging modalities. *Jpn. J. Radiol.* **2024**, *42*, 126–144. [CrossRef]
41. Bushra, F.; Chowdhury, M.E.H.; Sarmun, R.; Kabir, S.; Said, M.; Zoghoul, S.B.; Mushtak, A.; Al-Hashimi, I.; Alqahtani, A.; Hasan, A. Deep learning in computed tomography pulmonary angiography imaging: A dual-pronged approach for pulmonary embolism detection. *Expert Syst. Appl.* **2024**, *245*, 123029. [CrossRef]
42. Allena, N.; Khanal, S. The Algorithmic Lung Detective: Artificial Intelligence in the Diagnosis of Pulmonary Embolism. *Cureus* **2023**, *15*, e51006. [CrossRef]
43. Li, L.; Peng, M.; Zou, Y.; Li, Y.; Qiao, P. The promise and limitations of artificial intelligence in CTPA-based pulmonary embolism detection. *Front. Med.* **2025**, *12*, 1514931. [CrossRef]
44. Djahnine, A.; Lazarus, C.; Lederlin, M.; Mulé, S.; Wiemker, R.; Si-Mohamed, S.; Jupin-Delevaux, E.; Nempont, O.; Skandarani, Y.; De Craene, M.; et al. Detection and severity quantification of pulmonary embolism with 3D CT data using an automated deep learning-based artificial solution. *Diagn. Interv. Imaging* **2024**, *105*, 97–103. [CrossRef]
45. Das, M.; Mühlenbruch, G.; Helm, A.; Bakai, A.; Salganicoff, M.; Stanzel, S.; Liang, J.; Wolf, M.; Günther, R.W.; Wildberger, J.E. Computer-aided detection of pulmonary embolism: Influence on radiologists' detection performance with respect to vessel segments. *Eur. Radiol.* **2008**, *18*, 1350–1355. [CrossRef]
46. Cheikh, A.B.; Gorincour, G.; Nivet, H.; May, J.; Seux, M.; Calame, P.; Thomson, V.; Delabrousse, E.; Crombé, A. How artificial intelligence improves radiological interpretation in suspected pulmonary embolism. *Eur. Radiol.* **2022**, *32*, 5831–5842. [CrossRef]
47. Langius-Wiffen, E.; de Jong, P.A.; Hoesein, F.A.M.; Dekker, L.; van den Hoven, A.F.; Nijholt, I.M.; Boomsma, M.F.; Veldhuis, W.B. Retrospective batch analysis to evaluate the diagnostic accuracy of a clinically deployed AI algorithm for the detection of acute pulmonary embolism on CTPA. *Insights Imaging* **2023**, *14*, 102. [CrossRef]
48. Huang, G.; Liu, Z.; van der Maaten, L.; Weinberger, K.Q. Densely Connected Convolutional Networks. Available online: http://arxiv.org/abs/1608.06993 (accessed on 1 June 2025).
49. Liu, Z.; Yuan, H.; Wang, H. CAM-Wnet: An effective solution for accurate pulmonary embolism segmentation. *Med. Phys.* **2022**, *49*, 5294–5303. [CrossRef] [PubMed]

50. Zsarnoczay, E.; Rapaka, S.; Schoepf, U.J.; Gnasso, C.; Vecsey-Nagy, M.; Todoran, T.M.; Hagar, M.T.; Kravchenko, D.; Tremamunno, G.; Griffith, J.P.; et al. Accuracy of a deep neural network for automated pulmonary embolism detection on dedicated CT pulmonary angiograms. *Eur. J. Radiol.* **2025**, *187*, 112077. [CrossRef] [PubMed]
51. Huhtanen, H.; Nyman, M.; Mohsen, T.; Virkki, A.; Karlsson, A.; Hirvonen, J. Automated detection of pulmonary embolism from CT-angiograms using deep learning. *BMC Med. Imaging* **2022**, *22*, 43. [CrossRef]
52. Liu, W.; Liu, M.; Guo, X.; Zhang, P.; Zhang, L.; Zhang, R.; Kang, H.; Zhai, Z.; Tao, X.; Wan, J.; et al. Evaluation of acute pulmonary embolism and clot burden on CTPA with deep learning. *Eur. Radiol.* **2020**, *30*, 3567–3575. [CrossRef] [PubMed]
53. Kahraman, A.T.; Fröding, T.; Toumpanakis, D.; Gustafsson, C.J.; Sjöblom, T. Enhanced classification performance using deep learning based segmentation for pulmonary embolism detection in CT angiography. *Heliyon* **2024**, *10*, e38118. [CrossRef]
54. Mu, W.; Liang, Y.; Hall, L.O.; Tan, Y.; Balagurunathan, Y.; Wenham, R.; Wu, N.; Tian, J.; Gillies, R.J. 18F-FDG PET/CT Habitat Radiomics Predicts Outcome of Patients with Cervical Cancer Treated with Chemoradiotherapy. *Radiol. Artif. Intell.* **2020**, *2*, e190218. [CrossRef] [PubMed]
55. Soffer, S.; Klang, E.; Shimon, O.; Barash, Y.; Cahan, N.; Greenspan, H.; Konen, E. Deep learning for pulmonary embolism detection on computed tomography pulmonary angiogram: A systematic review and meta-analysis. *Sci. Rep.* **2021**, *11*, 15814. [CrossRef] [PubMed]
56. Lanza, E.; Ammirabile, A.; Francone, M. Meta-analysis of AI-based pulmonary embolism detection: How reliable are deep learning models? *Comput. Biol. Med.* **2025**, *193*, 110402. [CrossRef]
57. Ayobi, A.; Chang, P.D.; Chow, D.S.; Weinberg, B.D.; Tassy, M.; Franciosini, A.; Scudeler, M.; Quenet, S.; Avare, C.; Chaibi, Y. Performance and clinical utility of an artificial intelligence-enabled tool for pulmonary embolism detection. *Clin. Imaging* **2024**, *113*, 110245. [CrossRef]
58. Grenier, P.A.; Ayobi, A.; Quenet, S.; Tassy, M.; Marx, M.; Chow, D.S.; Weinberg, B.D.; Chang, P.D.; Chaibi, Y. Deep Learning-Based Algorithm for Automatic Detection of Pulmonary Embolism in Chest CT Angiograms. *Diagnostics* **2023**, *13*, 1324. [CrossRef]
59. Li, Y.; Zhang, L.; Liu, H.; Li, Y.; Liu, Z. Research progress of artificial intelligence and machine learning in pulmonary embolism. *Front. Med.* **2025**, *12*, 1577559. [CrossRef]
60. Naser, A.M.; Vyas, R.; Morgan, A.A.; Kalaiger, A.M.; Kharawala, A.; Nagraj, S.; Agarwal, R.; Maliha, M.; Mangeshkar, S.; Singh, N.; et al. Role of Artificial Intelligence in the Diagnosis and Management of Pulmonary Embolism: A Comprehensive Review. *Diagnostics* **2025**, *15*, 889. [CrossRef] [PubMed]
61. Huang, S.C.; Kothari, T.; Banerjee, I.; Chute, C.; Ball, R.L.; Borus, N.; Huang, A.; Patel, B.N.; Rajpurkar, P.; Irvin, J.; et al. PENet-a scalable deep-learning model for automated diagnosis of pulmonary embolism using volumetric CT imaging. *NPJ Digit. Med.* **2020**, *3*, 61, Erratum in *NPJ Digit. Med.* **2020**, *3*, 102. [CrossRef]
62. Wu, H.; Xu, Q.; He, X.; Xu, H.; Wang, Y.; Guo, L. SPE-YOLO: A deep learning model focusing on small pulmonary embolism detection. *Comput. Biol. Med.* **2025**, *184*, 109402. [CrossRef]
63. Hagen, F.; Vorberg, L.; Thamm, F.; Ditt, H.; Maier, A.; Brendel, J.M.; Ghibes, P.; Bongers, M.N.; Krumm, P.; Nikolaou, K.; et al. Improved detection of small pulmonary embolism on unenhanced computed tomography using an artificial intelligence-based algorithm—A single centre retrospective study. *Int. J. Cardiovasc. Imaging* **2024**, *40*, 2293–2304. [CrossRef]
64. Belkouchi, Y.; Lederlin, M.; Ben Afia, A.; Fabre, C.; Ferretti, G.; De Margerie, C.; Berge, P.; Liberge, R.; Elbaz, N.; Blain, M.; et al. Detection and quantification of pulmonary embolism with artificial intelligence: The SFR 2022 artificial intelligence data challenge. *Diagn. Interv. Imaging* **2023**, *104*, 485–489. [CrossRef] [PubMed]
65. Cho, S.U.; Cho, Y.D.; Choi, S.H.; Yoon, Y.H.; Park, J.H.; Park, S.J.; Lee, E.S. Assessing the severity of pulmonary embolism among patients in the emergency department: Utility of RV/LV diameter ratio. *PLoS ONE* **2020**, *15*, e0242340. [CrossRef]
66. Park, J.I.; Kim, D.; Lee, J.A.; Zheng, K.; Amin, A. Personalized Risk Prediction for 30-Day Readmissions with Venous Thromboembolism Using Machine Learning. *J. Nurs. Scholarsh.* **2021**, *53*, 278–287. [CrossRef] [PubMed]
67. Jin, Z.G.; Zhang, H.; Tai, M.H.; Yang, Y.; Yao, Y.; Guo, Y.T. Natural Language Processing in a Clinical Decision Support System for the Identification of Venous Thromboembolism: Algorithm Development and Validation. *J. Med. Internet. Res.* **2023**, *25*, e45139. [CrossRef]
68. Leidi, A.; Bex, S.; Righini, M.; Berner, A.; Grosgurin, O.; Marti, C. Risk Stratification in Patients with Acute Pulmonary Embolism: Current Evidence and Perspectives. *J. Clin. Med.* **2022**, *11*, 2533. [CrossRef] [PubMed]
69. Barca-Hernando, M.; Jara-Palomares, L. When should we involve interventional radiology in the management of acute pulmonary embolism? *Breathe* **2023**, *19*, 230085. [CrossRef]
70. Pruszczyk, P.; Klok, F.A.; Kucher, N.; Roik, M.; Meneveau, N.; Sharp, A.S.P.; Nielsen-Kudsk, J.E.; Obradović, S.; Barco, S.; Giannini, F.; et al. Percutaneous treatment options for acute pulmonary embolism: A clinical consensus statement by the ESC Working Group on Pulmonary Circulation and Right Ventricular Function and the European Association of Percutaneous Cardiovascular Interventions. *EuroIntervention* **2022**, *18*, e623–e638. [CrossRef]

71. Konstantinides, S.V.; Meyer, G.; Becattini, C.; Bueno, H.; Geersing, G.J.; Harjola, V.P.; Huisman, M.V.; Humbert, M.; Jennings, C.S.; Jiménez, D.; et al. ESC Scientific Document Group. 2019 ESC Guidelines for the diagnosis and management of acute pulmonary embolism developed in collaboration with the European Respiratory Society (ERS). *Eur. Heart J.* **2020**, *41*, 543–603. [CrossRef]
72. Stevens, S.M.; Woller, S.C.; Kreuziger, L.B.; Bounameaux, H.; Doerschug, K.; Geersing, G.J.; Huisman, M.V.; Kearon, C.; King, C.S.; Knighton, A.J.; et al. Antithrombotic Therapy for VTE Disease: Second Update of the CHEST Guideline and Expert Panel Report. *Chest* **2021**, *160*, e545–e608, Erratum in *Chest* **2022**, *162*, 269. [CrossRef] [PubMed]
73. Kucher, N.; Boekstegers, P.; Müller, O.J.; Kupatt, C.; Beyer-Westendorf, J.; Heitzer, T.; Tebbe, U.; Horstkotte, J.; Müller, R.; Blessing, E.; et al. Randomized, controlled trial of ultrasound-assisted catheter-directed thrombolysis for acute intermediate-risk pulmonary embolism. *Circulation* **2014**, *129*, 479–486. [CrossRef]
74. Tu, T.; Toma, C.; Tapson, V.F.; Adams, C.; Jaber, W.A.; Silver, M.; Khandhar, S.; Amin, R.; Weinberg, M.; Engelhardt, T.; et al. A Prospective, Single-Arm, Multicenter Trial of Catheter-Directed Mechanical Thrombectomy for Intermediate-Risk Acute Pulmonary Embolism: The FLARE Study. *JACC Cardiovasc. Interv.* **2019**, *12*, 859–869. [CrossRef]
75. Tapson, V.F.; Sterling, K.; Jones, N.; Elder, M.; Tripathy, U.; Brower, J.; Maholic, R.L.; Ross, C.B.; Natarajan, K.; Fong, P.; et al. A Randomized Trial of the Optimum Duration of Acoustic Pulse Thrombolysis Procedure in Acute Intermediate-Risk Pulmonary Embolism: The OPTALYSE PE Trial. *JACC Cardiovasc. Interv.* **2018**, *11*, 1401–1410. [CrossRef] [PubMed]
76. Avgerinos, E.D.; Jaber, W.; Lacomis, J.; Markel, K.; McDaniel, M.; Rivera-Lebron, B.N.; Ross, C.B.; Sechrist, J.; Toma, C.; Chaer, R. Randomized Trial Comparing Standard Versus Ultrasound-Assisted Thrombolysis for Submassive Pulmonary Embolism: The SUNSET sPE Trial. *JACC Cardiovasc. Interv.* **2021**, *14*, 1364–1373, Erratum in *JACC Cardiovasc. Interv.* **2021**, *14*, 2194. [CrossRef] [PubMed]
77. Netzel, A.; Iqbal, F.; Hansra, R.; Grier, L. Ekosonic endovascular system catheter for successful treatment of right atrial thrombus and pulmonary embolism: A case report. *Chest* **2022**, *162*, A798–A799. [CrossRef]
78. Toma, C.; Jaber, W.A.; Weinberg, M.D.; Bunte, M.C.; Khandhar, S.; Stegman, B.; Gondi, S.; Chambers, J.; Amin, R.; Leung, D.A.; et al. Acute outcomes for the full US cohort of the FLASH mechanical thrombectomy registry in pulmonary embolism. *EuroIntervention* **2023**, *18*, 1201–1212. [CrossRef]
79. Khandhar, S.; Jaber, W.; Bunte, M.C.; Cho, K.; Weinberg, M.D.; Mina, B.; Stegman, B.; Pollak, J.; Khosla, A.; Elmasri, F.; et al. Longer-Term Outcomes Following Mechanical Thrombectomy for Intermediate- and High-Risk Pulmonary Embolism: 6-Month FLASH Registry Results. *J. Soc. Cardiovasc. Angiogr. Interv.* **2023**, *2*, 101000. [CrossRef]
80. Silver, M.J.; Gibson, C.M.; Giri, J.; Khandhar, S.; Jaber, W.; Toma, C.; Mina, B.; Bowers, T.; Greenspon, L.; Kado, H.; et al. Outcomes in High-Risk Pulmonary Embolism Patients Undergoing FlowTriever Mechanical Thrombectomy or Other Contemporary Therapies: Results From the FLAME Study. *Circ. Cardiovasc. Interv.* **2023**, *16*, e013406. [CrossRef] [PubMed]
81. Jaber, W.A.; Gonsalves, C.F.; Stortecky, S.; Horr, S.; Pappas, O.; Gandhi, R.T.; Pereira, K.; Giri, J.; Khandhar, S.J.; Ammar, K.A.; et al. Large-Bore Mechanical Thrombectomy Versus Catheter-Directed Thrombolysis in the Management of Intermediate-Risk Pulmonary Embolism: Primary Results of the PEERLESS Randomized Controlled Trial. *Circulation* **2025**, *151*, 260–273. [CrossRef] [PubMed]
82. Sista, A.K.; Horowitz, J.M.; Tapson, V.F.; Rosenberg, M.; Elder, M.D.; Schiro, B.J.; Dohad, S.; Amoroso, N.E.; Dexter, D.J.; Loh, C.T.; et al. EXTRACT-PE Investigators. Indigo Aspiration System for Treatment of Pulmonary Embolism: Results of the EXTRACT-PE Trial. *JACC Cardiovasc. Interv.* **2021**, *14*, 319–329. [CrossRef]
83. Moriarty, J.M.; Dohad, S.Y.; Schiro, B.J.; Tamaddon, H.; Heithaus, R.E.; Iliadis, E.A.; Dexter, D.J., 2nd; Shavelle, D.M.; Leal, S.R.N.; Attallah, A.S.; et al. Clinical, Functional, and Quality-of-Life Outcomes after Computer Assisted Vacuum Thrombectomy for Pulmonary Embolism: Interim Analysis of the STRIKE-PE Study. *J. Vasc. Interv. Radiol.* **2024**, *35*, 1154–1165.e6. [CrossRef]
84. Angelini, G.; Maharaj, S.; McCarthy, A.; Martinez, A.; Gomez, J.; Rampersad, R. Thrombo-Aspiration in a High-Risk Case of Pulmonary Embolism. *J. Clin. Case Rep.* **2024**, *2*, 1011. [CrossRef]
85. Li, K.; Cui, M.; Zhang, K.; Liang, K.; Liu, H.; Zhai, S. Treatment of acute pulmonary embolism using rheolytic thrombectomy. *EuroIntervention* **2021**, *17*, E158–E166. [CrossRef]
86. Akbal, Ö.Y.; Keskin, B.; Tokgöz, H.C.; Hakgör, A.; Karagöz, A.; Tanyeri, S.; Kültürsay, B.; Külahçıoğlu, Ş.; Bayram, Z.; Efe, S.; et al. A seven-year single-center experience on AngioJet rheolytic thrombectomy in patients with pulmonary embolism at high risk and intermediate-high risk. *Anatol. J. Cardiol.* **2021**, *25*, 902–911. [CrossRef] [PubMed]
87. Bashir, R.; Foster, M.; Iskander, A.; Darki, A.; Jaber, W.; Rali, P.M.; Lakhter, V.; Gandhi, R.; Klein, A.; Bhatheja, R.; et al. Pharmacomechanical Catheter-Directed Thrombolysis with the Bashir Endovascular Catheter for Acute Pulmonary Embolism: The RESCUE Study. *JACC Cardiovasc. Interv.* **2022**, *15*, 2427–2436. [CrossRef]
88. Agnelli, G.; Becattini, C. Anticoagulant treatment for acute pulmonary embolism: A pathophysiology-based clinical approach. *Eur. Respir. J.* **2015**, *45*, 1142–1149. [CrossRef] [PubMed]
89. Konstantinides, S.; Geibel, A.; Heusel, G.; Heinrich, F.; Kasper, W. Heparin plus alteplase compared with heparin alone in patients with submassive pulmonary embolism. *N. Engl. J. Med.* **2002**, *347*, 1143–1150. [CrossRef]

90. Wan, S.; Quinlan, D.J.; Agnelli, G. Thrombolysis compared with heparin for the initial treatment of pulmonary embolism: A meta-analysis of the randomized controlled trials. *Circulation* **2004**, *110*, 744–749. [CrossRef] [PubMed]
91. Meyer, G.; Vicaut, E.; Danays, T.; Agnelli, G.; Becattini, C.; Beyer-Westendorf, J.; Bluhmki, E.; Bouvaist, H.; Brenner, B.; Couturaud, F.; et al. PEITHO Investigators. Fibrinolysis for patients with intermediate-risk pulmonary embolism. *N. Engl. J. Med.* **2014**, *370*, 1402–1411. [CrossRef] [PubMed]
92. Murguia, A.R.; Mukherjee, D.; Ojha, C. Reduced-dose thrombolysis in acute pulmonary embolism a systematic review. *Angiology* **2023**, *75*, 208–218. [CrossRef]
93. Rosa, A.; Murguia, A.R.; Brockman, M.J.; Mukherjee, D.; Rajachandran, M.; Nickel, N.P. Low-dose Systemic Tissue-type-plasminogen-activator Compared to Conventional Anti-coagulation for the Treatment of Intermediate-high Risk Pulmonary Embolism. *Cardiovasc. Hematol. Disord. Targets* **2025**, *25*, 46–53. [CrossRef] [PubMed]
94. Güner, A.; Güner, E.G.; Karakurt, S.; Kalçık, M. Efficacy and Safety of Low-Dose Systemic Fibrinolytic Therapy for Acute Submassive Pulmonary Embolism. *JACC Cardiovasc. Interv.* **2021**, *14*, 809. [CrossRef]
95. Zhang, L.Y.; Gao, B.A.; Jin, Z.; Xiang, G.M.; Gong, Z.; Zhang, T.T.; Lu, H.F.; Wang, Y.Q.; Gong, Y.; Lu, C.; et al. Clinical efficacy of low dose recombinant tissue-type plasminogen activator for the treatment of acute intermediate-risk pulmonary embolism. *Saudi Med. J.* **2018**, *39*, 1090–1095. [CrossRef]
96. Schultz, J.; Giordano, N.; Zheng, H.; Parry, B.A.; Barnes, G.D.; Heresi, G.A.; Jaber, W.; Wood, T.; Todoran, T.; Courtney, D.M.; et al. EXPRESS: A Multidisciplinary Pulmonary Embolism Response Team (PERT)—Experience from a national multicenter consortium. *Pulm. Circ.* **2019**, *9*, 1–10. [CrossRef] [PubMed]
97. Gardner, T.A.; Fuher, A.; Longino, A.; Sink, E.M.; Jurica, J.; Park, B.; Lindquist, J.; Bull, T.M.; Hountras, P. Reduced mortality associated with pulmonary embolism response team consultation for intermediate and high-risk pulmonary embolism: A retrospective cohort study. *Thromb. J.* **2024**, *22*, 38. [CrossRef]
98. Fleitas Sosa, D.; Lehr, A.L.; Zhao, H.; Roth, S.; Lakhther, V.; Bashir, R.; Cohen, G.; Panaro, J.; Maldonado, T.S.; Horowitz, J.; et al. Impact of pulmonary embolism response teams on acute pulmonary embolism: A systematic review and meta-analysis. *Eur. Respir. Rev.* **2022**, *31*, 220023. [CrossRef]
99. Sterling, K.M.; Goldhaber, S.Z.; Sharp, A.S.P.; Kucher, N.; Jones, N.; Maholic, R.; Meneveau, N.; Zlotnick, D.; Sayfo, S.; Konstantinides, S.V.; et al. Prospective Multicenter International Registry of Ultrasound-Facilitated Catheter-Directed Thrombolysis in Intermediate-High and High-Risk Pulmonary Embolism (KNOCOUT PE). *Circ. Cardiovasc. Interv.* **2024**, *17*, e013448. [CrossRef]
100. Sista, A.K.; Troxel, A.B.; Tarpey, T.; Parpia, S.; Goldhaber, S.Z.; Stringer, W.W.; Magnuson, E.A.; Cohen, D.J.; Kahn, S.R.; Rao, S.V.; et al. Rationale and design of the PE-TRACT trial: A multicenter randomized trial to evaluate catheter-directed therapy for the treatment of intermediate-risk pulmonary embolism. *Am. Heart J.* **2025**, *281*, 112–122. [CrossRef] [PubMed]

Journal of
*Cardiovascular
Development and Disease*

MDPI

Systematic Review

AI Applied to Cardiac Magnetic Resonance for Precision Medicine in Coronary Artery Disease: A Systematic Review

Cristina Jiménez-Jara [1,2,3,4], Rodrigo Salas [1,3,4], Rienzi Díaz-Navarro [2,4], Steren Chabert [1,3,4], Marcelo E. Andia [3,5], Julián Vega [6,7], Jesús Urbina [6,7,8], Sergio Uribe [9], Tetsuro Sekine [10], Francesca Raimondi [11,*] and Julio Sotelo [12,*]

1 School of Biomedical Engineering, Universidad de Valparaíso, Valparaíso 2362905, Chile; maria.jimenezj@postgrado.uv.cl (C.J.-J.); rodrigo.salas@uv.cl (R.S.); steren.chabert@uv.cl (S.C.)
2 Cardiovascular Physiology Laboratory, Department of Medicine, School of Medicine, Universidad de Valparaíso, Viña del Mar 2340000, Chile; rienzi.diaz@uv.cl
3 Millennium Institute for Intelligent Healthcare Engineering—iHealth, Valparaíso 2362905, Chile; meandia@uc.cl
4 Center of Interdisciplinary Biomedical and Engineering Research for Health—MEDING, Universidad de Valparaíso, Valparaíso 2362905, Chile
5 Biomedical Imaging Center and Department of Radiology, School of Medicine, Pontificia Universidad Católica de Chile, Santiago 8330023, Chile
6 Department of Radiology, Complejo Asistencial Dr. Sótero del Río, Santiago 8207257, Chile; julianvega@gmail.com (J.V.); jjesus.urbina@gmail.com (J.U.)
7 Chilean Institute of Cardiac Imaging —INCIC, Santiago 8320000, Chile
8 Department of Radiology, Clínica BUPA Santiago, Santiago 8240004, Chile
9 Department of Medical Imaging and Radiation Sciences, Monash University, Melbourne 3800, Australia; sergio.uribe@monash.edu
10 Department of Radiology, Nippon Medical School Musashi Kosugi Hospital, Kanagawa 211-8533, Japan; tetsuro.sekine@gmail.com
11 Congenital Heart Disease Unit, Papa Giovanni XXXIII Hospital, 24127 Bergamo, Italy
12 Departamento de Informática, Universidad Técnica Federico Santa María, Santiago 8940897, Chile
* Correspondence: francesca.raimondi@gmail.com (F.R.); julio.sotelo@usm.cl (J.S.)

Abstract: Cardiac magnetic resonance (CMR) imaging has become a key tool in evaluating myocardial injury secondary to coronary artery disease (CAD), providing detailed assessments of cardiac morphology, function, and tissue composition. The integration of artificial intelligence (AI), including machine learning and deep learning techniques, has enhanced the diagnostic capabilities of CMR by automating segmentation, improving image interpretation, and accelerating clinical workflows. Radiomics, through the extraction of quantitative imaging features, complements AI by revealing sub-visual patterns relevant to disease characterization. This systematic review analyzed AI applications in CMR for CAD. A structured search was conducted in MEDLINE, Web of Science, and Scopus up to 17 March 2025, following PRISMA guidelines and quality-assessed with the CLAIM checklist. A total of 106 studies were included: 46 on classification, 19 using radiomics, and 41 on segmentation. AI models were used to classify CAD vs. controls, predict major adverse cardiovascular events (MACE), arrhythmias, and post-infarction remodeling. Radiomics enabled differentiation of acute vs. chronic infarction and prediction of microvascular obstruction, sometimes from non-contrast CMR. Segmentation achieved high performance for myocardium (DSC up to 0.95), but scar and edema delineation were more challenging. Reported performance was moderate-to-high across tasks (classification AUC = 0.66–1.00; segmentation DSC = 0.43–0.97; radiomics AUC = 0.57–0.99). Despite promising results, limitations included small or overlapping datasets. In conclusion, AI and radiomics offer substantial potential to support diagnosis and prognosis of CAD through advanced CMR image analysis.

Keywords: AI; systematic review; artificial intelligence; CAD; coronary artery disease; CMR; cardiac magnetic resonance

1. Introduction

Coronary artery disease (CAD) is a pathological process characterized by atherosclerotic plaque accumulation in the epicardial arteries, whether obstructive or non-obstructive, and represents a range of clinical syndromes caused by insufficient coronary blood flow to the myocardium [1,2]. Angiography is the gold standard for characterizing CAD; however, angiography is invasive and patients are exposed to high radiation and contrast doses. Cardiac computed tomography angiogram (CTA) is the most commonly used method for the evaluation of the coronary arteries in children [3,4] and adults, particularly in patients with low to moderate risk of CAD [5]; however, patients are exposed to high doses of radiation and iodinated contrast agents. Cardiovascular magnetic resonance (CMR) imaging has gained widespread acceptance for its non-invasive global assessment, including evaluation of cardiac anatomy and function, and the coronary arteries, the characterization of tissue, and the quantification of flow [6–9]. A valuable tool for the cardiovascular diagnosis [10,11] and prognosis in patients with CAD, CMR imaging can be used to measure markers of cardiac structure and function, and myocardial perfusion and scarring, and to provide detailed insights about myocardial tissue [12]. CMR imaging findings have been shown to have prognostic values. In particular, left ventricular ejection fraction (LVEF) has been shown to be an independent predictor of future cardiovascular events in patients with a recent myocardial infarction (MI) and RWMA, inducible perfusion defects, and LVEF have been shown to identify patients with suspected or known CAD [13,14]. Recently, radiomics has become a promising method for medical imaging and for the extraction and analysis of quantitative metrics from medical images, the so-called radiomic features that can be used to convert images into mineable data [15,16]. Radiomics makes it possible to characterize information that is imperceptible to human vision and impossible to analyse using traditional imaging techniques [15]. Radiomics might allow the identification of new non-invasive imaging biomarkers that could be useful for predicting the prognosis and response to treatment in patients with CAD [15].

Traditional CMR image analysis methods have also evolved to include the use of artificial intelligence (AI). For example, through machine learning (ML) and deep learning (DL) [17,18]. AI enables the creation of models and automatic assessment of cardiovascular segmentation, which improve the reproducibility and accuracy of the analysis compared with the performance of expert radiologists and cardiologists [19]. Radiomics and AI are closely interconnected through the ability of AI to manage and analyse the huge amount of data extracted from medical images compared with traditional statistical methods [20]. This comprehensive review explores recent applications of AI that are gaining traction in the field of CMR, as well as the use of radiomics in patients with CAD. These tools offer varied approaches to CMR image analysis, which requires a synthesis of the different approaches and their purposes, identifying their potential applications, benefits, limitations, and knowledge gaps in the literature from the last 10 years. The aim of this review was to identify whether and how these methods have been implemented in clinical practice and whether they have transformative potential in this field.

2. Materials and Methods

The present systematic review follows the Preferred Reporting Items for Systematic reviews and Meta-Analyses (PRISMA) guidelines [21]. However, this systematic review was not registered in any public registry of reviews and a protocol was not prepared. The literature from the last 10 years was identified from the MEDLINE, Web of Science, and Scopus databases up to 17 March 2025. The search strategy used the following terms: "coronary artery disease", "ischemic heart disease", "myocardial infarction", "MRI", "magnetic resonance imaging", "CMR", "cardiac magnetic resonance", "artificial intelligence", "machine learning", and "deep learning". These terms of interest were used with Boolean operators (Table 1).

Table 1. Detailed search strategy.

Database	Search Parameters
Pubmed	((((coronary artery disease) OR (ischemic heart disease)) OR (myocardial infarction)) AND ((((MRI) OR (Magnetic resonance imaging)) OR (CMR)) OR (Cardiac Magnetic resonance))) AND (((artificial intelligence) OR (machine learning)) OR (deep learning))
WOS	(((ALL = (coronary artery disease)) OR ALL = (ischemic heart disease)) OR ALL = (myocardial infarction)) AND (((((ALL = (MRI)) OR ALL = (Magnetic resonance imaging))) OR ALL = (CMR)) OR ALL = (Cardiac Magnetic resonance)) AND (((ALL = (artificial intelligence)) OR ALL = (machine learning)) OR ALL = (deep learning))
Scopus	(coronary AND artery AND disease OR ischemic AND heart AND disease OR myocardial AND infarction) AND (mri OR magnetic AND resonance AND imaging OR cmr OR cardiac AND mag-netic AND resonance) AND (artificial AND intelligence OR machine AND learning OR deep AND learning)

All articles recovered from the systematic search were exported to the Rayyan web app [22], where duplicates were located and removed. The inclusion criteria used were as follows: original articles, studies based on humans, CAD population, AI, and English or Spanish language. Studies were excluded for the following reasons: duplicate studies, animal models, unpublished articles, grey literature, student dissertations or theses, book chapters, encyclopedias, or conference papers. Two independent reviewers (JS and MJ) performed two rounds of study selection: title and abstract screening followed by full-text review. Each article was screened by two independent reviewers, and disagreements were discussed with a third reviewer (RD) until consensus was achieved.

The authors extracted data that included general study information (author/s, study design, year of publication, country); clinical details (patient characteristics, age in years, sex, number of patients); AI models (ML and DL); targets; image acquisition details; and performance metrics according to the purpose of the study. The data extracted from the articles are presented in tables and analyzed by the authors. The quality of the included studies was assessed using the 44 verification criteria included in the Checklist for AI in Medical Imaging (CLAIM) [23].

3. Results

A total of 934 articles were found in the databases. After screening the titles and abstracts, 142 studies were considered relevant. Subsequently, a full-text assessment identified 106 studies that met the eligibility criteria (Figure 1). The studies showed a growing interest in the use of AI through ML and DL models over the past 10 years in the analysis of CMR images in CAD patients, with good diagnostic accuracy in the classification of CAD patients, as well as in the prediction of outcomes (CAD, arrhythmia, major adverse cardiovascular events "MACE", or death) (n = 46); the segmentation of cardiac structures (myocardium and myocardial infarct, scar, or edema) (n = 41); and the application of radiomics for texture analysis (n = 19). The following sub-sections describe the findings of the studies analysed.

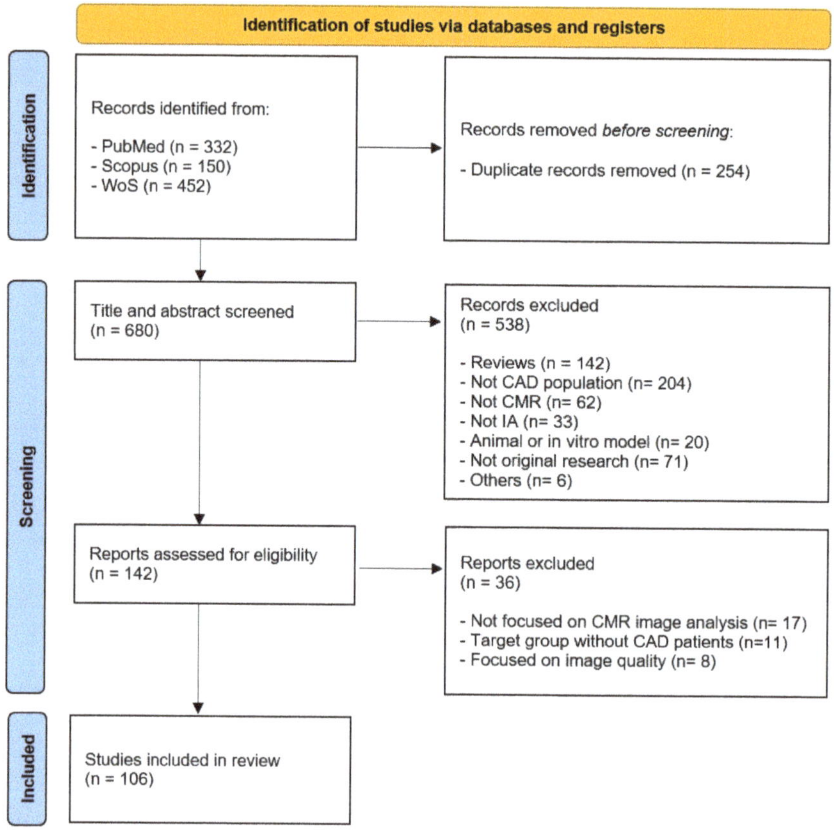

Figure 1. Flow diagram of study inclusion and exclusion criteria for this systematic review.

3.1. Classification

AI is attractive for clinical timescales wherein decisions must be made quickly on readily available computer systems. AI algorithms can learn outcomes based on key patient biomarkers using, for example traditional, ML techniques or even more sophisticated techniques such as DL/neural networks if distinguishing biomarkers are unknown, and these often provide superior accuracy and recall [24]. The steps used when applying AI algorithms of classification in CMR images are shown in Figure 2.

The characteristics of the forty-six included articles are provided in Table 2. The number of patients included in each study showed a high variability (range, 21–63,151). These articles included healthy volunteers and CAD patients, and the data came from both public and private databases. Thirty-four articles reported the number of subjects classified according to sex [25–58] and included a total of 35,916, men (65%) and 19,555 women (35%). Twenty-seven studies were conducted retrospectively [25,26,28,29,32,34–38,40,41,43–47,49–51,58–64] and eight prospectively [27,31,42,48,53–55,57]. Twelve were conducted across multiple centres, and 29 were performed at a single center. However, 15 articles did not provide a description of the databases used and the identification of aspects such as age, comorbidities, and clinical characteristics [24,33,51,52,59–69].

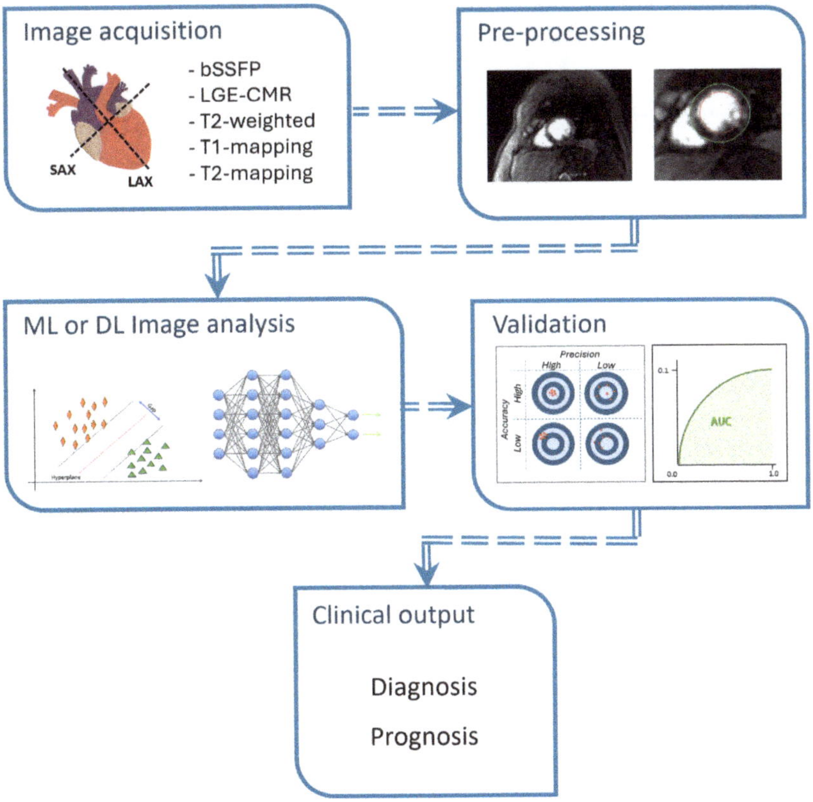

Figure 2. Classification steps for AI applications in CMR. (1) Acquisition of CMR images and clinical data. (2) Preprocessing of images through normalization, re-sizing for uniformity and data augmentation. (3) The data are split into training, validation, and test sets (e.g., 70/15/15). ML or DL models are trained on the training set for data analysis, and their performance is monitored using the vali-dation set. (4) The model is evaluated using the test set by calculating metrics such as accuracy (ACC) or area under the curve (AUC). (5) The output obtained is intended for diagnostic or prognostic purposes in CAD patients.

3.1.1. Classification Between Healthy Volunteers and Patients with Cardiovascular Diseases

In the period analysed, 15 studies focused on distinguishing between, healthy volunteers, CAD patients, and patients with other cardiac pathologies [29,32,38,40,44,49,55,56,58,60,63,68–70]. Joloudari et al. [63] and Iqbal et al. [68], used of DL and ML applications, respectively, and reported high accuracy (ACC = 99.91% and 99.35%, respectively) in distinguising healthy volunteers from CAD patients. However, the study by Iqbal et al. [68], reported a lower ACC and included 63151 subjects compared with Joloudari et al. [63] who included only 30. Neither of these two studies provided a description of the study subjects; both mentioned only the number of patients and healthy subjects without describing other characteristics that could be relevant to this pathology, such as age, gender, or comorbidities. The study conducted by Paciorek et al. [44], compared the classification of the normal and abnormal myocardium from late gadolinium enhancement (LGE) and T1-mapping images, and reported a higher ACC for LGE images (ACC = 88%) than for T1-mapping (ACC = 70%).

Table 2. Classification studies in CMR image in CAD.

Reference	# Subject (M/F)	Age(y) Mean ± Std	CMR Seq.	Target	(Category) AI Model	Performance
Bekheet, et al. [60]	1140 (NR)	NR	LGE	Myo Fibrosis +/−	(ML) MobileNetV2 GoogleNet ResNet50 FibrosisNet	ACC = 87.13 ACC = 88.60 ACC = 88.45 ACC = 96.05
Lalande, et al. [40]	150 (89/61)	MI 66 ± 14 HS 59 ± 12	LGE	MI +/−	(DL) Multi-input classification: CNN, RF.	ACC = 92.00 AUC = 0.96
Chen, et al. [32]	150 (89/61)	MI 66 ± 14 HS 59 ± 12	LGE	MI +/−	(ML) RF Regressor	Infarction: ACC = 88.67 PMVO: ACC = 77.33
Muthulakshmi, et al. [69]	21 (NR)	NR	bSSFP	MI +/−	(DL) Levenberg-Marquardt learning CNN	ACC = 86.39
Xu, et al. [56]	58 (36/22)	51 ± 16	LGE	MI +/−	(ML) SVM	ACC = 93.30
Attallah, et al [59]	100 (NR)	NR	LGE	MI +/−	(DL) Auto-MyIn	ACC = 98.40
Zhang, et al. [58]	299 (213/86)	HS 40 ± 13 CAD 56 ± 11	Non-contrast bSSFP	Chronic MI +/−	(DL) NR	AUC = 0.94
Joloudari, et al. [63]	30 (NR)	NR	NR	CAD +/−	(DL) FCM-DNN	ACC = 99.91 AUC = 1.00
Iqbal, et al. [68]	63151 (NR)	NR	LGE Perfusion T2w bSSFP	CAD +/−	(ML) LWNN (adapted version of LeNET5 model) NN	ACC = 99.35 AUC = 0.99
Wu, et al. [54]	64 (33/31)	59 ± 10	Non-contrast bSSFP	CAD +/−	(DL) CSAI	Patient: ACC = 87.50 Vessel: ACC = 91.10 Segment: ACC = 96.60
Chen [65]	120 (63/57)	Group A 64 ± 9 Group B 62 ± 8 Group C 62 ± 9	LGE	Myo injury	(DL) CNN	ACC = 91.04 AUC = 0.96

Table 2. *Cont.*

Reference	# Subject (M/F)	Age(y) Mean ± Std	CMR Seq.	Target	(Category) AI Model	Performance
Paciorek, et al. [44]	200 (132/68)	53 ± 19	LGE T1-mapping	Normal/ Abnormal	(DL) DenseNet-161 (LGE PSIR) DenseNet-161 (T1 mapping)	ACC = 88.00 AUC = 0.75 ACC = 70.00 AUC = 0.69
Backhaus, et al. [27]	1095 (820/275)	64	bSSFP	MACE +/−	(DL) Commercial software	Auto-GLS: AUC = 0.69 Auto-GCS: AUC = 0.66
Schuster, et al. [50]	1017 (763/254)	64	LGE	MACE +/−	(DL) Commercial software	Auto-mated: AUC = 0.67 Auto corrected: AUC = 0.68
Pezel, et al. [46]	2152 (1653/499)	66 ± 12	LGE	MACE +/−	(ML) U-net Dijkstra's algorithm	ICC = 0.83 (95% CI)
Knott, et al. [39]	1049 (702/347)	60 ± 13	Perfusion	Stress MBF and MPR associated with death or MACE	(NR) Commercial software	MBF: ICC = 0.68 (95%CI) MPR: ICC = 0.68 (95%CI)
Popescu, et al. [48]	269 (233/36)	61 ± 11	LGE	SCDA risk +/−	(DL) NN Architecture SSCAR	Internal: ACC = 77.00 External: ACC = 73.00
Pezel, et al. [45]	31762 (20,879/10,883)	63 ± 12	LGE	SCDA risk +/−	(ML) RSF	AUC = 0.75
Maleckar, et al. [24]	30 (NR)	NR	LGE	Arrhythmia risk +/−	(ML) NR	ACC = 86.00
Ghanbari, et al. [36]	761 (671/90)	65 ± 11	LGE	Arrhythmia risk +/−	(ML) Ternaus network (Multivariable Cox models–total scar) CNN	AUC = 0.67
Okada, et al. [43]	122 (106/16)	60 ± 11	LGE	Arrhythmia risk +/−	(ML) SVM+poly	ACC = 81.00
Zaidi, et al. [57]	397 (346/51)	64 ± 9	LGE	Major arrhythmic event +/−	(ML) Multivariate cox regression analysis	AUC = 0.81
Chen, et al. [30]	311 (294/17)	NR	T2w-STIR bSSFP T2-mapping LGE	Paradoxical pulsation +/−	(DL) CNN	Internal: ACC = 85.00 AUC = 0.91 External: ACC = 84.00 AUC = 0.83

Table 2. *Cont.*

Reference	# Subject (M/F)	Age(y) Mean ± Std	CMR Seq.	Target	(Category) AI Model	Performance
Paciorek, et al. [44]	200 (132/68)	53 ± 19	LGE T1-mapping	Normal/ Abnormal	(DL) DenseNet-161 (LGE PSIR) DenseNet-161 (T1 mapping)	ACC = 88.00 AUC = 0.75 ACC = 70.00 AUC = 0.69
Chen, et al. [31]	73 (51/22)	NR	LGE	Segment Infarct +/−	(DL) SDAE+SVM	ACC = 87.60
Feng, et al. [66]	30 (NR)	NR	bSSFP LGE	Segment Infarct +/−	(ML) SVM-RFE	Basal: ACC = 80.50 Middle: ACC = 87.90 Apical: ACC = 81.00
Kim, et al. [64]	170 (NR)	NR	LGE	Segment Infarct +/−	(DL) ResNet50	ACC = 81.10 AUC = 0.87
Wang, et al. [52]	301 (172/129)	57	LGE	Segment Infarct +/−	(DL) MI-ResNet50-AC CNN	AUC = 0.86
Hernández-Casillas, et al. [67]	35 (NR)	NR	LGE	Segment Infarct +/−	(ML) Naïve Bayes	AUC = 0.69
Mauger, et al. [42]	5098 (2451/2565)	HS 60 ± 9 CAD 66 ± 9	GRE	Relationship between LV 3D shape CMR and incident cardio-vascular events	(ML) Model 3 (model 1+30 event-specific remodeling signatures derived from the PLS analysis)	AUC = 0.77
Dieu, et al. [61]	443 (NR)	NR	NR	LV remodeling +/−	(ML) LR	AUC = 0.78
Böttcher, et al. [28]	50 (37/13)	57	bSSFP	Myo function	(DL) Commercially available software	LV EDV: ICC = 0.99 LV ESV: ICC = 0.99 LV SV: ICC = 0.89 LV EF: ICC = 0.97 LV mass: ICC = 0.99
Goldfarb, et al. [62]	64 (NR)	NR	bSSFP	Water–Fat	(DL) U-Net	$R2 \geq 0.97$ ($p < 0.001$)
Wu, et al. [53]	50 (15/35)	HS 24 ± 8 CAD 60 ± 12	Non-contrast bSSFP	Angiography	(DL) CSAI	Patient: ACC = 90.00 Vessel: ACC = 91.70 Segment: ACC = 97.30

Table 2. *Cont.*

Reference	# Subject (M/F)	Age(y) Mean ± Std	CMR Seq.	Target	(Category) AI Model	Performance
Paciorek, et al. [44]	200 (132/68)	53 ± 19	LGE T1-mapping	Normal/ Abnormal	(DL) DenseNet-161 (LGE PSIR) DenseNet-161 (T1 mapping)	ACC = 88.00 AUC = 0.75 ACC = 70.00 AUC = 0.69
Cau, et al. [29]	107 (72/35)	61	bSSFP	CAD +/−	(ML) GB-GAM	AUC = 0.82
Alskaf, et al. [25]	1286 (845/441)	<65 65–75 >75	Perfusion	Mortality risk +/−	(ML) HNN	AUC = 0.82
Alskaf, et al. [26]	2740 (1726/1014)	<65 65–75 >75	LGE	Mortality risk +/− Arrhythmia risk +/−	(ML) HNN	Mortality: AUC = 0.77 Arrhythmia: AUC = 0.75
Corral-Acero, et al. [33]	1021 (NR)	63	LGE T1-w	MACE +/−	(DL) UNet	AUC = 0.77
Li, et al. [41]	42 (33/9)	60 71 ± 11	LGE bSSFP	Remote Viable Unviable	(ML) SVM XGBoost NN	Remote vs. Viable: AUC = 0.65 Viable vs. Unviable: AUC = 0.77 Remote vs. Unviable: AUC = 0.89
Udin, et al. [51]	279 (168/111)	HS 58 CAD 63	LGE	MI +/−	(ML) ResNet50 ResNet152V2	Without LWP: AUC = 0.76 With LWP: AUC = 0.88 Without LWP: AUC = 0.76 With LWP: AUC = 0.90
Frøysa, et al. [34]	41 (33/8)	58 ± 12	LGE	MI +/−	(ML) Texture-based probability mapping	R2 ($p < 0.001$)
Ghaffari-Jolfayi, et al. [35]	79 (52/27)	47 ± 12	LGE, T1 mapping T2 mapping	Segment Infarct +/−	(ML) RF	LAD territory: AUC = 0.89 RCA territory: AUC = 0.90 LCX territory: AUC = 0.92
Jacob, et al. [38]	1337 (602/735)	HS 50 ± 16 CAD 63 ± 12	bSSFP	CAD +/−	(DL) RF XGBoost	ACC = 0.81 AUC = 0.85
Righetti, et al. [49]	206 (164/42)	67	bSSFP	CAD +/−	(DL) U-Net	ACC = 79.00

Table 2. *Cont.*

Reference	# Subject (M/F)	Age(y) Mean ± Std	CMR Seq.	Target	(Category) AI Model	Performance
Paciorek, et al. [44]	200 (132/68)	53 ± 19	LGE T1-mapping	Normal/ Abnormal	(DL) DenseNet-161 (LGE PSIR) DenseNet-161 (T1 mapping)	ACC = 88.00 AUC = 0.75 ACC = 70.00 AUC = 0.69
Wu, et al. [55]	99 (49/50)	HS 28 ± 11 CAD 59 ± 10	bSSFP	CAD +/−	(DL) DL-CS mDIXON	ACC = 84.10
Guglielmo, et al. [37]	730 (616/114)	63 ± 10	LGE	MACE +/−	(DL) FCN U-Net	HR = 1.08 (95% CI)
Pezel, et al. [47]	2038 (947/1091)	70 ± 12	LGE Perfusion	MACE +/−	(ML) XGBoost	Internal: AUC = 0.86 External: AUC = 0.84 AUC = 0.92

= number; CAD = coronary artery disease; HS = healthy subjects; MI = myocardial infarction; bSSFP = balanced steady-state free precession; Myo = myocardium; ML = machine learning; DL = deep learning; SVM = support vector machine; poly = polynomial kernel; RFE = recursive feature elimination; NN = neural network; LR = logistic regression; RF = random forest; RSF = random survival forest; LWNN = light-weight neural network; LGE = late gadolinium enhancement; CMR = cardiac magnetic resonance; LV = left ventricle; AUC = area under curve; ACC = accuracy (%); CNN = convolutional neural network; HNN = hybrid neural network; MACE = major adverse cardiac events; MBF = myocardial blood flow; MPR = myocardial perfusion reserve; PSIR = phase-sensitive inversion recovery; ICC = c-index; R2 = correlation; SDAE = stack denoising autoencoder; SCDA = arrhythmic sudden cardiac death; HR = hazard ratio; CSAI = compressed sensing artificial intelligence; FCM-DNN = fuzzy C-means clustering combined with deep neural network; DL-CS = deep learning-constrained compressed sensing; GB-GAM = gradient boosting generalized additive model; NR = Not reported.

3.1.2. Risk Stratification for Major Adverse Cardiovascular Events (MACE)

Four articles focused on the assessment of the risk of CAD patients developing MACE [27,33,37,39,46,47,50], which provides very useful prognostic information for the management of CAD patients. The study by Knott et al. [39] used cvi42 commercial software (Circle Cardiovascular Imaging, Calgary, Alberta, Canada), and the study by Backhaus et al. [27] used suiteHEART com-mercial software (v4.0.6; Neosoft, Pewaukee, WI, USA). Schuster et al. [50] used both software programs for their analysis. Both software programs perform the analysis fully automatically. These studies demonstrate the utility of different AI software programs in predicting MACE in CAD patients (see Table 2).

3.1.3. Risk Stratification for Arrhythmia-Induced Mortality in CAD Patients

Of the investigations targeting the prediction of arrhythmia and mortality in CAD patients [24–26,36,43,45,48,57], the study by Maleckar et al. [24] achieved the best performance with an ACC of 86%, based on a database of 30 patients by combining patient data and computational simulation-supported data augmentation using an ML model. By contrast, although the study by Pezel et al. [45], did not report superior performance (AUC = 0.75), it included clinical and stress CMR data for 31,762 patients and found a higher prognostic value for predicting death compared with all traditional clinical or CMR scores.

3.1.4. Early Identification of Left Ventricular Remodelling (LVR)

Left ventricular remodelling (LVR) is a risk in CAD [42,61]. Early detection of patients likely to undergo LVR can help to optimize therapeutic strategies aimed at preventing or reversing this condition and thereby reducing its subsequent clinical consequences [61].

Two studies using ML models aimed at predicting postinfarction LVR [42,61]. Although the study by Mauger et al. [42] included patients 10 or more years after the incident and the study by Dieu et al in 2022 was conducted 3 months after an MI both achieved similar performance values (AUC of 0.77 and 0.8, respectively).

3.1.5. Identification of Normal and Infarcted Myocardial Segments

An important factor when analysing CMR images of CAD patients is the differentiation of infarcted and non-infarcted remote myocardial segments (using the 16-segment American Heart Association (AHA) nomenclature [71]. Some research groups have aimed to identify infarcted segments in the left ventricular (LV) myocardium [31,35,41,52,64,66,67]. Chen et al. [31] reported the highest ACC (87.6%) in 73 patients using a DL model that combines a stack denoising autoencoder (SDAE) with a support vector machine (SVM). Wang et al. [52] found an ACC of 86%, using a DL model (CNN ResNet50-AC) in 301 patients. Li et al. [41] classified segments as viable, remote, or non-viable based on myocardial transmural extension.

LGE is the type of CMR imaging used most often in CAD patients because it provides better contrast between healthy and diseased. However, there some patients have contraindications for gadolinium-based contrast injection, and some authors have proposed using other types of CMR imaging, such as balanced steady state free precession (bSSFP), to detect MI [69] (ACC = 86.39%) or MACE [27] (AUC = 0.69 for automatic analysis of global longitudinal strain (GLS) and AUC = 0.66 for automatic analysis of global circumferential strain (GCS). Aiming to improve efficiency, other studies, such as those conducted by Iqbal et al. [68] and Chen et al. [30], have used models that integrate the analysis of different types of images to classify patients (see Table 2).

3.1.6. Other Classifications Findings

Other less-studied applications of CMR for CAD patients have been to identify LV paradoxical pulsation, such us in the study by Chen et al. [30], which achieved ACC values of 85% for the internal testing cohort and 84% for the external testing cohort. Goldfarb et al. [62] determined the viability and performance of water-fat separation by CMR imaging and parametric mapping using DL and found good correlations with the conventional model. Wu et al. [53] examined a compressed sensing AI framework to accelerate image acquisition in contrast-free wholeheart coronary MR bSSFP angiography and reported an ACC of 90% per patient. In the study by Chen et al. [65], the objective was to evaluate the myocardial protection of ivabradine (IBD) combined with trimetazidine (TMZ) in patients with CAD. For this purpose, Patients were randomized to groups A (treatment with TMZ), B (treatment with IBD), and C (combined treatment of IBD + TMZ), with 40 patients in each group. Following the study, the CNN algorithm obtained an accuracy of 91.04 and an AUC of 0.96 for the diagnosis of myocardial damage.

3.2. Classification Using Radiomics

Radiomics is a quantitative image analysis method that can be used to extract highly detailed information about ventricular shape and myocardial characteristics and thereby provides new information from existing standard-of-care images [72]. Radiomics and AI are closely linked given the ability of AI to handle and analyse the large volumes of data extracted from medical images, which surpasses traditional statistical methods [20]. Radiomics features classification steps for AI CMR applications are shown in Figure 3. In Table 3, we describe the studies that used radiomics in the analysis of CMR. In these studies, the cohort size ranged from 43 to 63,648 and included healthy volunteers and patients, from public and private databases [73–91]. However, the number of men and women included were reported in only 12 studies [74,76,78–80,83–89] and represent a total of 1.410 men

(75%) and 497 women (25%). Only one study was multicentric [89], 17 from a single medical centre [73–87,90,91], and one study did not report the location [90]. Twelve studies were conducted retrospectively [73,75,76,78–80,83–87,91] and four prospectively [74,81,88,90]. Seven studies did not report information about the database used [73,75,77,81,82,89,91], possibly because they used third-party databases.

The focus of the studies analysed varied. Three studies evaluated the ability of machine learning algorithms to use radiomic features extracted from cardiac magnetic resonance imaging (CMR) sequences for the differentiation of CAD patients [77,78,91]. Wang had the best ACC level (0.93), using the T1 + sBTFE imaging sequence. Six studies evaluated the extent of myocardial damage in CAD patients by identifying viable, non-viable, and remote tissue [73–75,80,84,86]. Ma et al. [86] evaluated the feasibility of texture analysis of non-contrast-enhanced T1 maps of CMR imaging for the diagnosis of myocardial injury in acute MI. They predicted various characteristics for the images, such as the presence of LGE, positive MVO segments, or non-irreversible injury at 6 months after MI and found the best results for identifying MVO when combining radiomics signatures and T1 values (AUC = 0.86). Larroza et al. [84] compared the accuracy of texture analysis on non-contrast MRI images with LGE MRI in a database of 50 subjects and obtained an AUC of 0.849, with showed that non-viable segments can be detected on cine MRI using texture analysis. However, another study by Abdulkareem et al. [73], which used a larger database of 272 subjects, yielded less promising results such as AUC values of 0.58 for SVM classification and 0.57 for decision tree (DT), which highlights the need for more robust studies on this topic.

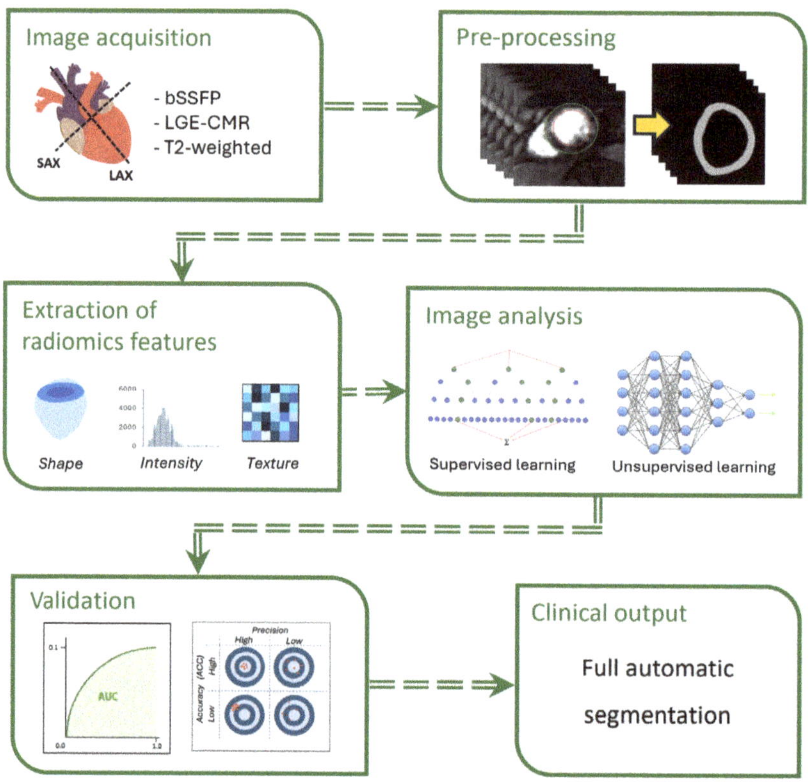

Figure 3. Radiomics features classification steps for AI CMR applications. (1) Acquisition of CMR images and clinical data. (2) Preprocessing of images through normalization, image resizing, and

segmentation of the structures of interest (e.g., LV myocardium). (3) Features are extracted from the images, such as pixel intensity, to calculate homogeneity and contrast, shape of the segmented structures, and transformation features to capture more complex patterns (using transformations such as wavelet or Fourier). (4) Feature selection is performed by applying techniques such as PCA to reduce dimensionality or decision trees (DT) to identify the most relevant features. (5) The data are divided into training, validation, and test sets (e.g., 70/15/15). ML or DL models are trained for data analysis on the training set, and their performance is monitored using the validation set. (6) The model is evaluated using the test set by calculating performance metrics such as the AUC. (7) The output obtained comprises of the fully automated analysis of cardiac structures in CAD patients.

The study by Durmaz et al. [79] was the only study aimed at predicting MACE in CAD patients using texture analysis combined with clinical variables and using various classification models, such as kNN, AdaBoost, random forest, SVM, naive Bayes, SGD, and neural networks (NN). They achieved the best results with NN (AUC = 0.965 and ACC = 0.894). Larroza et al. [83] and Baessler et al. [76] used radiomics to differentiate chronic and acute MI. The former compared the classification performance between LGE CMR images (AUC = 0.86) and cine CMR (AUC = 0.82). Baessler et al. [76] used only non-enhanced cine CMR and reported with very good results (AUC = 0.92). By contrast, Rauseo et al. [90], focused on defining the radiomic signatures that indicate the relationship between ischaemia processes occurring in the brain and heart. Radiomic signatures provided significantly better disease discrimination than conventional indices, as suggested by the AUCs: ischaemic heart disease: 0.82 vs. 0.75; cerebrovascular disease: 0.79 vs. 0.77; MI: 0.87 vs. 0.79; and ischemic stroke: 0.81 vs. 0.72.

Table 3. Radiomics studies in CMR image in CAD.

Reference	# Subject (M/F)	Age(y) Mean ± Std	CMR Seq.	Target	AI Model	Performance
Arian, et al. [74]	43 (34/39)	58 ± 11	LGE	Myo function	SCAD-penalized SVM RP algorithm	AUC = 0.78 AUC = 0.65
Avard, et al. [75]	72 (NR)	NR	non-contrast bSSFP	MI Viable Normal	LR SVM	AUC = 0.93 ACC = 86.00 AUC = 0.92 ACC = 85.00
Ma, et al. [86]	68 (57/11)	55 ± 10	non-contrast T1-maps	MVO SLS	T1values+ RS	MVO: AUC = 0.86 SLS: AUC = 0.77
Abdulkareem, et al. [73]	272 (NR)	NR	bSSFP LGE	Segment Myo+MIS	SVM DT	AUC = 0.58 AUC = 0.57
Larroza, et al. [84]	50 (45/5)	61 ± 12	bSSFP LGE (2D+t)	Nonviable Viable Remote segments	RBF-SVM classifier	AUC = 0.84
Liu, et al. [85]	167 (149/18)	52 ± 11	LGE	MVO +/−	LASSO	AUC = 0.78
Frøysa, et al. [80]	52 (40/12)	64	LGE	MIS size	The texture-based probability mapping method	DSC = 0.69

Table 3. *Cont.*

Reference	# Subject (M/F)	Age(y) Mean ± Std	CMR Seq.	Target	AI Model	Performance
Durmaz, et al. [79]	60 (55/5)	MACE: 57 ± 9 No MACE: 55 ± 9	LGE	MACE +/−	NN	AUC = 0.96 ACC = 89.40
Raisi-Estabragh, et al. [89]	92 (56/36)	NR	Perfusion	Rest and stress radiomics features	Model 4-Per territory (delta to histogram)	Sen = 53.00 Spec = 86.00
Khozeimeh, et al. [81]	63648 (NR)	NR	LGE Perfusion T2-w bSSFP	CAD +/−	Ensemble of CNNs and RF+Adam (optimizer)	AUC = 0.99 ACC = 99.18
Di Noto, et al. [87]	173 (153/20)	66 ± 9	LGE	MI Myo-carditis	SVM: (2D Features + RFE) LDA: (3D Features + PCA)	ACC = 88.00 ACC = 85.00
Kotu, et al. [82]	54 (NR)	NR	LGE	Arrhythmic risk	Several built-in classification schemes from matrix laboratory (matlab)	AUC = 0.96 ACC = 94.44
Rauseo, et al. [90]	2457 (NR)	HS 59 ± 7 CAD 67 ± 6	bSSFP	CAD CVD	SVM	IHD: AUC = 0.82 CVD: AUC = 0.79 MI: AUC = 0.87 IS: AUC = 0.81
Larroza, et al. [83]	44 (40/4)	61 ± 9	LGE bSSFP	Acute MI Chronic MI	SVM + poly	AUC = 0.86 AUC = 0.82
Baessler, et al. [76]	180 (138/42)	HS 48 ± 17 CAD 64 ± 10	Non-contrast bSSFP	Subacute MI Chronic MI	LR	Teta 1: AUC = 0.93 Perc.01: AUC = 0.92
Pujadas, et al. [88]	819 (NR)	66 ± 7	bSSFP	MI Other vascular pathologies	SVM	AUC = 0.76 ACC = 71.00
Wang, et al. [91]	115 (NR)	NR	LGE T1-w-transverse sBTFE T1+sBTFE	CAD +/−	Lasso RF/LR	AUC = 0.93 ACC = 0.93
Vande Berg, et al. [77]	148 (NR)	HS 48 ± 12 CAD 58 ± 12	Cine bSSFP T2w	CAD +/−	Lasso	ES: ACC = 0.84 ED: ACC = 0.76

Table 3. *Cont.*

Reference	# Subject (M/F)	Age(y) Mean ± Std	CMR Seq.	Target	AI Model	Performance
Deng, et al. [78]	115 (89/26)	58 ± 11	Cine	CAD +/−	GNB	AUC = 0.91

= number; CAD = coronary artery disease; HS = Healthy Subject; MI = myocardial infarction; MIS = myocardial infarction scar; HS = healthy subjects; Myo = myocardium; MVO = microvascular obstruction; MACE = major adverse cardiac events; bSSFP = balanced steady-state free precession; SVM = Support vector machine; poly = polynomial kernel; LR = logistic regression; DT = decision tree; LGE = late gadolinium enhancement; CMR = cardiac magnetic resonance; LV = left ventricle; AUC = area under curve; ACC = accuracy (%); DSC = dice similarity coefficient; Sen = sensitivity (%); Spec = specificity (%); RFE = recursive feature elimination; PCA = principal component analysis; CVD = cerebrovascular disease; IHD = ischemic heart dis-ease; SLS = segmental longitudinal strain; LDA = linear discriminant analysis; CNN = convolutional neural net-work; SCAD = smoothly clipped absolute deviation; RP = recursive partitioning; RS = radiomics signature; RBF = radial basis function; GNB = gaussian naive bayes; NR = Not reported.

3.3. Segmentation

Segmentation steps for AI CMR applications are shown in Figure 4. A total of 41 articles reported the segmentation of different cardiac structures such as the myocardium, myocardial infarction scar (MIS), myocardial edema (ME), coronary artery or adipose tissue on CMR images of CAD patients (see Table 4). The size of the cohort used in these studies varied widely from 20 to 1354, and included both patients and healthy volunteers from private and public databases. Sixteen articles reported the number of men and women included in the studies [30,92–100]:a total of 1986 men (75%) and 679 women (25%). Eighteen studies were retrospective [92–96,98,99,101–111], and only one mentioned being prospective [112]. Fifteen studies were multicentre [92,95,97,100,105,107–109,111–117], thirteen obtained data from a single medical centre [70,94,96,98,99,102–104,110,118–121], and 13 articles did not provide a description of the databases used.

The AI models were used for the segmentation of different cardiovascular structures. Generally, these studies used of Dice similarity coefficient (DSC) as an evaluation metric to evaluate the similarity between a predicted segmentation mask and the ground truth segmentation mask [122]. The DSC ranged from 0, indicating no overlap, to 1, indicating perfect overlap. Fourteen of the studies evaluated myocardium segmentation in CAD patients and healthy controls compared with the ground truth [92,95,99,102,103,106,111,113,115,118,119,121,123,124]. Yan et al. [121] studied a cohort of 1354 subjects and achieved the best results for myocardial segmentation with DSC values of 0.94 for training, 0.87 for validation, and 0.94 for testing. Ten studies segmented the Myo as well as the MI or MIS [70,96–98,100,107–110,112,120,125]. The studies by Lecesne et al. [125], and Heidenreich et al. [96] presented their segmentation accuracy results for Myo and MI or MIS separately. Lecesne et al reported better results with a DSC of 0.92 for Myo and 0.92 for MI for a database of 150 subjects. Other studies focused on the segmentation of MI or MIS. Zabihollahy et al. [100] obtained a DSC of 0.93 from an LGE MRI database of 34 subjects. This finding was similar to that of Xu et al. [109] (DSC of 0.65), who used a database for 165 subjects. The study by Xu et al. [109] was notable for using cine CMR images with no contrast, which is useful for patients for whom contrast agents cannot be administered [126].

Other studies have focused on segmenting MI and ME [104,116,126–129]. These studies performed segmentation using multisequence images, including bSSFP, LGE, T2-weighted, and T1- and T2-mapping images, and aimed to leverage the characteristics of each type of image. For example, LGE provides information about the infarcted region, T2 weighting allows the visualization of ME, and bSSFP CMR provides information about anatomical structural [129], and global or RWMA, which are complementary sequences when an-alysing CMR data. Only one study focused on automating coronary artery segmentation for CAD diagnosis [105].

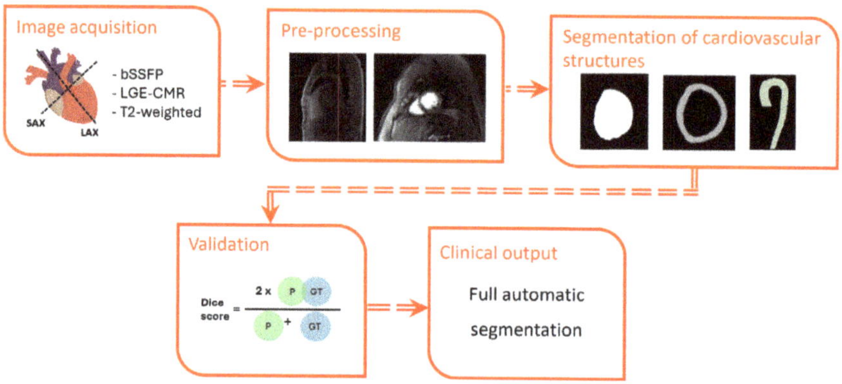

Figure 4. Segmentation steps for AI CMR applications. (1) Acquisition of CMR images. (2) Preprocessing of images through normalization, image resizing, and data augmentation. (3) The data are divided into training, validation, and test sets (e.g., 70/20/10). DL segmentation models (e.g., U-Net or SegNet) are trained for data analysis on the training set, and their performance is monitored using the validation set. (4) The model is evaluated using the test set by calculating segmentation-specific metrics such as the Dice score. (5) The output obtained comprises of the automatic segmentation of cardiac structures.

Studies of segmentation of myocardial infarction and microvascular obstruction (MVO) have been conducted by Brahim et al. [93], de la Rosa et al. [130], and Brahim et al. [131]. These authors used LGE CMR and DL models, and Brahim et al. [93] achieved the best results with DSC values of 0.95 for Myo, 0.78 for MI, and 0.77 for MVO. They also classified the regions based on whether they corresponded to Myo, MI, or MVO, with an ACC of 98%.

Chen et al. [94] studied segmented pericardial adipose tissue, which is associated with different cardiovascular diseases, including CAD. They used a different evaluation metric than DSC, called the Hausdorff distance (HD), whose use is increasing in medical image segmentation [132]. Unlike earlier metrics that examine every pixel, HD considers only the boundary pixels of every patch of pixels belonging to the same class. It calculates the distance between every corresponding point within one or two boundaries [133]. Chen et al. [94] obtained an HD of 15.62 ± 18.61 mm using a database of 150 LGE MRI images and concluded that these results are only an indicator but have potential in diagnosing cardiovascular pathologies, including CAD.

Table 4. Segmentation studies in CMR image in CAD.

Reference	# Subject (M/F)	Age(y) Mean ± Std	CMR Seq.	AI Model	Target	Performance
Gröschel, et al. [95]	136 (91/45)	HS 44 ± 16 CAD 68 ± 11	LGE	Deep CNN	LV-Myo	Healthy: DSC = 0.85 Patients: DSC = 0.80
Mosquera-Rojas, et al. [106]	274 (NR)	NR	LGE	DualUNet	LV-Myo	DSC = 0.84

Table 4. *Cont.*

Reference	#Subject (M/F)	Age(y) Mean ± Std	CMR Seq.	AI Model	Target	Performance
Barbaroux, et al. [92]	271 (197/73)	48 ± 14	LGE	DynU-Net	LV-Myo	SAx: DSC = 0.83 LAx: DSC = 0.82
Yan, et al. [121]	1354 (NR)	NR	LGE	SegNet model	LV-Myo	Train: DSC = 0.94 Validation: DSC = 0.87 Test: DSC = 0.94
Scannell, et al. [99]	175 (136/39)	64 ± 10	T1-w	U-Net	LV-Myo	DSC = 0.80
Ahmad, et al. [113]	56 (NR)	58	LGE	DL	LV-Myo	DSC = 0.85
Kim, et al. [115]	35 (NR)	NR	bSSFP	DL (CNN-U-Net)	LV-Myo	DSC = 0.80
Liu, et al. [123]	32 (NR)	NR	T2-w LGE	CLS	LV-Myo	DSC = 0.84 DSC = 0.78
Tan, et al. [124]	1340 (NR)	NR	bSSFP	CNN (three networks (LM, CTR, MB))	LV-Myo	DSC = 0.86
Chen, et al. [119]	150 (NR)	NR	T1-w LGE	Res-UNet	LV-ED LV-ES RV-ED RV-ES Myo ED Myo ES	DSC = 0.89 DSC = 0.81 DSC = 0.81 DSC = 0.70 DSC = 0.72 DSC = 0.76
Papetti, et al. [107]	144 (NR)	NR	LGE	CNN	LV-Myo MIS	DSC = 0.79 DSC = 0.78
Lecesne, et al. [125]	150 (NR)	NR	LGE	U-Net	LV-Myo MI	DSC = 0.92 DSC = 0.92
Lin, et al. [97]	34 (29/5)	NR	LGE	CTAEM-Net	MIS	DSC = 0.90
Mamalakis, et al. [120]	20 (NR)	NR	LGE	BZ-SOCRATIS	Myo Core Scar Border Scar Myo Core Scar Border Scar	Internal: DSC = 0.81 DSC = 0.60 DSC = 0.43 External: DSC = 0.70 DSC = 0.44 DSC = 0.54
Xu, et al. [110]	165 (NR)	NR	LGE	BMAnet	MI	Labeled 33: DSC = 0.59 Labeled 66: DSC = 0.65

Table 4. *Cont.*

Reference	#Subject (M/F)	Age(y) Mean ± Std	CMR Seq.	AI Model	Target	Performance
Chen, et al. [70]	195 (NR)	NR	LGE	U-Net	MI	DSC = 0.84
Heidenreich, et al. [96]	78 (64/14)	64	LGE	nnU-nets	Myo MIS	DSC = 0.83 DSC = 0.72
Xu, et al. [109]	165 (NR)	NR	bSSFP	DSTGAN	MIS	DSC = 0.92
Zabihollahy, et al. [100]	34 (29/5)	51 ± 12	LGE	CNN-based	MIS	DSC = 0.93
Moccia, et al. [98]	30 (26/4)	NR	LGE	FCNN	MIS	DSC = 0.71
Li, et al. [134]	NR (NR)	NR	bSSFP LGE T2-w	NVTrans-UNet	MI MI+ME	DSC = 0.64 DSC = 0.57
Qiu, et al. [116]	NR (NR)	NR	Multi-sequence: bSSFP LGE T2-w T1-mapping T2-mapping	MyoPS-Net		DSC = 0.65 DSC = 0.74
Cui, et al. [128]	45 (NR)	NR	LGE T2-w bSSFP	U-Net++ (Deep supervision) + EfficientSeg-B1 (Ours)	MIS MIS + ME Average MIS ME	DSC = 0.71 DSC = 0.74 DSC = 0.72
Li, et al. [129]	45 (NR)	NR	LGE T2-w bSSFP	TAUNet	LV RV Myo MIS ME	DSC = 0.94 DSC = 0.91 DSC = 0.91 DSC = 0.62 DSC = 0.78
Cui, et al. [127]	45 (NR)	NR	LGE T2-w bSSFP	Deep U-net Deep U-net+ DFM	MIS MIS+ME MIS MIS+ME	DSC = 0.68 DSC = 0.70 DSC = 0.69 DSC = 0.70
Brahim, et al. [93]	150 (89/61)	NR	LGE	ICPIU-Net	Myo MI MVO Classification	DSC = 0.95 DSC = 0.78 DSC = 0.77 ACC = 98,00
de la Rosa, et al. [130]	100 (NR)	NR	LGE	CNN	MI+MVO	DSC = 0.77
Brahim, et al. [131]	150 (NR)	NR	LGE	3D pretrained Autoencoder network and the 3D U-Net	Myo MI MVO	DSC = 0.95 DSC = 0.76 DSC = 0.73
Chen, et al. [94]	150 (92/58)	HS 32 ± 12 CAD 61 ± 12	LGE	3SUnet	Cardiac adipose tissue	HF = 15.62

Table 4. *Cont.*

Reference	#Subject (M/F)	Age(y) Mean ± Std	CMR Seq.	AI Model	Target	Performance
Arega, et al. [114]	295 (NR)	NR	T1-mapping (Native)	Swin-based U-Net	LV MYO RV	DSC = 0.97 DSC = 0.91 DSC = 0.92
			T1-mapping (Post-Contrast)		LV MYO RV	DSC = 0.95 DSC = 0.88 DSC = 0.89
			T1-mapping (Native)	CNN-based U-Net	LV MYO RV	DSC = 0.96 DSC = 0.90 DSC = 0.90
			T1-mapping (Post-Contrast)		LV MYO RV	DSC = 0.94 DSC = 0.85 DSC = 0.86
Popescu, et al. [135]	401 (NR)	NR	LGE bSSFP	DNN	LV Myo MIS	DSC = 0.93 DSC = 0.57
Mamalakis, et al [136]	60 (NR)	NR	LGE	MA-SOCRATIS	LV Myo	intra-observer: DSC = 0.81 inter-observer: DSC = 0.70
					MIS	intra-observer: DSC = 0.70 inter-observer: DSC = 0.70
Al-antari, et al. [101]	150 (89/61)	NR	LGE	ResU-Net	MI+MVO	ACC = 88.50
Jani, et al. [112]	501 (431/70)	59 ± 12	LGE	Cascaded U-Net	LV-Myo MIS	DSC = 0.66 DSC = 0.75
Qi, et al. [108]	415 (370/45)	59 ± 10	CGE	DGL	MIS	ACC = 0.92
Yalcinkaya, et al. [111]	150 (NR)	60 ± 14	LGE bSSFP	DNN	LV-Myo	Internal: DSC = 0.89 External: DSC = 0.88
Lin, et al. [105]	174 (119/55)	51 ± 12	Cine	U-Net	Coronary artery	Training: DSC = 0.95 Validation: DSC = 0.94
Ben Khalifa, et al. [103]	163 (40/123)	HS 42 ± 14 CAD 58 ± 11	LGE bSSFP	U-Net	LV-Myo Classification MI	DSC = 0.92 ACC = 0.96
Li, et al. [104]	45 (NR)	NR	LGE T2-w bSSFP	DNN (MPS-Mamba)	MIS ME	DSC = 0.71 DSC = 0.73
Bernardo, et al. [118]	171 (NR)	NR	NR	U-Net	LV	ED: DSC = 0.94 ES: DSC = 0.79
					Myo	ED: DSC = 0.81 ES: DSC = 0.69

Table 4. *Cont.*

Reference	#Subject (M/F)	Age(y) Mean ± Std	CMR Seq.	AI Model	Target	Performance
Jafari, et al. [102]	55 (37/18)	50 ± 17	DCE	U-Net	LV-Myo	DSC = 0.78

= number; MI = myocardial infarction; HS = Healthy Subject; MIS = myocardial infarction scar; ME = myocardial edema; Myo = myocardium; MVO = microvascular obstruction; bSSFP = balanced steady-state free precession; DL = deep learning; SVM = Support vector machine; LGE = late gadolinium enhancement; DCE = dynamic contrast enhanced; CMR = cardiac magnetic resonance; LV = left ventricle; RV = right ventricle; ED = end-diastolic; ES = end-systolic; ACC = accuracy; DSC = dice similarity coefficient; CNN = convolutional neural network; DNN = deep neural network; CLS = coupled level set; LM = landmarks network; DGL = Deep Generative Learning; CTR = center point network; CTAEM-Net = cascaded triplanar autoencoder M-Net; MB = myocardial boundaries network; FCNN = fully convolutional neural network; DSTGAN = deep spatio-temporal adversarial network; NR = Not reported.

3.4. *Quality Assessment*

Assessment of the studies using the Checklist for AI in Medical Images (CLAIM) [23] showed an overall compliance of 81%. However, many studies lacked a description of de-identification methods for clinical trial registration and explainability or interpretability methods (see Supplementary Material, CLAIM Quality).

4. Discussion

This analysis further supports the consolidated position of CMR as a non-invasive reference modality for the diagnostic and prognostic assessment of coronary artery disease, and how the use of AI and radiomics improves diagnostic accuracy and efficiency in clinical workflow.

In the classification between healthy volunteers and patients with cardiovascular diseases, one of the most developed areas has been the binary classification between healthy individuals and patients with CAD. Although some studies, such as those by Joloudari et al. [63] and Iqbal et al. [68], report extremely high accuracy values (>99%), their clinical validity is questionable due to the lack of transparency in population characterization. This absence of information may conceal biases in data collection or class composition. Moreover, other studies, such as that by Paciorek et al. [44], show that the choice of imaging sequence (LGE vs. T1-mapping) significantly influences model performance, highlighting the importance of selecting the appropriate imaging modality.

Studies aimed at predicting MACE and arrhythmias in CAD patients have demonstrated the potential clinical value of AI in personalised medicine. However, the investigations with the highest reported accuracy (e.g., Maleckar et al. [24]) often rely on small databases and artificial data augmentation, which limits their generalisability to real-world clinical settings. In contrast, studies such as that by Pezel et al. [45], though reporting lower performance (AUC = 0.75), are based on large clinical cohorts (>30,000 patients), thereby offering more robust and clinically relevant conclusions.

The prediction of post-infarction left ventricular remodelling represents a clinically relevant but still underexplored application. The few available studies, such as those by Mauger et al. [42] and Dieu et al. [61], show consistent performance (AUC = 0.78), yet they differ considerably in the time post-infarction at which patients were analysed (months vs. decades), suggesting the need for more longitudinal research and standardised cohort timelines.

Some innovative applications—such as the detection of left ventricular paradoxical pulsation, contrast-free imaging analysis, or the evaluation of combined pharmacological therapies—illustrate the potential of AI in less explored yet clinically meaningful areas. Although preliminary, these studies open up new research avenues, especially relevant in contexts where conventional methods present limitations in terms of time, cost, or accessibility.

The integration of radiomics has demonstrated its ability to identify quantitative information imperceptible to the human eye, even in non-contrast images. Some studies have shown its usefulness in distinguishing between acute and chronic infarction, predicting microvascular obstruction (MVO), and stratifying the risk of MACE.

Only three studies specifically investigated the use of radiomics features to differentiate CAD patients from healthy individuals. Among these, the work by Wang et al. [137] achieved the highest accuracy (ACC = 0.93) using a T1 + sBTFE imaging sequence, demonstrating the potential of radiomics in disease classification. Nevertheless, the small number of studies focused on this task calls for further research to validate and extend these findings.

Several other studies addressed the classification of myocardial tissue status—viable, non-viable, or remote—particularly in the context of infarction. These studies varied widely in their imaging sequences and computational approaches. For example, Ma et al. [86] demonstrated that combining radiomics signatures with T1 mapping yielded promising results for predicting microvascular obstruction (AUC = 0.86). Larroza et al. [84] also reported a high AUC (0.84) for detecting non-viable segments using cine MRI. However, the study by Abdulkareem et al. [73], which used a larger cohort, yielded substantially lower performance (AUC = 0.58), illustrating the current inconsistency and underscoring the need for more robust, standardised protocols and larger, better-characterised cohorts.

Only one study, conducted by Durmaz et al. [79], examined the use of radiomics for predicting major adverse cardiovascular events (MACE). Their findings, particularly the superior performance of neural networks (AUC = 0.96, ACC = 89.4), suggest that combining radiomic features with clinical data may significantly enhance predictive performance. This integrative approach could represent a future direction for risk stratification models.

Radiomics has also been used to differentiate between acute and chronic myocardial infarction. Larroza et al. [83] and Baessler et al. [76] demonstrated that both LGE and cine CMR sequences can be effective in this differentiation, with Baessler et. al achieving particularly high performance using only non-enhanced images (AUC = 0.92). These findings indicate that radiomics may offer alternatives to contrast-enhanced imaging in patients with contraindications to gadolinium administration.However, the accuracy and robustness of radiomics must be validated in larger, external, and multicenter cohorts, using standardized scanning parameters, to fully establish its reliability and added value in clinical practice.

Most studies evaluated segmentation performance using the Dice Similarity Coefficient (DSC), a standard metric that quantifies the spatial overlap between predicted and ground truth masks. Among the studies focused on myocardium segmentation, Yan et al. [121] achieved some of the highest DSC scores reported (up to 0.94 in both training and testing sets), which reflects strong agreement with manual annotations. Other studies, such as those by Lecesne et al. [125] and Zabihollahy et al. [100], also reported high DSC values for both Myo and infarcted regions, suggesting that AI models can perform comparably to human experts in segmenting key cardiac structures.

However, there is noticeable variability in segmentation accuracy across studies, which may relate to differences in imaging sequences (e.g., cine vs. LGE), dataset size, and model architecture. For example, Xu et al. [56] reported significantly lower DSCs (0.652) when using cine CMR without contrast, which highlights the challenges of achieving precise infarct segmentation in contrast-free protocols a relevant issue in patients contraindicated for gadolinium administration.

The quality assessment of the included studies, conducted using the Checklist for Artificial Intelligence in Medical Imaging (CLAIM) [23], revealed an overall compliance rate of 81%, suggesting that most studies adhered to key reporting standards. However, notable deficiencies were identified, particularly regarding the reporting of data de-identification procedures, clinical trial registration, and the inclusion of explainability or interpretability methods. These omissions are concerning given the increasing emphasis on transparency, reproducibility, and ethical use of AI in clinical practice. The limited attention to interpretability also raises questions about the clinical trustworthiness and usability of the models, especially in high-stakes decision-making scenarios. Addressing these gaps is essential to enhance the credibility and translational potential of AI applications in cardiac imaging.

On the other hand, of the 106 studies analysed, 49.1% were conducted in Europe, 24.5% in Asia—of which 69.2% were carried out in China—and 8.5% in North America. In contrast, Africa and Latin America were markedly underrepresented, accounting for only 2.8% and 0.9% of the studies, respectively. These findings highlight the need to promote research in underrepresented regions to generate contextually relevant evidence for these populations.

Furthermore, the studies analysed had several limitations. One of the main ones is the sample size. There is a repetitive use of similar databases, single-center studies, a lack of external validation, and a lack of prospective studies. Additionally, the imbalance between groups and the lack of population diversity make it difficult to generalize the results. This is reflected in the gender disparity, with a marked underrepresentation of female participants. Only three studies included a majority female population; however, these women were not part of the groups diagnosed with coronary artery disease (CAD). Some studies identified the use of commercial software, which limits transparency in data processing. Overall, the methodological quality of the studies is acceptable, but there are areas that require strengthening to ensure greater transparency and reproducibility. Finally, the quality of the ground truth was limited because several studies relied on a single expert.

Despite following a rigorous methodology for conducting this systematic review, several limitations were identified that should be considered when interpreting the results. First, the literature search was restricted to publications in English and Spanish, which may have led to the exclusion of relevant studies published in other languages. Second, although multiple databases were consulted (such as PubMed, Scopus, and Web of Science), there is a potential for publication bias, as studies with negative or non-significant results are less likely to be published. Additionally, some potentially relevant studies may have been omitted due to lack of access to full texts or limitations in the search terms used.

Another limitation was the process of quality assessment and data extraction. Although this was performed independently by two reviewers, it may still be subject to inevitable subjective bias.

Therefore, it is necessary to move toward multicenter, prospective studies that integrate relevant clinical variables, which will allow us to consolidate the clinical impact of these emerging tools, such AI and radiomics, in cardiovascular precision medicine.

5. Conclusions

This systematic review provides a synthesis of the use of AI tools described in the literature for CMR image analysis in patients with CAD. Various purposes for using these tools were identified, such as: diagnostic and/or prognostic prediction, segmentation of anatomical structures, and quantification of hemodynamic parameters. Although the number of studies has increased between 2015 and 2025 and these have generally shown very good results. However, they have limitations, including the use of common databases, some using small cohorts, and some not describing the population by identifying demographic or clinical characteristics. Therefore, to translate these studies into clinical practice, it is important that future studies expand the dataset, include a greater diversity of controls and healthy patients, and incorporate relevant clinical and demographic information to improve ACCs. Radiomics combined with AI models has been shown to have potential for improving the diagnostic and prognostic accuracy of CAD patients, even in non-contrast CMR images, though improvements and more valiation studies are necessary for clinical implementation.

Finally, the use of these applications is gaining ground in the field of CMR, and, together with their integration in future studies, could have a significant impact on the diagnosis, prognosis and management of CAD patients, and thereby support specialists in their work in this field.

Supplementary Materials: The following supporting information can be downloaded at: https://www.mdpi.com/article/10.3390/jcdd12090345/s1, Table S1: CLAIM Quality.

Author Contributions: C.J.-J., R.S., R.D.-N., F.R. and J.S., conceived the study aims and design, contributed to the systematic review and data extraction, performed the analysis, interpreted the results, and drafted the manuscript. S.C., M.E.A., J.V., J.U., S.U. and T.S., contributed to the interpretation of results, and the revision of the manuscript. All authors have read and agreed to the published version of the manuscript.

Funding: This work was funded by ANID—Millennium Science Initiative Program – ICN2021_004, and FONDECYT Regular No. 1221938 and No. 1231268, and FONDECYT de Iniciación No. 11200481.

Data Availability Statement: Data supporting the reported results are available from the corresponding author upon request.

Acknowledgments: All authors thank María Paula Montaña for the collaboration with the figures. J.S., thanks to Department of Medical Imaging and Radiation Sciences at Monash University, Melbourne, Australia.

Conflicts of Interest: The authors declare no conflicts of interest.

Abbreviations

The following abbreviations are used in this manuscript:

AI	Artificial intelligence
CAD	Coronary artery disease
MI	Myocardial infarction
CMR	Cardiac magnetic resonance
CTA	Computed tomography angiogram
LGE	Late gadolinium enhancement
LVEF	Left ventricular ejection fraction
ML	Machine learning
DL	Deep learning
SVM	Support vector machine
MACE	Major adverse cardiovascular events
ACC	Accuracy
AUC	Area under curve
LVR	Left ventricular remodelling
AHA	American Heart Association
SDAE	Stack denoising autoencode
CNN	Convolutional neural network

References

1. Halle, M.; Papadakis, M. Correction to: 2023 ESC Guidelines for the management of acute coronary syndromes: Developed by the task force on the management of acute coronary syndromes of the European Society of Cardiology (ESC). *Eur. Heart J.* **2024**, *45*, 1145–1145. [CrossRef]
2. Knuuti, J.; Wijns, W.; Saraste, A.; Capodanno, D.; Barbato, E.; Funck-Brentano, C.; Prescott, E.; Storey, R.F.; Deaton, C.; Cuisset, T.; et al. 2019 ESC Guidelines for the diagnosis and management of chronic coronary syndromes: The Task Force for the diagnosis and management of chronic coronary syndromes of the European Society of Cardiology (ESC). *Eur. Heart J.* **2019**, *41*, 407–477. [CrossRef] [PubMed]
3. Habib, B.; Calmon, R.; Khraiche, D.; Boddaert, N.; Bonnet, D.; Raimondi, F. Radiation dose reduction in paediatric coronary computed tomography: Assessment of effective dose and image quality. *Eur. Radiol.* **2016**, *26*, 2030–2038. [CrossRef]
4. Habib, B.; Calmon, R.; Donciu, V.; Khraiche, D.; Warin-Fresse, K.; Bonnet, D.; Boddaert, N.; Raimondi, F. Low-dose paediatric cardiac and thoracic computed tomography with prospective triggering: Is it possible at any heart rate? *Phys. Medica* **2018**, *49*, 99–104. [CrossRef] [PubMed]
5. Guo, W.; Zhao, S.; Xu, H.; He, W.; Yin, L.; Yao, Z.; Xu, Z.; Jin, H.; Wu, D.; Li, C.; et al. Comparison of machine learning-based CT fractional flow reserve with cardiac MR perfusion mapping for ischemia diagnosis in stable coronary artery disease. *Eur. Radiol.* **2024**, *34*, 5654–5665. [CrossRef]
6. Ali, L.A.; Marrone, C.; Martins, D.S.; Khraiche, D.; Festa, P.; Martini, N.; Santoro, G.; Todiere, G.; Panaioli, E.; Bonnet, D.; et al. Prognostic factors in hypertrophic cardiomyopathy in children: An MRI based study. *Int. J. Cardiol.* **2022**, *364*, 141–147. [CrossRef]
7. Martins, D.; Khraiche, D.; Legendre, A.; Boddaert, N.; Raisky, O.; Bonnet, D.; Raimondi, F. Aortic angle is associated with neo-aortic root dilatation and regurgitation following arterial switch operation. *Int. J. Cardiol.* **2019**, *280*, 53–56. [CrossRef] [PubMed]
8. Martins, D.S.; Ait-Ali, L.; Khraiche, D.; Festa, P.; Barison, A.; Martini, N.; Benadjaoud, Y.; Anjos, R.; Boddaert, N.; Bonnet, D.; et al. Evolution of acute myocarditis in a pediatric population: An MRI based study. *Int. J. Cardiol.* **2021**, *329*, 226–233. [CrossRef]
9. Raimondi, F.; Martins, D.; Coenen, R.; Panaioli, E.; Khraiche, D.; Boddaert, N.; Bonnet, D.; Atkins, M.; El-Said, H.; Alshawabkeh, L.; et al. Prevalence of Venovenous Shunting and High-Output State Quantified with 4D Flow MRI in Patients with Fontan Circulation. *Radiol. Cardiothorac. Imaging* **2021**, *3*, e210161. [CrossRef]
10. von Knobelsdorff-Brenkenhoff, F.; Schulz-Menger, J. Cardiovascular magnetic resonance in the guidelines of the European Society of Cardiology: A comprehensive summary and update. *J. Cardiovasc. Magn. Reson.* **2023**, *25*, 42. [CrossRef]
11. Kramer, C.M.; Barkhausen, J.; Bucciarelli-Ducci, C.; Flamm, S.D.; Kim, R.J.; Nagel, E. Standardized cardiovascular magnetic resonance imaging (CMR) protocols: 2020 update. *J. Cardiovasc. Magn. Reson.* **2020**, *22*, 1–18. [CrossRef]
12. Hajhosseiny, R.; Bustin, A.; Munoz, C.; Rashid, I.; Cruz, G.; Manning, W.J.; Prieto, C.; Botnar, R.M. Coronary Magnetic Resonance Angiography: Technical Innovations Leading Us to the Promised Land? *JACC Cardiovasc. Imaging* **2020**, *13*, 2653–2672. [CrossRef]
13. Aidi, H.E.; Adams, A.; Moons, K.G.; Ruijter, H.M.D.; Mali, W.P.M.; Doevendans, P.A.; Nagel, E.; Schalla, S.; Bots, M.L.; Leiner, T. Cardiac Magnetic Resonance Imaging Findings and the Risk of Cardiovascular Events in Patients With Recent Myocardial Infarction or Suspected or Known Coronary Artery Disease: A Systematic Review of Prognostic Studies. *J. Am. Coll. Cardiol.* **2014**, *63*, 1031–1045. [CrossRef]
14. Gronda, E.; Vanoli, E.; Sacchi, S.; Grassi, G.; Ambrosio, G.; Napoli, C. Risk of heart failure progression in patients with reduced ejection fraction: Mechanisms and therapeutic options. *Heart Fail. Rev.* **2020**, *25*, 295–303. [CrossRef]
15. Mayerhoefer, M.E.; Materka, A.; Langs, G.; Häggström, I.; Szczypiński, P.; Gibbs, P.; Cook, G. Introduction to Radiomics. *J. Nucl. Med.* **2020**, *61*, 488. [CrossRef]
16. Polidori, T.; Santis, D.D.; Rucci, C.; Tremamunno, G.; Piccinni, G.; Pugliese, L.; Zerunian, M.; Guido, G.; Pucciarelli, F.; Bracci, B.; et al. Radiomics applications in cardiac imaging: A comprehensive review. *Radiol. Medica* **2023**, *128*, 922–933. [CrossRef]
17. Hani, S.H.B.; Ahmad, M.M. Machine-learning Algorithms for Ischemic Heart Disease Prediction: A Systematic Review. *Curr. Cardiol. Rev.* **2022**, *19*, 87–99. [CrossRef]
18. Zhang, Q.; Fotaki, A.; Ghadimi, S.; Wang, Y.; Doneva, M.; Wetzl, J.; Delfino, J.G.; O'Regan, D.P.; Prieto, C.; Epstein, F.H. Improving the efficiency and accuracy of cardiovascular magnetic resonance with artificial intelligence—review of evidence and proposition of a roadmap to clinical translation. *J. Cardiovasc. Magn. Reson.* **2024**, *26*, 101051. [CrossRef] [PubMed]
19. Moradi, A.; Olanisa, O.O.; Nzeako, T.; Shahrokhi, M.; Esfahani, E.; Fakher, N.; Tabari, M.A.K. Revolutionizing Cardiac Imaging: A Scoping Review of Artificial Intelligence in Echocardiography, CTA, and Cardiac MRI. *J. Imaging* **2024**, *10*, 193. [CrossRef] [PubMed]
20. Infante, T.; Cavaliere, C.; Punzo, B.; Grimaldi, V.; Salvatore, M.; Napoli, C. Radiogenomics and Artificial Intelligence Approaches Applied to Cardiac Computed Tomography Angiography and Cardiac Magnetic Resonance for Precision Medicine in Coronary Heart Disease: A Systematic Review. *Circ. Cardiovasc. Imaging* **2021**, *14*, 1133–1146. [CrossRef] [PubMed]

21. Page, M.J.; McKenzie, J.E.; Bossuyt, P.M.; Boutron, I.; Hoffmann, T.C.; Mulrow, C.D.; Shamseer, L.; Tetzlaff, J.M.; Akl, E.A.; Brennan, S.E.; et al. The PRISMA 2020 statement: An updated guideline for reporting systematic reviews. *BMJ* **2021**, *372*, n71. [CrossRef] [PubMed]
22. Ouzzani, M.; Hammady, H.; Fedorowicz, Z.; Elmagarmid, A. Rayyan—A web and mobile app for systematic reviews. *Syst. Rev.* **2016**, *5*, 210. [CrossRef] [PubMed]
23. Tejani, A.S.; Klontzas, M.E.; Gatti, A.A.; Mongan, J.T.; Moy, L.; Park, S.H.; Kahn, C.E. Checklist for Artificial Intelligence in Medical Imaging (CLAIM): 2024 Update. *Radiol. Artif. Intell.* **2024**, *6*, e240300. [CrossRef] [PubMed]
24. Maleckar, M.M.; Myklebust, L.; Uv, J.; Florvaag, P.M.; Strøm, V.; Glinge, C.; Jabbari, R.; Vejlstrup, N.; Engstrøm, T.; Ahtarovski, K.; et al. Combined In-silico and Machine Learning Approaches Toward Predicting Arrhythmic Risk in Post-infarction Patients. *Front. Physiol.* **2021**, *12*, 745349. [CrossRef]
25. Alskaf, E.; Crawley, R.; Scannell, C.M.; Suinesiaputra, A.; Young, A.; Masci, P.G.; Perera, D.; Chiribiri, A. Hybrid artificial intelligence outcome prediction using features extraction from stress perfusion cardiac magnetic resonance images and electronic health records. *J. Med. Artif. Intell.* **2024**, *7*, 3. [CrossRef]
26. Alskaf, E.; Scannell, C.M.; Suinesiaputra, A.; Crawley, R.; Masci, P.; Young, A.; Perera, D.; Chiribiri, A. Qualitative American Heart Association plot of late gadolinium enhancement with mortality and ventricular arrhythmia prediction using artificial intelligence. *J. Med. Artif. Intell.* **2025**, *8*, 2. [CrossRef]
27. Backhaus, S.J.; Aldehayat, H.; Kowallick, J.T.; Evertz, R.; Lange, T.; Kutty, S.; Bigalke, B.; Gutberlet, M.; Hasenfuß, G.; Thiele, H.; et al. Artificial intelligence fully automated myocardial strain quantification for risk stratification following acute myocardial infarction. *Sci. Rep.* **2022**, *12*, 12220. [CrossRef]
28. Böttcher, B.; Beller, E.; Busse, A.; Cantré, D.; Yücel, S.; Öner, A.; Ince, H.; Weber, M.A.; Meinel, F.G. Fully automated quantification of left ventricular volumes and function in cardiac MRI: Clinical evaluation of a deep learning-based algorithm. *Int. J. Cardiovasc. Imaging* **2020**, *36*, 2239–2247. [CrossRef]
29. Cau, R.; Pisu, F.; Pintus, A.; Palmisano, V.; Montisci, R.; Suri, J.S.; Salgado, R.; Saba, L. Cine-cardiac magnetic resonance to distinguish between ischemic and non-ischemic cardiomyopathies: A machine learning approach. *Eur. Radiol.* **2024**, *34*, 5691–5704. [CrossRef]
30. Chen, B.H.; Wu, C.W.; An, D.A.; Zhang, J.L.; Zhang, Y.H.; Yu, L.Z.; Watson, K.; Wesemann, L.; Hu, J.; Chen, W.B.; et al. A deep learning method for the automated assessment of paradoxical pulsation after myocardial infarction using multicenter cardiac MRI data. *Eur. Radiol.* **2023**, *33*, 8477–8487. [CrossRef]
31. Chen, M.; Fang, L.; Zhuang, Q.; Liu, H. Deep Learning Assessment of Myocardial Infarction from MR Image Sequences. *IEEE Access* **2019**, *7*, 5438–5446. [CrossRef]
32. Chen, Z.; Shi, J.; Pommier, T.; Cottin, Y.; Salomon, M.; Decourselle, T.; Lalande, A.; Couturier, R. Prediction of Myocardial Infarction From Patient Features With Machine Learning. *Front. Cardiovasc. Med.* **2022**, *9*, 754609. [CrossRef]
33. Acero, J.C.; Lamata, P.; Eitel, I.; Zacur, E.; Evertz, R.; Lange, T.; Backhaus, S.J.; Stiermaier, T.; Thiele, H.; Bueno-Orovio, A.; et al. Comprehensive characterization of cardiac contraction for improved post-infarction risk assessment. *Sci. Rep.* **2024**, *14*, 8951. [CrossRef] [PubMed]
34. Frøysa, V.; Berg, G.J.; Singsaas, E.; Eftestøl, T.; Woie, L.; Ørn, S. Texture-based probability mapping for automatic assessment of myocardial injury in late gadolinium enhancement images after revascularized STEMI. *Int. J. Cardiol.* **2025**, *427*, 133107. [CrossRef] [PubMed]
35. GhaffariJolfayi, A.; Salmanipour, A.; Heshmat-Ghahdarijani, K.; MozafaryBazargany, M.H.; Azimi, A.; Pirouzi, P.; Mohammadzadeh, A. Machine learning-based interpretation of non-contrast feature tracking strain analysis and T1/T2 mapping for assessing myocardial viability. *Sci. Rep.* **2025**, *15*, 753. [CrossRef]
36. Ghanbari, F.; Joyce, T.; Lorenzoni, V.; Guaricci, A.I.; Pavon, A.G.; Fusini, L.; Andreini, D.; Rabbat, M.G.; Aquaro, G.D.; Abete, R.; et al. AI Cardiac MRI Scar Analysis Aids Prediction of Major Arrhythmic Events in the Multicenter DERIVATE Registry. *Radiology* **2023**, *307*, e222239. [CrossRef]
37. Guglielmo, M.; Penso, M.; Carerj, M.L.; Giacari, C.M.; Volpe, A.; Fusini, L.; Baggiano, A.; Mushtaq, S.; Annoni, A.; Cannata, F.; et al. DEep LearnIng-based QuaNtification of epicardial adipose tissue predicts MACE in patients undergoing stress CMR. *Atherosclerosis* **2024**, *397*, 117549. [CrossRef]
38. Jacob, A.J.; Chitiboi, T.; Schoepf, U.J.; Sharma, P.; Aldinger, J.; Baker, C.; Lautenschlager, C.; Emrich, T.; Varga-Szemes, A. Deep-Learning-Based Disease Classification in Patients Undergoing Cine Cardiac MRI. *J. Magn. Reson. Imaging JMRI* **2025**, *61*, 1635–1647. [CrossRef] [PubMed]
39. Knott, K.D.; Seraphim, A.; Augusto, J.B.; Xue, H.; Chacko, L.; Aung, N.; Petersen, S.E.; Cooper, J.A.; Manisty, C.; Bhuva, A.N.; et al. The Prognostic Significance of Quantitative Myocardial Perfusion: An Artificial Intelligence-Based Approach Using Perfusion Mapping. *Circulation* **2020**, *141*, 1282–1291. [CrossRef]

40. Lalande, A.; Chen, Z.; Pommier, T.; Decourselle, T.; Qayyum, A.; Salomon, M.; Ginhac, D.; Skandarani, Y.; Boucher, A.; Brahim, K.; et al. Deep learning methods for automatic evaluation of delayed enhancement-MRI. The results of the EMIDEC challenge. *Med. Image Anal.* **2022**, *79*, 102428. [CrossRef]
41. Li, G.; Zheng, C.; Cui, Y.; Si, J.; Yang, Y.; Li, J.; Lu, J. Diagnostic efficacy of complexity metrics from cardiac MRI myocardial segmental motion curves in detecting late gadolinium enhancement in myocardial infarction patients. *Heliyon* **2024**, *10*, e31889. [CrossRef]
42. Mauger, C.A.; Gilbert, K.; Suinesiaputra, A.; Bluemke, D.A.; Wu, C.O.; Lima, J.A.; Young, A.A.; Ambale-Venkatesh, B. Multi-Ethnic Study of Atherosclerosis: Relationship between Left Ventricular Shape at Cardiac MRI and 10-year Outcomes. *Radiology* **2023**, *306*, e220122. [CrossRef] [PubMed]
43. Okada, D.R.; Miller, J.; Chrispin, J.; Prakosa, A.; Trayanova, N.; Jones, S.; Maggioni, M.; Wu, K.C. Substrate Spatial Complexity Analysis for the Prediction of Ventricular Arrhythmias in Patients With Ischemic Cardiomyopathy. *Circ. Arrhythmia Electrophysiol.* **2020**, *13*, E007975. [CrossRef] [PubMed]
44. Paciorek, A.M.; von Schacky, C.E.; Foreman, S.C.; Gassert, F.G.; Gassert, F.T.; Kirschke, J.S.; Laugwitz, K.L.; Geith, T.; Hadamitzky, M.; Nadjiri, J. Automated assessment of cardiac pathologies on cardiac MRI using T1-mapping and late gadolinium phase sensitive inversion recovery sequences with deep learning. *BMC Med. Imaging* **2024**, *24*, 43. [CrossRef]
45. Pezel, T.; Sanguineti, F.; Garot, P.; Unterseeh, T.; Champagne, S.; Toupin, S.; Morisset, S.; Hovasse, T.; Faradji, A.; Ah-Sing, T.; et al. Machine-Learning Score Using Stress CMR for Death Prediction in Patients With Suspected or Known CAD. *JACC Cardiovasc. Imaging* **2022**, *15*, 1900–1913. [CrossRef] [PubMed]
46. Pezel, T.; Garot, P.; Toupin, S.; Hovasse, T.; Sanguineti, F.; Champagne, S.; Morisset, S.; Chitiboi, T.; Jacob, A.J.; Sharma, P.; et al. Prognostic impact of artificial intelligence-based fully automated global circumferential strain in patients undergoing stress CMR. *Eur. Heart J. Cardiovasc. Imaging* **2023**, *24*, 1269–1279. [CrossRef]
47. Pezel, T.; Toupin, S.; Bousson, V.; Hamzi, K.; Hovasse, T.; Lefevre, T.; Chevalier, B.; Unterseeh, T.; Sanguineti, F.; Champagne, S.; et al. A Machine Learning Model Using Cardiac CT and MRI Data Predicts Cardiovascular Events in Obstructive Coronary Artery Disease. *Radiology* **2025**, *314*, e233030. [CrossRef]
48. Popescu, D.M.; Shade, J.K.; Lai, C.; Aronis, K.N.; Ouyang, D.; Moorthy, M.V.; Cook, N.R.; Lee, D.C.; Kadish, A.; Albert, C.M.; et al. Arrhythmic sudden death survival prediction using deep learning analysis of scarring in the heart. *Nat. Cardiovasc. Res.* **2022**, *1*, 334–343. [CrossRef]
49. Righetti, F.; Rubiu, G.; Penso, M.; Moccia, S.; Carerj, M.L.; Pepi, M.; Pontone, G.; Caiani, E.G. Deep learning approaches for the detection of scar presence from cine cardiac magnetic resonance adding derived parametric images. *Med. Biol. Eng. Comput.* **2024**, *63*, 59–73. [CrossRef]
50. Schuster, A.; Lange, T.; Backhaus, S.J.; Strohmeyer, C.; Boom, P.C.; Matz, J.; Kowallick, J.T.; Lotz, J.; Steinmetz, M.; Kutty, S.; et al. Fully Automated Cardiac Assessment for Diagnostic and Prognostic Stratification Following Myocardial Infarction. *J. Am. Heart Assoc.* **2020**, *9*, 18. [CrossRef]
51. Udin, M.H.; Armstrong, S.; Kai, A.; Doyle, S.; Ionita, C.N.; Pokharel, S.; Sharma, U.C. Lightweight preprocessing and template matching facilitate streamlined ischemic myocardial scar classification. *J. Med. Imaging* **2024**, *11*, 024503. [CrossRef]
52. Wang, S.; Abdelaty, A.M.; Parke, K.; Arnold, J.R.; McCann, G.P.; Tyukin, I.Y. MyI-Net: Fully Automatic Detection and Quantification of Myocardial Infarction from Cardiovascular MRI Images. *Entropy* **2023**, *25*, 431. [CrossRef]
53. Wu, X.; Tang, L.; Li, W.; He, S.; Yue, X.; Peng, P.; Wu, T.; Zhang, X.; Wu, Z.; He, Y.; et al. Feasibility of accelerated non-contrast-enhanced whole-heart bSSFP coronary MR angiography by deep learning–constrained compressed sensing. *Eur. Radiol.* **2023**, *33*, 8180–8190. [CrossRef] [PubMed]
54. Wu, X.; Deng, L.; Li, W.; Peng, P.; Yue, X.; Tang, L.; Pu, Q.; Ming, Y.; Zhang, X.; Huang, X.; et al. Deep Learning-Based Acceleration of Compressed Sensing for Noncontrast-Enhanced Coronary Magnetic Resonance Angiography in Patients With Suspected Coronary Artery Disease. *J. Magn. Reson. Imaging* **2023**, *58*, 1521–1530. [CrossRef]
55. Wu, X.; Yue, X.; Peng, P.; Tan, X.; Huang, F.; Cai, L.; Li, L.; He, S.; Zhang, X.; Liu, P.; et al. Accelerated 3D whole-heart non-contrast-enhanced mDIXON coronary MR angiography using deep learning-constrained compressed sensing reconstruction. *Insights Imaging* **2024**, *15*, 224. [CrossRef] [PubMed]
56. Xu, C.; Xu, L.; Zhang, H.; Zhang, Y.; Du, X.; Li, S. A novel machine-learning algorithm to estimate the position and size of myocardial infarction for MRI sequence. *Computing* **2018**, *101*, 653–665. [CrossRef]
57. Zaidi, H.A.; Jones, R.E.; Hammersley, D.J.; Hatipoglu, S.; Balaban, G.; Mach, L.; Halliday, B.P.; Lamata, P.; Prasad, S.K.; Bishop, M.J. Machine learning analysis of complex late gadolinium enhancement patterns to improve risk prediction of major arrhythmic events. *Front. Cardiovasc. Med.* **2023**, *10*, 1082778. [CrossRef]
58. Zhang, N.; Yang, G.; Gao, Z.; Xu, C.; Zhang, Y.; Shi, R.; Keegan, J.; Xu, L.; Zhang, H.; Fan, Z.; et al. Deep learning for diagnosis of chronic myocardial infarction on nonenhanced cardiac cine MRI. *Radiology* **2019**, *291*, 606–607. [CrossRef]
59. Attallah, O.; Ragab, D.A. Auto-MyIn: Automatic diagnosis of myocardial infarction via multiple GLCMs, CNNs, and SVMs. *Biomed. Signal Process. Control* **2023**, *80*, 104273. [CrossRef]

60. Bekheet, M.; Sallah, M.; Alghamdi, N.S.; Rusu-Both, R.; Elgarayhi, A.; Elmogy, M. Cardiac Fibrosis Automated Diagnosis Based on FibrosisNet Network Using CMR Ischemic Cardiomyopathy. *Diagnostics* **2024**, *14*, 255. [CrossRef]
61. Dieu, X.; Chabrun, F.; Prunier, F.; Angoulvant, D.; Mewton, N.; Roubille, F.; Reynier, P.; Ferre, M.; Moal, V.; Cottin, L.; et al. Post-infarct cardiac remodeling predictions with machine learning. *Int. J. Cardiol.* **2022**, *355*, 1–4. [CrossRef]
62. Goldfarb, J.W.; Craft, J.; Cao, J.J. Water–fat separation and parameter mapping in cardiac MRI via deep learning with a convolutional neural network. *J. Magn. Reson. Imaging* **2019**, *50*, 655–665. [CrossRef] [PubMed]
63. Joloudari, J.H.; Saadatfar, H.; Gol, M.G.; Alizadehsani, R.; Sani, Z.A.; Hasanzadeh, F.; Hassannataj, E.; Sharifrazi, D.; Mansor, Z. FCM-DNN: Diagnosing coronary artery disease by deep accuracy fuzzy C-means clustering model. *Math. Biosci. Eng. MBE* **2022**, *19*, 3609–3635. [CrossRef]
64. Kim, Y.C.; Chung, Y.; Choe, Y.H. Deep learning for classification of late gadolinium enhancement lesions based on the 16-segment left ventricular model. *Phys. Medica* **2024**, *117*, 103193. [CrossRef]
65. Chen, C. Protection of Ivabradine Combined with Trimetazidine on Myocardial Injury after Percutaneous Coronary Intervention in Patients with Coronary Artery Disease Evaluated by Magnetic Resonance Image under Convolutional Neural Network. *Contrast Media Mol. Imaging* **2021**, *2021*, 3150938. [CrossRef]
66. Feng, Y.; Xulei, Y.; Kng, T.S.; Lee, G.; Liang, Z.; Tan, R.S.; Yi, S. Multi-dimensional proprio-proximus machine learning for assessment of myocardial infarction. *Comput. Med. Imaging Graph.* **2018**, *70*, 63–72. [CrossRef]
67. Hernandez-Casillas, A.; Del-Canto, I.; Ruiz-Espana, S.; Lopez-Lereu, M.P.; Monmeneu, J.V.; Moratal, D. Detection and Classification of Myocardial Infarction Transmurality Using Cardiac MR Image Analysis and Machine Learning Algorithms. In Proceedings of the Annual International Conference of the IEEE Engineering in Medicine and Biology Society. IEEE Engineering in Medicine and Biology Society. Annual International Conference, Scotland, UK, 11–15 July 2022; Volume 2022, pp. 1686–1689. [CrossRef]
68. Iqbal, T.; Khalid, A.; Ullah, I. Explaining decisions of a light-weight deep neural network for real-time coronary artery disease classification in magnetic resonance imaging. *J. Real-Time Image Process.* **2024**, *21*, 31. [CrossRef] [PubMed]
69. Muthulakshmi, M.; Kavitha, G. Deep CNN with LM learning based myocardial ischemia detection in cardiac magnetic resonance images. In Proceedings of the Annual International Conference of the IEEE Engineering in Medicine and Biology Society. IEEE Engineering in Medicine and Biology Society. Annual International Conference, Berlin, Germany, 23–27 July 2019; Volume 2019, pp. 824–827. [CrossRef]
70. Chen, Z.; Lalande, A.; Salomon, M.; Decourselle, T.; Pommier, T.; Qayyum, A.; Shi, J.; Perrot, G.; Couturier, R. Automatic deep learning-based myocardial infarction segmentation from delayed enhancement MRI. *Comput. Med. Imaging Graph.* **2022**, *95*, 102014. [CrossRef] [PubMed]
71. Cerqueira, M.D.; Weissman, N.J.; Dilsizian, V.; Jacobs, A.K.; Kaul, S.; Laskey, W.K.; Pennell, D.J.; Rumberger, J.A.; Ryan, T.; Verani, M.S. Standardized Myocardial Segmentation and Nomenclature for Tomographic Imaging of the Heart. *Circulation* **2002**, *105*, 539–542. [CrossRef]
72. Raisi-Estabragh, Z.; Izquierdo, C.; Campello, V.M.; Martin-Isla, C.; Jaggi, A.; Harvey, N.C.; Lekadir, K.; Petersen, S.E. Cardiac magnetic resonance radiomics: Basic principles and clinical perspectives. *Eur. Heart J. Cardiovasc. Imaging* **2020**, *21*, 349–356. [CrossRef]
73. Abdulkareem, M.; Kenawy, A.A.; Rauseo, E.; Lee, A.M.; Sojoudi, A.; Amir-Khalili, A.; Lekadir, K.; Young, A.A.; Barnes, M.R.; Barckow, P.; et al. Predicting post-contrast information from contrast agent free cardiac MRI using machine learning: Challenges and methods. *Front. Cardiovasc. Med.* **2022**, *9*, 894503. [CrossRef] [PubMed]
74. Arian, F.; Amini, M.; Mostafaei, S.; Kalantari, K.R.; Avval, A.H.; Shahbazi, Z.; Kasani, K.; Rajabi, A.B.; Chatterjee, S.; Oveisi, M.; et al. Myocardial Function Prediction After Coronary Artery Bypass Grafting Using MRI Radiomic Features and Machine Learning Algorithms. *J. Digit. Imaging* **2022**, *35*, 1708–1718. [CrossRef] [PubMed]
75. Avard, E.; Shiri, I.; Hajianfar, G.; Abdollahi, H.; Kalantari, K.R.; Houshmand, G.; Kasani, K.; Bitarafan-rajabi, A.; Deevband, M.R.; Oveisi, M.; et al. Non-contrast Cine Cardiac Magnetic Resonance image radiomics features and machine learning algorithms for myocardial infarction detection. *Comput. Biol. Med.* **2022**, *141*, 105145. [CrossRef]
76. Baessler, B.; Mannil, M.; Oebel, S.; Maintz, D.; Alkadhi, H.; Manka, R. Subacute and Chronic Left Ventricular Myocardial Scar: Accuracy of Texture Analysis on Nonenhanced Cine MR Images. *Radiology* **2018**, *286*, 103–112. [CrossRef]
77. Berg, B.V.; Keyzer, F.D.; Cernicanu, A.; Claus, P.; Masci, P.G.; Bogaert, J.; Dresselaers, T. Radiomics-based detection of acute myocardial infarction on noncontrast enhanced midventricular short-axis cine CMR images. *Int. J. Cardiovasc. Imaging* **2024**, *40*, 1211–1220. [CrossRef]
78. Deng, J.; Zhou, L.; Li, Y.; Yu, Y.; Zhang, J.; Liao, B.; Luo, G.; Tian, J.; Zhou, H.; Tang, H. Integration of Cine-cardiac Magnetic Resonance Radiomics and Machine Learning for Differentiating Ischemic and Dilated Cardiomyopathy. *Acad. Radiol.* **2024**, *31*, 2704–2714. [CrossRef]

79. Durmaz, E.S.; Karabacak, M.; Ozkara, B.B.; Kargın, O.A.; Raimoglu, U.; Tokdil, H.; Durmaz, E.; Adaletli, I. Radiomics-based machine learning models in STEMI: A promising tool for the prediction of major adverse cardiac events. *Eur. Radiol.* **2023**, *33*, 4611–4620. [CrossRef]
80. Frøysa, V.; Berg, G.J.; Eftestøl, T.; Woie, L.; Ørn, S. Texture-based probability mapping for automatic scar assessment in late gadolinium-enhanced cardiovascular magnetic resonance images. *Eur. J. Radiol. Open* **2021**, *8*, 100387. [CrossRef]
81. Khozeimeh, F.; Sharifrazi, D.; Izadi, N.H.; Joloudari, J.H.; Shoeibi, A.; Alizadehsani, R.; Tartibi, M.; Hussain, S.; Sani, Z.A.; Khodatars, M.; et al. RF-CNN-F: Random forest with convolutional neural network features for coronary artery disease diagnosis based on cardiac magnetic resonance. *Sci. Rep.* **2022**, *12*, 11178. [CrossRef] [PubMed]
82. Kotu, L.P.; Engan, K.; Borhani, R.; Katsaggelos, A.K.; Ørn, S.; Woie, L.; Eftestøl, T. Cardiac magnetic resonance image-based classification of the risk of arrhythmias in post-myocardial infarction patients. *Artif. Intell. Med.* **2015**, *64*, 205–215. [CrossRef]
83. Larroza, A.; Materka, A.; López-Lereu, M.P.; Monmeneu, J.V.; Bodí, V.; Moratal, D. Differentiation between acute and chronic myocardial infarction by means of texture analysis of late gadolinium enhancement and cine cardiac magnetic resonance imaging. *Eur. J. Radiol.* **2017**, *92*, 78–83. [CrossRef] [PubMed]
84. Larroza, A.; López-Lereu, M.P.; Monmeneu, J.V.; Gavara, J.; Chorro, F.J.; Bodí, V.; Moratal, D. Texture analysis of cardiac cine magnetic resonance imaging to detect nonviable segments in patients with chronic myocardial infarction. *Med. Phys.* **2018**, *45*, 1471–1480. [CrossRef] [PubMed]
85. Liu, X.; Xu, T.; Peng, Y.; Yuan, J.; Wang, S.; Xu, W.; Gong, J. Non-contrast cine cardiovascular magnetic resonance-based radiomics nomogram for predicting microvascular obstruction after reperfusion in ST-segment elevation myocardial infarction. *Front. Cardiovasc. Med.* **2023**, *10*, 1274267. [CrossRef]
86. Ma, Q.; Ma, Y.; Yu, T.; Sun, Z.; Hou, Y. Radiomics of Non-Contrast-Enhanced T1 Mapping: Diagnostic and Predictive Performance for Myocardial Injury in Acute ST-Segment-Elevation Myocardial Infarction. *Korean J. Radiol.* **2021**, *22*, 535. [CrossRef] [PubMed]
87. Noto, T.D.; von Spiczak, J.; Mannil, M.; Gantert, E.; Soda, P.; Manka, R.; Alkadhi, H. Radiomics for distinguishing myocardial infarction from myocarditis at late gadolinium enhancement at mri: Comparison with subjective visual analysis. *Radiol. Cardiothorac. Imaging* **2019**, *1*, e180026. [CrossRef]
88. Pujadas, E.R.; Raisi-Estabragh, Z.; Szabo, L.; McCracken, C.; Morcillo, C.I.; Campello, V.M.; Martín-Isla, C.; Atehortua, A.M.; Vago, H.; Merkely, B.; et al. Prediction of incident cardiovascular events using machine learning and CMR radiomics. *Eur. Radiol.* **2023**, *33*, 3488–3500. [CrossRef]
89. Raisi-Estabragh, Z.; Martin-Isla, C.; Nissen, L.; Szabo, L.; Campello, V.M.; Escalera, S.; Winther, S.; Bøttcher, M.; Lekadir, K.; Petersen, S.E. Radiomics analysis enhances the diagnostic performance of CMR stress perfusion: A proof-of-concept study using the Dan-NICAD dataset. *Front. Cardiovasc. Med.* **2023**, *10*, 1141026. [CrossRef]
90. Rauseo, E.; Morcillo, C.I.; Raisi-Estabragh, Z.; Gkontra, P.; Aung, N.; Lekadir, K.; Petersen, S.E. New Imaging Signatures of Cardiac Alterations in Ischaemic Heart Disease and Cerebrovascular Disease Using CMR Radiomics. *Front. Cardiovasc. Med.* **2021**, *8*, 716577. [CrossRef]
91. Wang, D.; Taher, H.J.; Al-Fatlawi, M.; Abdullah, B.A.; Ismailova, M.K.; Abedi-Firouzjah, R. Multi-parametric assessment of cardiac magnetic resonance images to distinguish myocardial infarctions: A tensor-based radiomics feature. *J. X-Ray Sci. Technol.* **2024**, *32*, 735–749. [CrossRef]
92. Barbaroux, H.; Kunze, K.P.; Neji, R.; Nazir, M.S.; Pennell, D.J.; Nielles-Vallespin, S.; Scott, A.D.; Young, A.A. Automated segmentation of long and short axis DENSE cardiovascular magnetic resonance for myocardial strain analysis using spatio-temporal convolutional neural networks. *J. Cardiovasc. Magn. Reson.* **2023**, *25*, 16. [CrossRef] [PubMed]
93. Brahim, K.; Arega, T.W.; Boucher, A.; Bricq, S.; Sakly, A.; Meriaudeau, F. An Improved 3D Deep Learning-Based Segmentation of Left Ventricular Myocardial Diseases from Delayed-Enhancement MRI with Inclusion and Classification Prior Information U-Net (ICPIU-Net). *Sensors* **2022**, *22*, 2084. [CrossRef]
94. Chen, S.; An, D.; Feng, C.; Bian, Z.; Wu, L.M. Segmentation of Pericardial Adipose Tissue in CMR Images: A Benchmark Dataset MRPEAT and a Triple-Stage Network 3SUnet. *IEEE Trans. Med. Imaging* **2023**, *42*, 2386–2399. [CrossRef] [PubMed]
95. Gröschel, J.; Kuhnt, J.; Viezzer, D.; Hadler, T.; Hormes, S.; Barckow, P.; Schulz-Menger, J.; Blaszczyk, E. Comparison of manual and artificial intelligence based quantification of myocardial strain by feature tracking—A cardiovascular MR study in health and disease. *Eur. Radiol.* **2024**, *34*, 1003–1015. [CrossRef] [PubMed]
96. Heidenreich, J.F.; Gassenmaier, T.; Ankenbrand, M.J.; Bley, T.A.; Wech, T. Self-configuring nnU-net pipeline enables fully automatic infarct segmentation in late enhancement MRI after myocardial infarction. *Eur. J. Radiol.* **2021**, *141*, 109817. [CrossRef] [PubMed]
97. Lin, M.; Jiang, M.; Zhao, M.; Ukwatta, E.; White, J.A.; Chiu, B. Cascaded Triplanar Autoencoder M-Net for Fully Automatic Segmentation of Left Ventricle Myocardial Scar From Three-Dimensional Late Gadolinium-Enhanced MR Images. *IEEE J. Biomed. Health Inform.* **2022**, *26*, 2582–2593. [CrossRef]

98. Moccia, S.; Banali, R.; Martini, C.; Muscogiuri, G.; Pontone, G.; Pepi, M.; Caiani, E.G. Development and testing of a deep learning-based strategy for scar segmentation on CMR-LGE images. *Magn. Reson. Mater. Phys. Biol. Med.* **2019**, *32*, 187–195. [CrossRef]
99. Scannell, C.M.; Veta, M.; Villa, A.D.; Sammut, E.C.; Lee, J.; Breeuwer, M.; Chiribiri, A. Deep-Learning-Based Preprocessing for Quantitative Myocardial Perfusion MRI. *J. Magn. Reson. Imaging JMRI* **2020**, *51*, 1689–1696. [CrossRef]
100. Zabihollahy, F.; White, J.A.; Ukwatta, E. Convolutional neural network-based approach for segmentation of left ventricle myocardial scar from 3D late gadolinium enhancement MR images. *Med. Phys.* **2019**, *46*, 1740–1751. [CrossRef]
101. Al-antari, M.A.; Shaaf, Z.F.; Jamil, M.M.A.; Samee, N.A.; Alkanhel, R.; Talo, M.; Al-Huda, Z. Deep learning myocardial infarction segmentation framework from cardiac magnetic resonance images. *Biomed. Signal Process. Control* **2024**, *89*, 105710. [CrossRef]
102. Jafari, R.; Verma, R.; Aggarwal, V.; Gupta, R.K.; Singh, A. Deep learning-based segmentation of left ventricular myocardium on dynamic contrast-enhanced MRI: A comprehensive evaluation across temporal frames. *Int. J. Comput. Assist. Radiol. Surg.* **2024**, *19*, 2055–2062. [CrossRef]
103. Khalifa, A.B.; Mili, M.; Maatouk, M.; Abdallah, A.B.; Abdellali, M.; Gaied, S.; Ali, A.B.; Lahouel, Y.; Bedoui, M.H.; Zrig, A. Deep Transfer Learning for Classification of Late Gadolinium Enhancement Cardiac MRI Images into Myocardial Infarction, Myocarditis, and Healthy Classes: Comparison with Subjective Visual Evaluation. *Diagnostics* **2025**, *15*, 207. [CrossRef]
104. Li, S.; Li, X.; Wang, P.; Liu, K.; Wei, B.; Cong, J. An enhanced visual state space model for myocardial pathology segmentation in multi-sequence cardiac MRI. *Med. Phys.* **2025**, *52*, 4355–4370. [CrossRef]
105. Lin, L.; Zheng, Y.; Li, Y.; Jiang, D.; Cao, J.; Wang, J.; Xiao, Y.; Mao, X.; Zheng, C.; Wang, Y. Automatic vessel segmentation and reformation of non-contrast coronary magnetic resonance angiography using transfer learning-based three-dimensional U-net with attention mechanism. *J. Cardiovasc. Magn. Reson.* **2025**, *27*, 101126. [CrossRef]
106. Mosquera-Rojas, G.; Ouadah, C.; Hadadi, A.; Lalande, A.; Leclerc, S. Automatic Myocardium Segmentation in Delayed-Enhancement MRI with Pathology-Specific Data Augmentation and Deep Learning Architectures. *Algorithms* **2023**, *16*, 488. [CrossRef]
107. Papetti, D.M.; Abeelen, K.V.; Davies, R.; Menè, R.; Heilbron, F.; Perelli, F.P.; Artico, J.; Seraphim, A.; Moon, J.C.; Parati, G.; et al. An accurate and time-efficient deep learning-based system for automated segmentation and reporting of cardiac magnetic resonance-detected ischemic scar. *Comput. Methods Programs Biomed.* **2023**, *229*, 107321. [CrossRef] [PubMed]
108. Qi, H.; Qian, P.; Tang, L.; Chen, B.; An, D.; Wu, L.M. Predicting Late Gadolinium Enhancement of Acute Myocardial Infarction in Contrast-Free Cardiac Cine MRI Using Deep Generative Learning. *Circ. Cardiovasc. Imaging* **2024**, *17*, 16786. [CrossRef] [PubMed]
109. Xu, C.; Howey, J.; Ohorodnyk, P.; Roth, M.; Zhang, H.; Li, S. Segmentation and quantification of infarction without contrast agents via spatiotemporal generative adversarial learning. *Med. Image Anal.* **2020**, *59*, 101568. [CrossRef]
110. Xu, C.; Wang, Y.; Zhang, D.; Han, L.; Zhang, Y.; Chen, J.; Li, S. BMAnet: Boundary Mining With Adversarial Learning for Semi-Supervised 2D Myocardial Infarction Segmentation. *IEEE J. Biomed. Health Inform.* **2023**, *27*, 87–96. [CrossRef]
111. Yalcinkaya, D.M.; Youssef, K.; Heydari, B.; Wei, J.; Merz, N.B.; Judd, R.; Dharmakumar, R.; Simonetti, O.P.; Weinsaft, J.W.; Raman, S.V.; et al. Improved robustness for deep learning-based segmentation of multi-center myocardial perfusion cardiovascular MRI datasets using data-adaptive uncertainty–guided space-time analysis. *J. Cardiovasc. Magn. Reson.* **2024**, *26*, 101082. [CrossRef]
112. Jani, V.P.; Ostovaneh, M.; Chamera, E.; Kato, Y.; Lima, J.A.; Ambale-Venkatesh, B. Deep learning for automatic volumetric segmentation of left ventricular myocardium and ischaemic scar from multi-slice late gadolinium enhancement cardiovascular magnetic resonance. *Eur. Heart J. Cardiovasc. Imaging* **2024**, *25*, 829–838. [CrossRef]
113. Ahmad, I.; Qayyum, A.; Gupta, B.B.; Alassafi, M.O.; Alghamdi, R.A. Ensemble of 2D Residual Neural Networks Integrated with Atrous Spatial Pyramid Pooling Module for Myocardium Segmentation of Left Ventricle Cardiac MRI. *Mathematics* **2022**, *10*, 627. [CrossRef]
114. Arega, T.W.; Bricq, S.; Legrand, F.; Jacquier, A.; Lalande, A.; Meriaudeau, F. Automatic uncertainty-based quality controlled T1 mapping and ECV analysis from native and post-contrast cardiac T1 mapping images using Bayesian vision transformer. *Med. Image Anal.* **2023**, *86*, 102773. [CrossRef]
115. Kim, Y.C.; Kim, K.R.; Choe, Y.H. Automatic myocardial segmentation in dynamic contrast enhanced perfusion MRI using Monte Carlo dropout in an encoder-decoder convolutional neural network. *Comput. Methods Programs Biomed.* **2020**, *185*, 105150. [CrossRef] [PubMed]
116. Qiu, J.; Li, L.; Wang, S.; Zhang, K.; Chen, Y.; Yang, S.; Zhuang, X. MyoPS-Net: Myocardial pathology segmentation with flexible combination of multi-sequence CMR images. *Med. Image Anal.* **2023**, *84*, 102694. [CrossRef]
117. Tan, X.W.; Zheng, Q.; Shi, L.; Gao, F.; Allen, J.C.J.; Coenen, A.; Baumann, S.; Schoepf, U.J.; Kassab, G.S.; Lim, S.T.; et al. Combined diagnostic performance of coronary computed tomography angiography and computed tomography derived fractional flow reserve for the evaluation of myocardial ischemia: A meta-analysis. *Int. J. Cardiol.* **2017**, *236*, 100–106. [CrossRef]
118. Bernardo, A.; Mato, G.; Calandrelli, M.; Medus, J.; Curiale, A. A novel deep learning based method for myocardial strain quantification. *Biomed. Phys. Eng. Express* **2024**, *11*. [CrossRef] [PubMed]

119. Chen, Y.; Xie, W.; Zhang, J.; Qiu, H.; Zeng, D.; Shi, Y.; Yuan, H.; Zhuang, J.; Jia, Q.; Zhang, Y.; et al. Myocardial Segmentation of Cardiac MRI Sequences With Temporal Consistency for Coronary Artery Disease Diagnosis. *Front. Cardiovasc. Med.* **2022**, *9*, 804442. [CrossRef]
120. Mamalakis, M.; Garg, P.; Nelson, T.; Lee, J.; Swift, A.J.; Wild, J.M.; Clayton, R.H. Automatic development of 3D anatomical models of border zone and core scar regions in the left ventricle. *Comput. Med. Imaging Graph.* **2023**, *103*, 102152. [CrossRef] [PubMed]
121. Yan, Z.; Su, Y.; Sun, H.; Yu, H.; Ma, W.; Chi, H.; Cao, H.; Chang, Q. SegNet-based left ventricular MRI segmentation for the diagnosis of cardiac hypertrophy and myocardial infarction. *Comput. Methods Programs Biomed.* **2022**, *227*, 107197. [CrossRef]
122. Yeung, M.; Rundo, L.; Nan, Y.; Sala, E.; Schönlieb, C.B.; Yang, G. Calibrating the Dice Loss to Handle Neural Network Overconfidence for Biomedical Image Segmentation. *J. Digit. Imaging* **2023**, *36*, 739–752. [CrossRef]
123. Liu, J.; Xie, H.; Zhang, S.; Gu, L. Multi-sequence myocardium segmentation with cross-constrained shape and neural network-based initialization. *Comput. Med. Imaging Graph.* **2019**, *71*, 49–57. [CrossRef]
124. Tan, L.K.; McLaughlin, R.A.; Lim, E.; Aziz, Y.F.A.; Liew, Y.M. Fully automated segmentation of the left ventricle in cine cardiac MRI using neural network regression. *J. Magn. Reson. Imaging JMRI* **2018**, *48*, 140–152. [CrossRef]
125. Lecesne, E.; Simon, A.; Garreau, M.; Barone-Rochette, G.; Fouard, C. Segmentation of cardiac infarction in delayed-enhancement MRI using probability map and transformers-based neural networks. *Comput. Methods Programs Biomed.* **2023**, *242*, 107841. [CrossRef]
126. Li, X.; Guo, Y.; Lin, L.; Wang, Y.; Liu, P.; Wang, Q.; Chen, W.; Wang, W.; Xia, Q.; Huang, N.; et al. Identification of Myocardial Scarring Using Contrast-Free Cardiac MRI in Patients With Autoimmune Rheumatic Diseases. *J. Magn. Reson. Imaging JMRI* **2023**, *60*, 979–987. [CrossRef] [PubMed]
127. Cui, H.; Jiang, L.; Yuwen, C.; Xia, Y.; Zhang, Y. Deep U-Net architecture with curriculum learning for myocardial pathology segmentation in multi-sequence cardiac magnetic resonance images. *Knowl.-Based Syst.* **2022**, *249*, 108942. [CrossRef]
128. Cui, H.; Li, Y.; Jiang, L.; Wang, Y.; Xia, Y.; Zhang, Y. Improving myocardial pathology segmentation with U-Net++ and EfficientSeg from multi-sequence cardiac magnetic resonance images. *Comput. Biol. Med.* **2022**, *151*, 106218. [CrossRef]
129. Li, D.; Peng, Y.; Guo, Y.; Sun, J. TAUNet: A triple-attention-based multi-modality MRI fusion U-Net for cardiac pathology segmentation. *Complex Intell. Syst.* **2022**, *8*, 2489–2505. [CrossRef]
130. de la Rosa, E.; Sidibé, D.; Decourselle, T.; Leclercq, T.; Cochet, A.; Lalande, A. Myocardial Infarction Quantification from Late Gadolinium Enhancement MRI Using Top-Hat Transforms and Neural Networks. *Algorithms* **2021**, *14*, 249. [CrossRef]
131. Brahim, K.; Qayyum, A.; Lalande, A.; Boucher, A.; Sakly, A.; Meriaudeau, F. A 3D Network Based Shape Prior for Automatic Myocardial Disease Segmentation in Delayed-Enhancement MRI. *IRBM* **2021**, *42*, 424–434. [CrossRef]
132. Karimi, D.; Salcudean, S.E. Reducing the Hausdorff Distance in Medical Image Segmentation with Convolutional Neural Networks. *IEEE Trans. Med. Imaging* **2020**, *39*, 499–513. [CrossRef]
133. Nawaz, M.; Uvaliyev, A.; Bibi, K.; Wei, H.; Abaxi, S.M.D.; Masood, A.; Shi, P.; Ho, H.P.; Yuan, W. Unraveling the complexity of Optical Coherence Tomography image segmentation using machine and deep learning techniques: A review. *Comput. Med. Imaging Graph.* **2023**, *108*, 102269. [CrossRef]
134. Li, B.; Yang, T.; Zhao, X. NVTrans-UNet: Neighborhood vision transformer based U-Net for multi-modal cardiac MR image segmentation. *J. Appl. Clin. Med. Phys.* **2023**, *24*. [CrossRef]
135. Popescu, D.M.; Abramson, H.G.; Yu, R.; Lai, C.; Shade, J.K.; Wu, K.C.; Maggioni, M.; Trayanova, N.A. Anatomically informed deep learning on contrast-enhanced cardiac magnetic resonance imaging for scar segmentation and clinical feature extraction. *Cardiovasc. Digit. Health J.* **2022**, *3*, 2–13. [CrossRef] [PubMed]
136. Mamalakis, M.; Garg, P.; Nelson, T.; Lee, J.; Wild, J.M.; Clayton, R.H. MA-SOCRATIS: An automatic pipeline for robust segmentation of the left ventricle and scar. *Comput. Med. Imaging Graph.* **2021**, *93*, 101982. [CrossRef] [PubMed]
137. Wang, Z.; Zhang, J.; Fan, G.; Zhao, H.; Wang, X.; Zhang, J.; Zhang, P.; Wang, W. Imaging transparent intact cardiac tissue with single-cell resolution. *Biomed. Opt. Express* **2018**, *9*, 423–436. [CrossRef] [PubMed]

MDPI AG
Grosspeteranlage 5
4052 Basel
Switzerland
Tel.: +41 61 683 77 34

Journal of Cardiovascular Development and Disease Editorial Office
E-mail: jcdd@mdpi.com
www.mdpi.com/journal/jcdd

www.ingramcontent.com/pod-product-compliance
Lightning Source LLC
Chambersburg PA
CBHW061625210926
51850CB00009B/2440
* 9 7 8 3 7 2 5 8 5 5 9 7 1 *